Novel Therapeutic Considerations in Bone and Soft Tissue Sarcoma

Novel Therapeutic Considerations in Bone and Soft Tissue Sarcoma

Editors

Joanna Szkandera
Dimosthenis Andreou

MDPI • Basel • Beijing • Wuhan • Barcelona • Belgrade • Manchester • Tokyo • Cluj • Tianjin

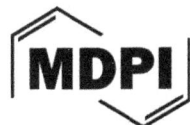

Editors
Joanna Szkandera
Division of Oncology
Medical University of Graz
Graz
Austria

Dimosthenis Andreou
Department of Orthopaedics
and Trauma
Medical University of Graz
Graz
Austria

Editorial Office
MDPI
St. Alban-Anlage 66
4052 Basel, Switzerland

This is a reprint of articles from the Special Issue published online in the open access journal *Cancers* (ISSN 2072-6694) (available at: www.mdpi.com/journal/cancers/special_issues/sarcoma_therapy).

For citation purposes, cite each article independently as indicated on the article page online and as indicated below:

LastName, A.A.; LastName, B.B.; LastName, C.C. Article Title. *Journal Name* **Year**, *Volume Number*, Page Range.

ISBN 978-3-0365-7015-0 (Hbk)
ISBN 978-3-0365-7014-3 (PDF)

© 2023 by the authors. Articles in this book are Open Access and distributed under the Creative Commons Attribution (CC BY) license, which allows users to download, copy and build upon published articles, as long as the author and publisher are properly credited, which ensures maximum dissemination and a wider impact of our publications.

The book as a whole is distributed by MDPI under the terms and conditions of the Creative Commons license CC BY-NC-ND.

Contents

Preface to "Novel Therapeutic Considerations in Bone and Soft Tissue Sarcoma" vii

Alexander Klein, Theresa Fell, Christof Birkenmaier, Julian Fromm, Volkmar Jansson and Thomas Knösel et al.
Relative Sensitivity of Core-Needle Biopsy and Incisional Biopsy in the Diagnosis of Musculoskeletal Sarcomas
Reprinted from: *Cancers* **2021**, *13*, 1393, doi:10.3390/cancers13061393 1

Zeger Rijs, A. Naweed Shifai, Sarah E. Bosma, Peter J. K. Kuppen, Alexander L. Vahrmeijer and Stijn Keereweer et al.
Candidate Biomarkers for Specific Intraoperative Near-Infrared Imaging of Soft Tissue Sarcomas: A Systematic Review
Reprinted from: *Cancers* **2021**, *13*, 557, doi:10.3390/cancers13030557 11

Mateusz Jacek Spałek, Aneta Maria Borkowska, Maria Telejko, Michał Wagrodzki, Daria Niebyłowska and Aldona Uzar et al.
The Feasibility Study of Hypofractionated Radiotherapy with Regional Hyperthermia in Soft Tissue Sarcomas
Reprinted from: *Cancers* **2021**, *13*, 1332, doi:10.3390/cancers13061332 39

Christoph Theil, Kristian Nikolaus Schneider, Georg Gosheger, Ralf Dieckmann, Niklas Deventer and Jendrik Hardes et al.
Does the Duration of Primary and First Revision Surgery Influence the Probability of First and Subsequent Implant Failures after Extremity Sarcoma Resection and Megaprosthetic Reconstruction?
Reprinted from: *Cancers* **2021**, *13*, 2510, doi:10.3390/cancers13112510 53

Richard E. Evenhuis, Ibtissam Acem, Anja J. Rueten-Budde, Diederik S. A. Karis, Marta Fiocco and Desiree M. J. Dorleijn et al.
Survival Analysis of 3 Different Age Groups and Prognostic Factors among 402 Patients with Skeletal High-Grade Osteosarcoma. Real World Data from a Single Tertiary Sarcoma Center
Reprinted from: *Cancers* **2021**, *13*, 486, doi:10.3390/cancers13030486 63

Daniel Pink, Dimosthenis Andreou, Sebastian Bauer, Thomas Brodowicz, Bernd Kasper and Peter Reichardt et al.
Treatment of Angiosarcoma with Pazopanib and Paclitaxel: Results of the EVA (Evaluation of Votrient® in Angiosarcoma) Phase II Trial of the German Interdisciplinary Sarcoma Group (GISG-06)
Reprinted from: *Cancers* **2021**, *13*, 1223, doi:10.3390/cancers13061223 77

Andrea P. Espejo-Freire, Andrew Elliott, Andrew Rosenberg, Philippos Apolinario Costa, Priscila Barreto-Coelho and Emily Jonczak et al.
Genomic Landscape of Angiosarcoma: A Targeted and Immunotherapy Biomarker Analysis
Reprinted from: *Cancers* **2021**, *13*, 4816, doi:10.3390/cancers13194816 87

Luana Madalena Sousa, Jani Sofia Almeida, Tânia Fortes-Andrade, Manuel Santos-Rosa, Paulo Freitas-Tavares and José Manuel Casanova et al.
Tumor and Peripheral Immune Status in Soft Tissue Sarcoma: Implications for Immunotherapy
Reprinted from: *Cancers* **2021**, *13*, 3885, doi:10.3390/cancers13153885 101

Gemma Di Pompo, Margherita Cortini, Nicola Baldini and Sofia Avnet
Acid Microenvironment in Bone Sarcomas
Reprinted from: *Cancers* **2021**, *13*, 3848, doi:10.3390/cancers13153848 123

Georgia Karpathiou, Maroa Dridi, Lila Krebs-Drouot, François Vassal, Emmanuel Jouanneau and Timothée Jacquesson et al.
Autophagic Markers in Chordomas: Immunohistochemical Analysis and Comparison with the Immune Microenvironment of Chordoma Tissues
Reprinted from: *Cancers* **2021**, *13*, 2169, doi:10.3390/cancers13092169 . . . . **145**

Preface to "Novel Therapeutic Considerations in Bone and Soft Tissue Sarcoma"

Sarcomas are a group of rare cancers that arise in connective tissues of the body. These tumours exhibit a wide range of different behaviours and underlying molecular pathologies. The two main types of sarcoma are soft tissue and bone sarcomas, but there are more than 70 different entities within these two categories.

There is a limited medical understanding of this type of rare malignancy. The natural history of these aggressive tumours is characterised by a strong tendency toward local recurrence and metastatic spreading. Despite advances in therapeutic approaches over the last several decades, the outcome for metastatic patients remains poor. Therefore, it is important to identify patients who are at high risk for tumour recurrence and dissemination, which has resulted in an increasing interest in the investigation of prognostic biomarkers that help to guide treatment decisions.

Surgical resection is pivotal for the management of locoregional disease. In locally advanced or metastatic disease settings, systemic therapy has an important role in the multidisciplinary management of sarcoma. Cytotoxic therapy has been the mainstay of treatment for many years. However, recent advances in molecular pathogenesis, the investigation of the tumour microenvironment, changes in clinical trial design, and increased international collaboration have led to the development of histology-driven therapy. Furthermore, genomic profiling has highlighted that, while some sarcomas have complex karyotypes, others are driven by translocation, amplification, and mutation, representing targets for the development of novel therapies. Checkpoint inhibitors have been used as single agents or in combination in clinical sarcoma trials. This progress will move the therapeutic modality in sarcoma patients from the "one-size-fits-all" approach towards a more personalized therapeutic algorithm and better outcomes soon

In this Special Issue, we present original research and review articles highlighting novel therapeutic approaches in the treatment of sarcoma patients.

Joanna Szkandera and Dimosthenis Andreou
Editors

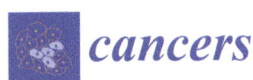

Article

Relative Sensitivity of Core-Needle Biopsy and Incisional Biopsy in the Diagnosis of Musculoskeletal Sarcomas

Alexander Klein [1,*], Theresa Fell [1], Christof Birkenmaier [1], Julian Fromm [1], Volkmar Jansson [1], Thomas Knösel [2] and Hans Roland Dürr [1]

[1] Musculoskeletal Oncology, Department of Orthopaedics, Physical Medicine and Rehabilitation, University Hospital, LMU Munich, 81377 Munich, Germany; t.fell@campus.lmu.de (T.F.); christof.birkenmaier@med.uni-muenchen.de (C.B.); julian.fromm@med.uni-muenchen.de (J.F.); volkmar.jansson@med.uni-muenchen.de (V.J.); hans_roland.duerr@med.uni-muenchen.de (H.R.D.)

[2] Institute of Pathology, University Hospital, LMU Munich, 81377 Munich, Germany; thomas.knoesel@med.uni-muenchen.de

* Correspondence: alexander.klein@med.uni-muenchen.de

Simple Summary: A precise diagnosis is key in the correct treatment of sarcomas. However, which kind of biopsy should be done: A minimal invasive core needle biopsy (CNB) or an incisional biopsy (IB), yielding more tissue but requiring surgery? We compared the results of both methods after resection of musculoskeletal sarcomas in respect to the accuracy of the diagnosis. In total, 417 patients with 472 biopsies and final sarcoma diagnoses were included. The rate of unequivocal sarcoma diagnoses was 84.9% with CNB vs. 87.6% with IB ($p = 0.465$). The rate of repeat biopsies was higher with CNB as compared to IB ($p = 0.003$). There was no difference in the determination of the sarcoma subtype or the grade of malignancy. Sarcoma subtype, bone vs. soft tissue, and the biopsy technique utilized did not influence the sensitivity. The single exception to this was with chondrosarcomas, where IB was significantly superior to CNB ($p = 0.024$). Based on our data, the minimal invasive technique can be used without disadvantages in the majority of patients.

Abstract: Background: There is no evidence as to the diagnostic value of the two most frequently used methods of biopsies in sarcomas: Incisional or core needle biopsy. The aim of our study was to evaluate the diagnostic sensitivity of the incisional and the core needle biopsy techniques in the diagnosis of bone and soft tissue sarcomas. Methods: We included 417 patients with a definitive diagnosis of bone or soft tissue sarcoma in whom a total of 472 biopsies had been performed. We correlated the results of the biopsies with the result of the definitive histopathological examination of the resected tumor. Dignity, entity, and grading (whenever possible) of the tissue samples were evaluated. Results: A total of 258 biopsies (55%) were performed in order to diagnose a soft tissue tumor and 351 biopsies (74.4%) were core needle biopsies. The number of repeat core needle biopsies, necessitated because of inconclusive histopathological results, was significantly higher (50 vs. 5; $p = 0.003$). We observed no significant difference regarding dignity, entity, and grading between the 2 different types of biopsies. Only with regards to the determination of dignity and entity of chondroid tumors, incisional biopsy was superior with statistical significance ($p = 0.024$). Conclusions: This study represents the largest study on biopsies for bone and soft tissue sarcomas. Based only on our results, we are unable to favor one method of biopsy and found high accuracy with both methods. Considering the potential complications, the added oncological risks of incisional biopsies and the ready availability of core needle biopsies, the latter, in our assessment, represents a valid and favourable method for bone and soft tissue sarcomas.

Keywords: sarcoma; incisional biopsy; core needle biopsy; sensitivity; bone; soft tissue

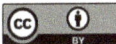

Citation: Klein, A.; Fell, T.; Birkenmaier, C.; Fromm, J.; Jansson, V.; Knösel, T.; Dürr, H.R. Relative Sensitivity of Core-Needle Biopsy and Incisional Biopsy in the Diagnosis of Musculoskeletal Sarcomas. *Cancers* **2021**, *13*, 1393. https://doi.org/10.3390/cancers13061393

Academic Editor: Maria Smolle

Received: 8 January 2021
Accepted: 16 March 2021
Published: 19 March 2021

Publisher's Note: MDPI stays neutral with regard to jurisdictional claims in published maps and institutional affiliations.

Copyright: © 2021 by the authors. Licensee MDPI, Basel, Switzerland. This article is an open access article distributed under the terms and conditions of the Creative Commons Attribution (CC BY) license (https://creativecommons.org/licenses/by/4.0/).

1. Background

Sarcomas are comparatively rare bone or soft tissue tumors, representing about 3% of all malignancies in adults [1]. Because of their rarity, diagnosis is often delayed. However, an accurate and timely diagnosis is essential for the timely start of the appropriate therapy [2,3]. Dependent on the location of the lesion, core needle biopsies (CNB) and incisional biopsies (IB) are the two main options for securing a diagnosis. Excisional biopsy should be only used in cases of small (<3 cm.) and epifascially located tumors [4].

While IB is considered the "gold standard" by many sarcoma experts, there is little evidence to support this standard [5]. An IB offers certain advantages, since a larger volume of tissue can be obtained and precise control of the incisional tract is possible, especially near vessels or nerves. The disadvantages of IB are the more frequent necessity for inpatient treatment with this procedure, higher cost, a higher risk of complications (e.g., hematoma), and a higher risk of potential contamination of the surrounding tissues [6]. In the case of CNB, ultrasound-, CT- or MRI-guidance is possible [7,8]. Already in 1991, Stoker et al. showed with 97% of primary correct diagnosis a very high sensitivity with CNB in the diagnosis of musculoskeletal lesions [9]. In addition, CNB can easily be performed on an outpatient basis. However, the diagnostic value of CNB is still being discussed controversially [10–12]. The decision for one of these two types of biopsy frequently depends on the infrastructure of a medical facility and/or the personal experience of its surgeons [6].

At our institution, CNB has traditionally played an important role in diagnosing musculoskeletal lesions. They have been and still are the primary method in our diagnostic and therapy algorithm.

The aim of this mono-centric retrospective study was to compare the sensitivity of CNB and IB in the diagnosis of soft tissue and bone sarcomas regarding a correct diagnosis of entity, dignity, and grading.

2. Methods

Inclusion criteria were:

- Focusing on sarcomas the definitive diagnosis of a primary or locally recurrent soft tissue or bone sarcoma of the extremities, the pelvis, and the trunk after resection at our center. All benign and intermediate lesions had been excluded;
- Biopsy performed at our musculoskeletal oncology center.

The key criterion for the inclusion of the patients in our cohort was the final diagnosis of a sarcoma. Our rationale for employing this kind of selection was that we intended to identify a homogenous cohort of sarcoma patients. Most of the published case series based their analysis on the complete patient collective, including suspected lesions [13–15]. The diagnostic algorithm of our Sarcoma Center requires a repeat biopsy in all suspicious lesions, whenever the first or the second tissue sample cannot confirm the diagnosis of a sarcoma. The interdisciplinary sarcoma board, including an experienced musculoskeletal radiologist, allows for the reassessment of the imaging studies and their correlation with histopathological findings. If the biopsy was negative, repeat imaging by means of MRI was repeated after an interval of 6–10 weeks. A new biopsy was then initiated in cases with a changing lesion. This algorithm ensures that the rate of false-negative diagnoses of sarcomas is reduced to a minimum.

Two experienced orthopedic oncologic surgeons performed all biopsies. We included 417 patients, treated between 2003 and 2017. These patients underwent a total of 472 biopsies. All patients received either magnetic resonance imaging or computed tomography. The patients with bone tumors (BT) received radiographs in addition. In our biopsy workflow, the feasibility of a CNB is generally assessed first. In cases with a close anatomical relationship of the tumor to vessels or nerves, we used CT- or ultrasound- guidance for obtaining a representative tissue sample. In cases with extended tumor necrosis or after failure of a CNB to provide a reliable diagnosis, we used an IB. In addition, in cases where some differential diagnoses were established beforehand and where more material was deemed necessary, a primary IB was performed.

After exact planning based on the cross-sectional imaging and palpation of the tumor, local anesthesia was applied. After performing a small stab incision of the skin, a core needle (14 G; 2.0 mm; MEDAX s.r.l. Unipersonale; San Possidonio, Italy) was used for soft tissue lesions. A Jamshidi needle (11 G; 3.1 mm; Fa. CareFusion LTD, San Diego, CA, USA) and fluoroscopic guidance was used in bone tumors. Then 2–3 tissue cylinders were sent for histopathological examination.

IB was performed under general anesthesia after identical planning. The skin incision was as small as reasonably possible with straight preparation to the lesion. For bone lesions, a guided 8–12-mm large core drill was used. Careful hemostasis was performed using a resorbable gelatin sponge (Fa. Aegis Lifesciences, Gujarat, India) to fill the bone defect. The majority of patients received a suction drain and an elasto-compressive bandage.

The term "entity" was defined as the type or group of musculoskeletal tumor according to the WHO classification. The term "dignity" refers to the differentiation between the benign and malignant tumors in the histopathological evaluation, also according to the WHO classification. The classification of "grading" was performed based on the classification of the FNCLCC (Fédération nationale des Centres de lutte contre le cancer, Paris, France); G1 corresponds to low-grade, G2 and 3 to high-grade, respectively). The grading of sarcoma was not feasible for every sarcoma subtype according to WHO classification. The classification of grading was not possible in sarcomas that had undergone neoadjuvant therapy. These cases were excluded from the sensitivity evaluation of grading.

In this retrospective study, the histopathology results obtained by biopsy and the final histopathological results after tumor resection were correlated. The histopathological evaluation was performed by 2 experienced pathologists. Every histopathological finding was discussed on the background of the imaging studies in the interdisciplinary board. In cases of inconclusive histopathological findings, an indication for repetition of CNB or an IB was discussed and performed accordingly.

The final histological findings were the basis of the database. The case of patient was graded as false-negative and non-sarcoma diagnosis for the statistical evaluation in case of inconclusive (benign or semimalignant) entity as result of histopathological examination. For statistical analysis, the data of all patients were included. Significance analyses were performed using the Mann–Whitney test, with a 95% confidence interval. The level of significance was set at less than 0.05. The data analysis software used was IBM® SPSS® Statistics 25.

3. Results

In total, 417 consecutive patients underwent 472 biopsies: 409 (86.7%) in primary tumors, 63 (13.3%) because of recurrent sarcomas. Of the patients, 224 (53.8%) were male, and 193 (46.2%) were female. The mean age was 52.3 years. Regarding the biopsies, 258 (55%) were performed in soft tissues, and 214 (45%) in bones. In total, 351 (74.4%) biopsies were CNB and 121 were IB (25.6%). Figure 1 shows the distribution of the sarcoma entities.

3.1. Failure Rate in Dependence of the Kind of Biopsy

In 352 of 417 patients (84.4%), a diagnosis of sarcoma was established with the first attempt (Figure 2). In total, 51 patients needed one repetition of biopsy, 2 patients repetitions. The percentage of repeat CNB, necessitated because of inconclusive results, was significantly higher ($n = 50$ of 351 (14.2%) vs. $n = 5$ of 121 (4.1%); $p = 0.003$) in comparison to repeat IB. In 404 (96.9%) cases, the biopsy finally showed a sarcoma. In 13 cases (3.1%), there were no signs of a malignant tumor in the histopathological examination of the tissue sample. In an interdisciplinary discussion based on clinical, radiological, and pathological findings, a malignant diagnosis was suspected. These cases underwent primary wide resection with the final diagnosis of a sarcoma.

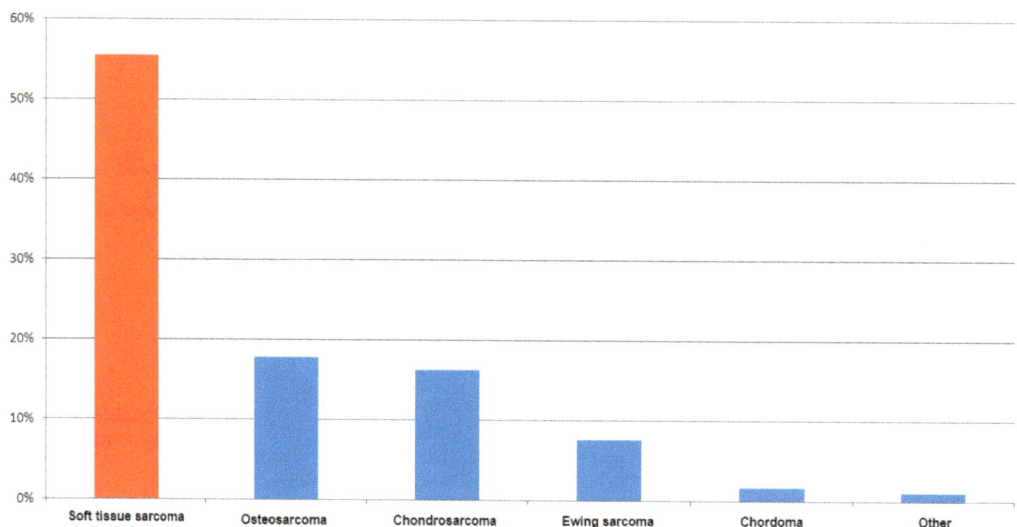

Figure 1. Tumor entities in 417 patients.

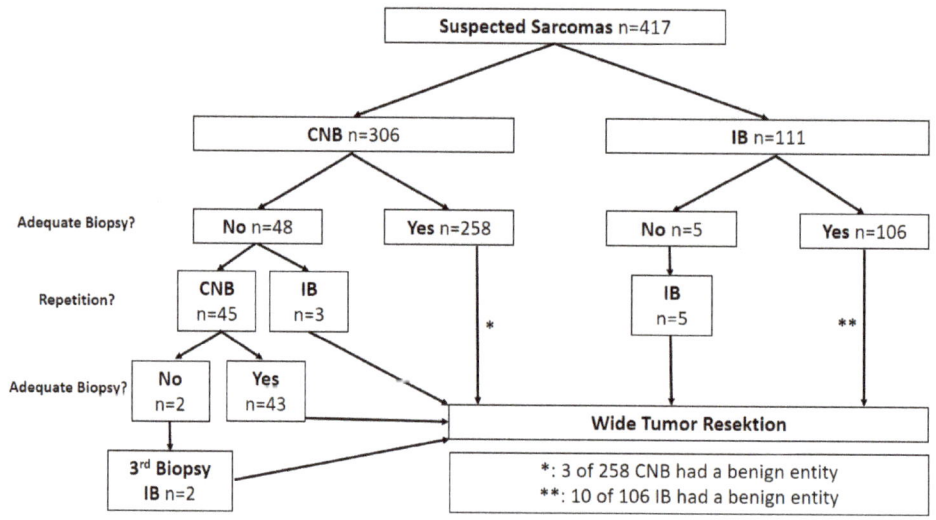

Figure 2. Characteristics of biopsies (CNB: Core needle biopsy, IB: Incisional biopsy).

3.2. Determination of Dignity

Comparing primary CNB and IB regarding their sensitivity with respect to the definitive malignant diagnosis, a rate of 83.3% (255/306 cases CNB) vs. 86.5% (96/111 cases IB) (p = 0.482) was found (Figure 2). In 53 cases with a non-malignant diagnosis or absence of tumor tissue from the first biopsy but with radiological characteristics of a malignant tumor, a repeat biopsy was performed. A second CNB was done in 45 cases (93.3% malignant results) and in 8 cases, an IB was performed as a second biopsy, 3 of which had undergone a primary CNB. All 8 showed malignant results with IB. Two patients with a second CNB required a third biopsy as an IB in order to arrive at a diagnosis. The analysis of false-negative biopsies showed no relevant specific factors, such as entity, location, or kind of tissue.

Included repeat biopsies, the total rate of correct CNB results was 84.9% (298/351 biopsies) vs. 87.6% with IB (106/121 biopsies; $p = 0.465$).

During the observational period, there were no patients with a malignant biopsy and a final diagnosis of a non-malignant tumor in the resection specimen.

3.3. Determination of Entity and Grading

Overall, in 472 biopsy samples, the entity determination was correct in 84.3% (102/121 biopsies) of the IB group compared to 80.1% (281/351 biopsies) in the CNB group ($p = 0.304$). A total of 187 of 472 biopsies (39.6%) were excluded from the grading evaluation because of neoadjuvant therapy. A correct grading, as well as the possibility, depending on the entity, was found in 53.4% of CNB (110/206 biopsies) vs. 65.8% of IB (52/79) ($p = 0.058$). An analysis of the different sarcoma subtypes also did not show any significant differences in the determination of dignity, entity, and grading (if feasible for the entity) between CNB and IB with a single exception (Table 1). This was the determination of dignity of chondroid tumors (enchondroma vs. chondrosarcoma) by means of CNB. IB had a significantly higher specificity in those cases (88.9% (18/20 cases) vs. 66.7% (38/57; $p = 0.024$).

Table 1. Sensitivity of biopsy kinds in different subtypes of sarcomas (CNB: Core needle biopsy; IB: Incisional biopsy; bolded p-value is a significant difference, $p < 0.05$).

Subtypes of Sarcomas	Dignity			Entity			Grading		
	CNB	IB	p	CNB	IB	p	CNB	IB	p
Osteosarcoma	39/52 (75%)	26/32 (81.3%)	0.506	45/52 (86.5%)	28/32 (87.5%)	0.899			
Chondrosarcoma	38/57 (66.7%)	18/20 (88.9%)	**0.024**	45/57 (78.9%)	18/20 (88.9%)	0.270	29/57 (50.8%)	14/20 (70.0%)	0.181
Ewing Sarcoma	26/32 (81.3%)	4/4 (100%)	0.343	26/32 (81.3%)	4/4 (100%)	0.343			
Myxofibrosarcoma	14/19 (73.7%)	5/6 (83.3%)	0.629	14/19 (73.7%)	5/6 (83.3%)	0.629	6/13 (46.2%)	2/4 (50.0%)	0.893
Liposarcoma	27/37 (73.0%)	17/21 (81.0%)	0.495	30/37 (81.1%)	17/21 (81.0%)	0.990	16/26 (61.5%)	12/19 (63.2%)	0.912
MPNST	13/15 (86.7%)	3/5 (60.0%)	0.197	13/15 (86.7%)	4/5 (80.0%)	0.718	2/7 (28.7%)	1/2 (50.0%)	0.571
Synovialsarcoma	6/6 (100%)	8/9 (88.9%)	0.398	6/6 (100%)	9/9 (100%)		2/2 (100%)	2/3 (100%)	
Leiomyo-/Rhabdomyosarcoma	21/23 (91.3%)	5/5 (100%)	0.494	21/23 (91.3%)	5/5 (100%)	0.494	6/10 (60%)	3/3 (100%)	0.188
Epithelioid Sarcoma	7/9 (77.8%)	2/2 (100%)		8/9 (88.9%)	2/2 (100%)	0.621	5/6 (88.3%)	0	

3.4. Differences between Bone and Soft Tissue Sarcomas

The type of tissue did not influence a correct diagnosis of malignancy (83.6%; 179/214 biopsies) in bone sarcoma vs. 87.2%; 225/258 biopsies in soft tissue sarcoma; $p = 0.272$). 196 biopsies in soft tissue sarcomas (STS) were performed as CNB. In 171 (87.2%), a correct result regarding malignancy was made. In bone sarcomas 155 (72.4%) of 214 biopsies were performed as CNB (Table 2). In 127 (81.9%), a correct result regarding malignancy was established.

In soft tissue sarcomas, the rate of primarily correct histopathologic diagnoses was identical between CNB and IB (79% in both groups), and also dignity or grading were not different within this group between both types of biopsy. In bone sarcomas, we also did not observe significant differences between CNB and IB regarding a correct diagnosis of entity and dignity. The evaluation of grading was done after exclusion of osteosarcomas and Ewing sarcomas because of neoadjuvant therapies and was hence limited to chondrosarcomas with significantly higher sensitivity for IB ($p = 0.024$).

Table 2. Characteristics of biopsies and their result (STS: Soft tissue sarcoma; BS: Bone sarcoma; CNB: Core needle biopsy; IB: Incisional biopsy).

	Kind of Biopsy	n	p
Total Number of Biopsies		472	
Kind of Tissue	STS BS	258 (55%) 214 (45%)	
Kind of Biopsy	CNB IB	351 (74.4%) 121 (25.6%)	
Dignity Clarified	CNB IB	84.9% 87.6%	0.465
Biopsy Repeated	CNB IB	50 (14.2%) 5 (4.1%)	0.003
STS Confirmed Dignity	CNB IB	73% 76.4%	0.976
STS Confirmed Entity	CNB IB	79.1% 79%	0.824
STS Confirmed Grading	CNB IB	60% 64.1%	0.610
BS Confirmed Dignity	CNB IB	81.9% 88.1%	0.273
BS Confirmed Entity	CNB IB	76.8% 84.7%	0.201

In cases of local recurrence, the biopsy was significantly more sensitive in comparison to primary diagnosis of sarcoma (95.2 vs. 84.1%; $p = 0.019$) with CNB and IB showing the same results.

Thus, in total, 65 (of 417 cases; 15.6%) of all primary biopsies returned false-negative results (i.e., benign or no tumor tissue) and in these cases, a second or even a third biopsy was necessary to establish the correct diagnosis. There were no significant differences between CNB and IB with regards to the determination of malignancy, entity, and grading of the sarcomas, with one exception: In cases of chondrosarcoma, IB was superior to CNB.

4. Discussion

It is essential to obtain an adequate amount of tumor tissue when performing a biopsy in order to establish the correct histopathological diagnosis. There is general consensus that, in this sense, a fine needle aspiration biopsy is not a reliable method in bone sarcomas [16]. In this context, IB has been considered the gold standard for decades [17]. However, good results of CNB in the diagnosis of sarcomas are described. A number of publications describe the accuracy of CNB in bone and soft tissue lesions. Two large series include several hundred cases: Yong et al. achieved a diagnostic accuracy (entity) of 89% in 509 cases of bone and soft tissue tumors [18]; Ng et al. 77.2% in 432 soft tissue tumors [13]. CNB is easily available and less invasive than IB.

4.1. Patient Selection

Other studies have compared CNB and IB in the diagnosis of bone tumors of different dignities [6,19]. Our study included 417 cases with 472 consecutive biopsies in sarcomas only. Patient inclusion into our study was based on the final sarcoma diagnosis. This kind of cohort selection is not commonly used. However, this strategy allows for the building of a homogeneous study group. The infrastructure of a Sarcoma Center with highly specialized radiologists, surgeons and pathologists and regular case reviews leads to a differentiated and detailed approach to findings with sarcoma-suspicious lesions and negative histopathological results [20,21]. This workflow reduces the risk of false-negative biopsy results in sarcoma patients to the practically achievable minimum.

4.2. Disadvantages of Core Needle Biopsy

The authors are well aware of the fact that due to the small sample sizes obtained with CNB, a major disadvantage of this strategy was a loss of vital tissue for research, i.e., storage in a tissue bank. CNB (14.2%) had a significantly higher failure rate, when compared to IB (4.1%) in our cohort. The most common reason for failure was a non-representative tissue sample from the periphery of the lesion. Other authors have described the difficulties with the technical implementation of CNB as a frequent cause of the failed biopsy [15]. Our standard instrument for CNB is a 14-gauge Tru-Cut needle, according to the recommended guidelines [4]. In addition, and in order to improve the accuracy of CNB, currently we perform these biopsies under ultra-sound guidance more frequently in selected cases (small tumor, non-palpable location). Andreou et al. reported the inferior results (higher rate of local recurrences: 4.2% vs. 10.1%; $p = 0.001$) in patients, who underwent biopsies outside experienced centers [22]. The repetition of a biopsy could adversely affect the outcomes of treated patients according to these results. However, this result is mainly based on IB with a higher risk of contamination. The argument of a faster diagnostic procedure by CNB is put into perspective in 14% of patients needing a second biopsy. However, repetition of the new biopsy is normally within one week possible. There is no evidence for the influence of symptom duration on the oncologic outcome: None of cited studies was able to show a negative effect of longer symptom duration on overall survival of sarcoma patients [23–25].

4.3. Results in Respect to Tissue Type and Entity

The comparison between bone and soft tissue sarcomas showed similar results in both groups (83.6% vs. 83.3%). Some studies suggested a worse sensitivity for malignancy in bone tumors with CNB as opposed to IB [26,27]. In another study, the diagnostic accuracy of CNB's was 100% in bone tumors [14]. Our results as compared to other authors [11,15] were less convincing (15% rate of false-negatives). The only exception was the subgroup of chondrosarcoma patients. Initially, 18% of chondrosarcomas were incorrectly diagnosed as benign tumors: 33.3% in the CNB group and 11.1% in the IB group. In cartilaginous tumors, IB therefore seems to be the better choice, whereas in all other bone lesions, CNB and IB are equivalent [28]. Similar results have already been indicated by other authors [29,30]: Roitman et al. demonstrated an impressive failure rate of CNB with the grading of chondrosarcomas (64% in pelvic bones). This makes the imaging all the more important in assessing chondroid tumors [31].

The comparison of CNB and IB in the subgroup of STS shows a homogenous result. The accuracy rate of IB and CNB (76.4% vs. 73%) is comparable with the international literature [32,33] and does not show any significant differences. Some authors have reported difficulties with the diagnostic procedure in certain soft tissue sarcomas, like angiosarcoma and synovial sarcoma [19,34]. In total, 258 biopsies in STS were done in our cohort. We were unable to identify subgroups of STS, which had a higher probability of correct diagnosis by one particular kind of biopsy. The inclusion of local recurrences in this study has to be discussed. Knowing the primary tumor might facilitate the final diagnosis. The diagnosis of the entity in recurrent tumor might be easier. However, in some cases we observed changes from a more distinct lesion to an undifferentiated sarcoma. in addition, systemic therapy might induce a change in the tumor's biology during the course of treatment, so that the secondary tumor can differ from the primary sarcoma. The biopsy of the suspected recurred tumor is recommended for these reasons [35].

4.4. Advantages of CNB Regarding Local Recurrence

The risk of local recurrence in dependence of the type of biopsy is also of significant importance. Barrientos–Ruiz at al. analyzed the oncological outcomes of 180 sarcoma patients with different kinds of biopsies and the contaminations of biopsy tracts. Their results were: The contamination of the biopsy tracts was significantly higher in the cases of IB (32% vs. 0.8%) [36] and these were associated with a higher number of local recurrences [37]. The lower risk of local recurrence after CNB was confirmed in other studies [38,39]. At many musculoskeletal oncology centers, CNB is therefore favored over IB [6,12,36].

4.5. Study Design and Quality

The retrospective non-randomized design of this study limits the power of our findings. As stated in the method section due to the preselection of cases with difficult differential diagnosis to IB a certain degree of selection bias has to be acknowledged. Despite these limitations, this study is the largest mono-centric series comparing CNB to IB in sarcoma patients. Due to only two surgeons performing all procedures, the techniques are comparable and the patient group is very homogenous. The recently published meta-analysis from Birgin et al. essentially confirms our results [5]: The evaluation of biopsies in 2680 patients with sarcomas (17 studies analyzing CNB and IB) ranges CNB superior to IB.

4.6. Summary

In summary, CNB is at least equivalent to IB. As the higher risk of complications in IB vs. CNB is well known [40], in consideration of a higher risk of complications and possibly worse oncological outcome with IB, CNB is a valid and favorable method of biopsy in the diagnostics of bone and soft tissue sarcomas. The only exception are cases of cartilaginous tumors, where IB should be preferred. A comparison of local recurrence and complications in both types of biopsies is necessary in future studies.

Based on these and previous findings, we have established an internal algorithm for the diagnostic workup in sarcoma cases: The primary biopsy method is CNB, when appropriately guided by sonography or computed tomography. Only in cases of cartilaginous tumors, should IB be preferred.

5. Conclusions

Based on our results, both CNB and IB have a high diagnostic accuracy in suspected sarcomas of the musculoskeletal system. Considering the potential complication and the oncological risks of IB and the better availability of CNB, the latter could be a more favorable method in the diagnosis of musculoskeletal sarcomas, even if in 15% of patients a second CNB was necessary.

Author Contributions: Conceptualization: A.K., T.F., H.R.D.; methodology: A.K., C.B., H.R.D.; software: A.K., J.F.; validation: A.K., C.B., T.K., H.R.D.; writing—original draft preparation: A.K.; writing—review and editing: C.B., H.R.D.; visualization: A.K., J.F.; supervision: H.R.D., T.K., V.J.; project administration: H.R.D., V.J. Each author has contributed significantly to, and is willing to take public responsibility for this study: Its design, data acquisition, and analysis and interpretation of data. All authors have been actively involved in the drafting and critical revision of the manuscript. All authors read and approved the final manuscript. All authors have read and agreed to the published version of the manuscript.

Funding: This research received no external funding.

Institutional Review Board Statement: The study was conducted in accordance with the guidelines of the Declaration of Helsinki, and approved by the Ethics Committee of the Medical Faculty, University of Munich (ID 17-89; Date of approval 2 July 2018).

Informed Consent Statement: Informed consent was obtained from all subjects involved in the study.

Data Availability Statement: The data presented in this study are available by corresponding author of this study.

Conflicts of Interest: None of the authors has financial or personal relationships with other people or organizations that could inappropriately influence (bias) this work. This study was not supported by any grants or external funding. The authors declare that they have no competing interests.

References

1. Stiller, C.; Trama, A.; Serraino, D.; Rossi, S.; Navarro, C.; Chirlaque, M.; Casali, P. Descriptive epidemiology of sarcomas in Europe: Report from the RARECARE project. *Eur. J. Cancer* **2013**, *49*, 684–695. [CrossRef]
2. Nakamura, T.; Matsumine, A.; Matsubara, T.; Asanuma, K.; Uchida, A.; Sudo, A. The symptom-to-diagnosis delay in soft tissue sarcoma influence the overall survival and the development of distant metastasis. *J. Surg. Oncol.* **2011**, *104*, 771–775. [CrossRef]
3. Soomers, V.; Husson, O.; Young, R.; Desar, I.; Van Der Graaf, W. The sarcoma diagnostic interval: A systematic review on length, contributing factors and patient outcomes. *ESMO Open* **2020**, *5*, e000592. [CrossRef]
4. Casali, P.G.; Blay, J.-Y. Soft tissue sarcomas: ESMO Clinical Practice Guidelines for diagnosis, treatment and follow-up. *Ann. Oncol.* **2010**, *21*, v198–v203. [CrossRef]
5. Birgin, E.; Yang, C.; Hetjens, S.; Reissfelder, C.; Hohenberger, P.; Rahbari, N.N. Core needle biopsy versus incisional biopsy for differentiation of soft-tissue sarcomas: A systematic review and meta-analysis. *Cancer* **2020**, *126*, 1917–1928. [CrossRef] [PubMed]
6. Traina, F.; Errani, C.; Toscano, A.; Pungetti, C.; Fabbri, D.; Mazzotti, A.; Donati, D.; Faldini, C. Current Concepts in the Biopsy of Musculoskeletal Tumors: AAOS exhibit selection. *J. Bone Jt. Surg. Am. Vol.* **2015**, *97*, e7. [CrossRef] [PubMed]
7. Kiatisevi, P.; Thanakit, V.; Sukunthanak, B.; Boonthatip, M.; Bumrungchart, S.; Witoonchart, K. Computed Tomography-Guided Core Needle Biopsy versus Incisional Biopsy in Diagnosing Musculoskeletal Lesions. *J. Orthop. Surg.* **2013**, *21*, 204–208. [CrossRef]
8. Issakov, J.; Flusser, G.; Kollender, Y.; Merimsky, O.; Lifschitz-Mercer, B.; Meller, I. Computed tomography-guided core needle biopsy for bone and soft tissue tumors. *Isr. Med Assoc. J. IMAJ* **2003**, *5*, 28–30.
9. Stoker, D.J.; Cobb, J.P.; Pringle, J.A. Needle biopsy of musculoskeletal lesions. A review of 208 procedures. *J. Bone Joint Surg. Br. Vol.* **1991**, *73*, 498–500. [CrossRef] [PubMed]
10. Rougraff, B.T.; Aboulafia, A.; Biermann, S.J.; Healey, J. Biopsy of Soft Tissue Masses: Evidence-based Medicine for the Musculoskeletal Tumor Society. *Clin. Orthop. Relat. Res.* **2009**, *467*, 2783–2791. [CrossRef]
11. Skrzynski, M.C.; Biermann, J.S.; Montag, A.; Simon, M.A. Diagnostic Accuracy and Charge-Savings of Outpatient Core Needle Biopsy Compared with Open Biopsy of Musculoskeletal Tumors. *J. Bone Jt. Surg. Am. Vol.* **1996**, *78*, 644–649. [CrossRef] [PubMed]
12. Kubo, T.; Furuta, T.; Johan, M.P.; Sakuda, T.; Ochi, M.; Adachi, N. A meta-analysis supports core needle biopsy by radiologists for better histological diagnosis in soft tissue and bone sarcomas. *Medicine* **2018**, *97*, e11567. [CrossRef] [PubMed]
13. Hau, M.A.; Kim, J.I.; Kattapuram, S.; Hornicek, F.J.; Rosenberg, A.E.; Gebhardt, M.C.; Mankin, H.J. Accuracy of CT-guided biopsies in 359 patients with musculoskeletal lesions. *Skelet. Radiol.* **2002**, *31*, 349–353. [CrossRef] [PubMed]
14. Pohlig, F.; Kirchhoff, C.; Lenze, U.; Schauwecker, J.; Burgkart, R.; Rechl, H.; Von Eisenhart-Rothe, R. Percutaneous core needle biopsy versus open biopsy in diagnostics of bone and soft tissue sarcoma: A retrospective study. *Eur. J. Med Res.* **2012**, *17*, 29. [CrossRef] [PubMed]
15. Mitsuyoshi, G.; Naito, N.; Kawai, A.; Kunisada, T.; Yoshida, A.; Yanai, H.; Dendo, S.; Yoshino, T.; Kanazawa, S.; Ozaki, T. Accurate diagnosis of musculoskeletal lesions by core needle biopsy. *J. Surg. Oncol.* **2006**, *94*, 21–27. [CrossRef] [PubMed]
16. Casali, P.; Abecassis, N.; Bauer, S.; Biagini, R.; Bielack, S.; Bonvalot, S.; Boukovinas, I.; Bovee, J.V.M.G.; Brodowicz, T.; Broto, J.; et al. Soft tissue and visceral sarcomas: ESMO–EURACAN Clinical Practice Guidelines for diagnosis, treatment and follow-up. *Ann. Oncol.* **2018**, *29*, iv51–iv67. [CrossRef] [PubMed]
17. Bickels, J.; Jelinek, J.S.; Shmookler, B.M.; Neff, R.S.; Malawer, M.M. Biopsy of musculoskeletal tumors. Current concepts. *Clin. Orthop. Relat. Res.* **1999**, *2*, 212–219.
18. Yang, J.; Frassica, F.J.; Fayad, L.; Clark, D.P.; Weber, K.L. Analysis of Nondiagnostic Results after Image-guided Needle Biopsies of Musculoskeletal Lesions. *Clin. Orthop. Relat. Res.* **2010**, *468*, 3103–3111. [CrossRef]
19. Sung, K.-S.; Seo, S.-W.; Shon, M.-S. The diagnostic value of needle biopsy for musculoskeletal lesions. *Int. Orthop.* **2009**, *33*, 1701–1706. [CrossRef] [PubMed]
20. Hoekstra, H.J.; Haas, R.L.M.; Verhoef, C.; Suurmeijer, A.J.H.; Van Rijswijk, C.S.P.; Bongers, B.G.H.; Van Der Graaf, W.T.; Hoekstra, H.J. Adherence to Guidelines for Adult (Non-GIST) Soft Tissue Sarcoma in the Netherlands: A Plea for Dedicated Sarcoma Centers. *Ann. Surg. Oncol.* **2017**, *24*, 3279–3288. [CrossRef]
21. Trautmann, F.; Reißfelder, C.; Pecqueux, M.; Weitz, J.; Schmitt, J. Evidence-based quality standards improve prognosis in colon cancer care. *Eur. J. Surg. Oncol.* **2018**, *44*, 1324–1330. [CrossRef] [PubMed]
22. Andreou, D.; Bielack, S.S.; Carrle, D.; Kevric, M.; Kotz, R.; Winkelmann, W.; Jundt, G.; Werner, M.; Fehlberg, S.; Kager, L.; et al. The influence of tumor- and treatment-related factors on the development of local recurrence in osteosarcoma after adequate surgery. An analysis of 1355 patients treated on neoadjuvant Cooperative Osteosarcoma Study Group protocols. *Ann. Oncol.* **2010**, *22*, 1228–1235. [CrossRef] [PubMed]
23. Rougraff, B.T.; Davis, K.; Lawrence, J. Does Length of Symptoms Before Diagnosis of Sarcoma Affect Patient Survival? *Clin. Orthop. Relat. Res.* **2007**, *462*, 181–189. [CrossRef] [PubMed]
24. Lawrenz, J.M.; Styron, J.F.; Parry, M.; Grimer, R.J.; Mesko, N.W. Longer duration of symptoms at the time of presentation is not associated with worse survival in primary bone sarcoma. *Bone Jt. J.* **2018**, *100-B*, 652–661. [CrossRef] [PubMed]

25. Saithna, A.; Pynsent, P.B.; Grimer, R.J. Retrospective analysis of the impact of symptom duration on prognosis in soft tissue sarcoma. *Int. Orthop.* **2007**, *32*, 381–384. [CrossRef]
26. Adams, S.C.; Potter, B.K.; Pitcher, D.J.; Temple, T.H. Office-based Core Needle Biopsy of Bone and Soft Tissue Malignancies: An Accurate Alternative to Open Biopsy with Infrequent Complications. *Clin. Orthop. Relat. Res.* **2010**, *468*, 2774–2780. [CrossRef]
27. Wu, J.S.; Goldsmith, J.D.; Horwich, P.J.; Shetty, S.K.; Hochman, M.G. Bone and Soft-Tissue Lesions: What Factors Affect Diagnostic Yield of Image-guided Core-Needle Biopsy? *Radiology* **2008**, *248*, 962–970. [CrossRef] [PubMed]
28. Hogendoorn, P.C.W.; Athanasou, N.; Bielack, S.; De Alava, E.; Tos, A.P.D.; Ferrari, S.; Gelderblom, H.; Grimer, R.; Hall, K.S.; Hassan, B.; et al. Bone sarcomas: ESMO Clinical Practice Guidelines for diagnosis, treatment and follow-up. *Ann. Oncol.* **2010**, *21*, v204–v213. [CrossRef]
29. Roitman, P.D.; Farfalli, G.L.; Ayerza, M.A.; Múscolo, L.D.; Milano, F.E.; Aponte-Tinao, L.A. Is Needle Biopsy Clinically Useful in Preoperative Grading of Central Chondrosarcoma of the Pelvis and Long Bones? *Clin. Orthop. Relat. Res.* **2017**, *475*, 808–814. [CrossRef]
30. Brown, M.T.; Gikas, P.D.; Bhamra, J.S.; Skinner, J.A.; Aston, W.J.S.; Pollock, R.C.; Saifuddin, A.; Briggs, T.W.R. How safe is curettage of low-grade cartilaginous neoplasms diagnosed by imaging with or without pre-operative needle biopsy? *Bone Jt. J.* **2014**, *96-B*, 1098–1105. [CrossRef]
31. Fritz, B.; Müller, D.A.; Sutter, R.; Wurnig, M.C.; Wagner, M.W.; Pfirrmann, C.W.; Fischer, M.A. Magnetic Resonance Imaging–Based Grading of Cartilaginous Bone Tumors: Added Value of Quantitative Texture Analysis. *Investig. Radiol.* **2018**, *53*, 663–672. [CrossRef]
32. Heslin, M.J.; Lewis, J.J.; Woodruff, J.M.; Brennan, M.F. Core needle biopsy for diagnosis of extremity soft tissue sarcoma. *Ann. Surg. Oncol.* **1997**, *4*, 425–431. [CrossRef]
33. Kasraeian, S.; Allison, D.C.; Ahlmann, E.R.; Fedenko, A.N.; Menendez, L.R. A Comparison of Fine-needle Aspiration, Core Biopsy, and Surgical Biopsy in the Diagnosis of Extremity Soft Tissue Masses. *Clin. Orthop. Relat. Res.* **2010**, *468*, 2992–3002. [CrossRef]
34. Strauss, D.; Qureshi, Y.; Hayes, A.; Thway, K.; Fisher, C.; Thomas, J. The role of core needle biopsy in the diagnosis of suspected soft tissue tumours. *J. Surg. Oncol.* **2010**, *102*, 523–529. [CrossRef]
35. Trans-Atlantic RPS Working Group. Management of Recurrent Retroperitoneal Sarcoma (RPS) in the Adult: A Consensus Approach from the Trans-Atlantic RPS Working Group. *Ann. Surg. Oncol.* **2016**, *23*, 3531–3540. [CrossRef] [PubMed]
36. Barrientos-Ruiz, I.; Ortiz-Cruz, E.J.; Serrano-Montilla, J.; Bernabeu-Taboada, D.; Pozo-Kreilinger, J.J. Are Biopsy Tracts a Concern for Seeding and Local Recurrence in Sarcomas? *Clin. Orthop. Relat. Res.* **2017**, *475*, 511–518. [CrossRef] [PubMed]
37. Oliveira, M.P.; Lima, P.M.D.A.; De Mello, R.J.V. Tumor contamination in the biopsy path of primary malignant bone tumors. *Rev. Bras. Ortop.* **2012**, *47*, 631–637. [CrossRef] [PubMed]
38. Berger-Richardson, D.; Swallow, C.J. Needle tract seeding after percutaneous biopsy of sarcoma: Risk/benefit considerations. *Cancer* **2017**, *123*, 560–567. [CrossRef]
39. Schaffler-Schaden, D.; Birsak, T.; Zintl, R.; Lorber, B.; Schaffler, G. Risk of needle tract seeding after coaxial ultrasound-guided percutaneous biopsy for primary and metastatic tumors of the liver: Report of a single institution. *Abdom. Radiol.* **2020**, *45*, 3301–3306. [CrossRef]
40. Mankin, H.J.; Mankin, C.J.; Simon, M.A. The Hazards of the Biopsy, Revisited. For the Members of the Musculoskeletal Tumor Society. *J. Bone Jt. Surg. Am. Vol.* **1996**, *78*, 656–663. [CrossRef]

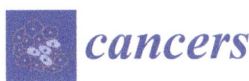

Systematic Review

Candidate Biomarkers for Specific Intraoperative Near-Infrared Imaging of Soft Tissue Sarcomas: A Systematic Review

Zeger Rijs [1,*], A. Naweed Shifai [1], Sarah E. Bosma [1], Peter J. K. Kuppen [2], Alexander L. Vahrmeijer [2], Stijn Keereweer [3], Judith V. M. G. Bovée [4], Michiel A. J. van de Sande [1], Cornelis F. M. Sier [2,5] and Pieter B. A. A. van Driel [6]

1. Department of Orthopedic Surgery, Leiden University Medical Center, Albinusdreef 2, 2333 ZA Leiden, The Netherlands; A.N.Shifai@lumc.nl (A.N.S.); S.E.Bosma@lumc.nl (S.E.B.); M.A.J.van_de_Sande@lumc.nl (M.A.J.v.d.S.)
2. Department of Surgery, Leiden University Medical Center, Albinusdreef 2, 2333 ZA Leiden, The Netherlands; P.J.K.Kuppen@lumc.nl (P.J.K.K.); A.L.Vahrmeijer@lumc.nl (A.L.V.); C.F.M.Sier@lumc.nl (C.F.M.S.)
3. Department of Otorhinolaryngology Head and Neck Surgery, Erasmus Medical Center Cancer Institute, Wytemaweg 80, 3015 CN Rotterdam, The Netherlands; S.Keereweer@erasmusmc.nl
4. Department of Pathology, Leiden University Medical Center, Albinusdreef 2, 2333 ZA Leiden, The Netherlands; J.V.M.G.Bovee@lumc.nl
5. Percuros BV, Zernikedreef 8, 2333 CL Leiden, The Netherlands
6. Department of Orthopedic Surgery, Isala Hospital, Dokter van Heesweg 2, 8025 AB Zwolle, The Netherlands; p.b.a.a.van.driel@isala.nl
* Correspondence: Z.Rijs@lumc.nl; Tel.: +31-641637074

Simple Summary: Near-infrared imaging of tumors during surgery facilitates the oncologic surgeon to distinguish malignant from healthy tissue. The technique is based on fluorescent tracers binding to tumor biomarkers on malignant cells. Currently, there are no clinically available fluorescent tracers that specifically target soft tissue sarcomas. This review searched the literature to find candidate biomarkers for soft tissue sarcomas, based on clinically used therapeutic antibodies. The search revealed 7 biomarkers: TEM1, VEGFR-1, EGFR, VEGFR-2, IGF-1R, PDGFRα, and CD40. These biomarkers are abundantly present on soft tissue sarcoma tumor cells and are already being targeted with humanized monoclonal antibodies. The conjugation of these antibodies with a fluorescent dye will yield in specific tracers for image-guided surgery of soft tissue sarcomas to improve the success rates of tumor resections.

Abstract: Surgery is the mainstay of treatment for localized soft tissue sarcomas (STS). The curative treatment highly depends on complete tumor resection, as positive margins are associated with local recurrence (LR) and prognosis. However, determining the tumor margin during surgery is challenging. Real-time tumor-specific imaging can facilitate complete resection by visualizing tumor tissue during surgery. Unfortunately, STS specific tracers are presently not clinically available. In this review, STS-associated cell surface-expressed biomarkers, which are currently already clinically targeted with monoclonal antibodies for therapeutic purposes, are evaluated for their use in near-infrared fluorescence (NIRF) imaging of STS. Clinically targeted biomarkers in STS were extracted from clinical trial registers and a PubMed search was performed. Data on biomarker characteristics, sample size, percentage of biomarker-positive STS samples, pattern of biomarker expression, biomarker internalization features, and previous applications of the biomarker in imaging were extracted. The biomarkers were ranked utilizing a previously described scoring system. Eleven cell surface-expressed biomarkers were identified from which 7 were selected as potential biomarkers for NIRF imaging: TEM1, VEGFR-1, EGFR, VEGFR-2, IGF-1R, PDGFRα, and CD40. Promising biomarkers in common and aggressive STS subtypes are TEM1 for myxofibrosarcoma, TEM1, and PDGFRα for undifferentiated soft tissue sarcoma and EGFR for synovial sarcoma.

Keywords: TEM1; VEGFR-1; EGFR; VEGFR-2; IGF-1R; PDGFRα; CD40; image guided surgery; near-infra red fluorescence; soft tissue sarcomas

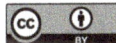

1. Introduction

Soft tissue sarcomas (STS) are a heterogeneous group of mesenchymal tumors that represent 1% of all malignancies [1]. The incidence in Europe is estimated at 4–5/100,000 per year, accumulating to approximately 18,000 new patients in Europe per year [2,3]. While most STS are diagnosed in the extremities (60%), they can arise anywhere in the body [4]. There are over 50 histological subtypes of STS, each with distinct behavioral, clinical, and prognostic features [5]. Surgery of STS is the mainstay of treatment for localized disease. For the aim of curative surgery, a tumor needs to be removed with a margin of normal tissue as the tumor pseudocapsule and reactive zone are expected to contain tumor cells [6]. Clinical outcome after surgical treatment is highly dependent on surgical resection margins, as tumor-positive margins are clearly associated with local recurrence (LR), and indirectly associated with overall survival [7–10]. Further, close or positive margins often necessitate the need for adjuvant radiotherapy to reduce the risk for LR with about 50%, but this increases the risk for local complications [11,12]. However, determining the surgical margin is challenging, particularly when tumor tissue is surrounded by vital structures or in STS subtypes with a highly infiltrative growth pattern, such as myxofibrosarcoma (MFS), undifferentiated soft tissue sarcoma (USTS, previously called undifferentiated pleomorphic sarcoma), and synovial sarcoma (SS). In these specific tumors, preoperative surgical planning is complicated by current limitations in preoperative radiological imaging. The infiltrative growth of sarcoma with long slender tails, clearly diagnosed by histology after surgical resection, is sometimes difficult to detect with preoperative imaging [13]. Consequently, despite centralizing STS treatment and (neo)adjuvant treatment modalities, positive margins and LR are still common. Positive margins are 13%, 20% and 28%, with LR rates of 12% (5-year follow up), 40% (10-year follow up), and 45% (5-year follow up) in SS, MFS, and USTS respectively [14–18]. The real-time intraoperative tumor-specific imaging of STS could help the surgeon to discriminate tumor from normal tissue, improving complete tumor resections and reducing LR rates. Near-infrared fluorescence (NIRF) imaging is one of the most upcoming technologies in real-time targeted imaging as it facilitates surgeons to visualize tumor tissue during surgery. It has been explored for various tumor types with promising results and is expected to play an important role in future surgery of STS [19].

Three important parameters define successful NIRF tumor-specific imaging: a tumor-specific biomarker, a targeting moiety conjugated to a fluorescent dye/fluorophore (tracer), and a NIRF camera system. In NIRF imaging, light in the near-infrared (NIR) wavelength is used (650–900 nm). In this region, tissue penetration of light is relatively high, due to low tissue absorption, and the autofluorescence of normal tissue is limited [20]. Light in the NIR region is invisible to the human eye and therefore a dedicated NIRF camera system is needed, which has the advantage that the surgical field is not altered by the fluorescence from the tracer. Clinical NIRF cameras of various companies are available [21].

The search for a tumor-specific biomarker for NIRF imaging of STS is complex, because of the rarity and heterogeneity of the disease. The ideal biomarker should be highly and homogenously expressed on tumor cells of most subtypes of STS, while being absent on adjacent healthy tissue. Like for other cancers, the biomarker should preferably be located on the cell surface of malignant cells to permit direct targeting and have the possibility of internalization (endocytosis of an extracellular molecule upon binding to a specific protein on the cell surface) to facilitate a long-lasting fluorescence signal. Ideally, this biomarker is still present on residual cells after neoadjuvant therapy.

Fluorescent tracers for tumor biomarkers are generated by the conjugation of a fluorescent dye/fluorophore to a targeting moiety. Various fluorophores are available and some are clinically approved [22]. Targeting moieties consist of proteins, like monoclonal antibodies or fragments thereof, peptides, RNA aptamers, or other small synthetic molecules. Monoclonal antibodies are the most widely used targeting moieties in biotherapy and imaging. The advantages of antibodies are their specificity, affinity, flexibility, and relatively long plasma half-life. To minimize immune reactions, human(ized) versions are mostly used. A disadvantage of antibodies for the use of imaging is the relatively high costs of development, which is particularly relevant for rare diseases like STS. In the past decade, therapeutic antibodies have been equipped with NIRF dyes and evaluated for imaging of common cancer types, like breast and colorectal cancer [19].

Elaborating on this approach, the aim of this systematic review is to select candidate biomarkers for specific intraoperative NIRF imaging of soft tissue sarcomas. STS are a rare and heterogeneous group of tumors. The development of a specific tracer for NIRF imaging that is not already clinically used in therapy would be very challenging as it would be costly and time consuming. Therefore, the search is restricted to clinically available monoclonal antibodies of which the safety profiles are already demonstrated and a translation towards a tracer for NIRF imaging can be expected. The overall purpose of this evaluation is to find optimal biomarkers for the three most common and aggressive STS subtypes MFS, USTS, and SS, which account for challenging resections and currently result in high rates of local recurrences.

2. Materials and Methods

2.1. Search Strategy

An initial search was performed to find clinically available monoclonal antibodies targeting STS. The EU Clinical Trials Register (www.clinicaltrialsregister.eu/) and clinical trials.gov (clinicaltrials.gov/) databases were searched with the keyword "Soft tissue sarcoma", and all clinically available monoclonal antibodies targeting STS were listed. Next, a PubMed search with the respective biomarkers targeted by those monoclonal antibodies was created with the assistance of a medical librarian (Appendix A). The search was done in August 2019 and updated in September 2020 due to the publication of multiple relevant articles between August 2019 and September 2020. This systematic review was performed following the Preferred Reporting Items for Systematic Reviews and Meta-Analysis (PRISMA) guidelines of 2009 (registration ID: CRD42020206473) [23].

2.2. Eligibility Criteria

Studies were eligible for inclusion if they met the following criteria: (1) report of expression of cell surface-expressed biomarkers in STS for which a clinically available antibody was present, (2) at least 95% of the included tumor samples were primary STS, (3) sample size of at least 4, (4) published in the English language, and (5) full text was available. The eligibility of the studies was assessed by two authors (Z.R. and A.N.S.). Disagreements were discussed with a third reviewer (P.B.A.A.v.D.). Animal studies, xenograft studies, cell line studies, articles without positive and negative control samples, case reports, reviews, viewpoints, conference reports, meeting abstracts, letters to journals, or editors were excluded.

2.3. Data Extraction

The following data were extracted from eligible studies: target characteristics, sample size, type of sample, percentage of positive STS samples, localization of expression, pattern of expression, positive and negative controls, internalization, and previously imaged. A second tumor type-independent search was performed for data on internalization and previous imaging of targets where no information was found after the first search (Appendix B). Data on safety profiles of monoclonal antibodies was acquired through the search of Appendix A.

2.4. Biomarker Selection Scoring System

In order to select the optimal biomarkers for tumor specific NIRF imaging in STS, we developed a target selection scoring system. The scoring system is based on the modified version of the Target Selection Criteria (TASC), developed by Bosma et al. [24]. The scoring system is based on five domains (see Table 1).

1. Sample size. The number of samples indicate how much evidence is acquired.
2. Percentage of biomarker-positive STS samples. This is calculated based on the amount of STS samples that positively showed presence of the biomarker in each included article, independent of the percentage of positive tumor cells within each sample. Immunohistochemistry was used to assess the percentage of positive STS in tissue samples.
3. Pattern of expression. Ideally, the target is expressed diffusely by all tumor cells (particularly at the tumor border) to guide surgical resection. The pattern of expression is defined as diffuse when expression is randomly spread throughout the tumor sample and focal when expression is located in a specific region of the tumor sample. When different samples show variable expression patterns (diffuse and focal), the expression pattern for the whole cohort is defined as heterogeneous. No distinction was made based on exact location of expression within tumor samples. While this review included studies evaluating tissue samples and tissue microarrays, data regarding the pattern of expression was extracted from studies including tissue samples.
4. Internalization. This is important because internalization after binding of the tracer creates a long-lasting signal for tumor-specific imaging.
5. Previously imaged. If there is prove that imaging is possible, it has more potential to be translated to the clinics. The distinction between imaging with or without NIRF is important for its applicability in NIRF imaging. This criterium was tumor type independent.

The maximum score for a target is 9 points, 7 was chosen as the cut-off value for promising targets for tumor specific NIRF imaging in STS.

Table 1. Target selection scoring system.

Score	0	1	2
Sample size	0–100	101–500	>500
Percentage of positive STS samples	0–33%	33–67%	>67%
Pattern of expression *	Focal	Heterogeneous	Diffuse
Internalization	not described	Yes	
Previously imaged	not described	Yes, but not with NIRF imaging	Yes, NIRF imaging

Note. * Pattern of expression is focal when the expression is located in a specific region of the tumor sample and diffuse when expression is randomly spread throughout the tumor sample. When different samples show variable expression patterns (diffuse and focal), the expression pattern is defined as heterogeneous.

3. Results

3.1. Study Selection

Our analysis of the EU Clinical Trials Register (https://www.clinicaltrialsregister.eu/) and clinical trials.gov (https://clinicaltrials.gov/) revealed the following clinically available monoclonal antibodies targeting STS-associated cell surface-expressed biomarkers (Table 2): Ontuxizumab (MORAb-004) [trial number: NCT01574716] targeting tumor endothelial marker 1 (TEM1), recombinant monoclonal antibody Aflibercept [NCT00390234], and humanized monoclonal antibody Bevacizumab [NCT03913806] targeting vascular endothelial growth factor A (VEGF-A), thereby indirectly targeting vascular endothelial growth factor receptor-1 (VEGFR-1) and vascular endothelial growth factor receptor-2 (VEGFR-2), Ramucirumab [NCT04145700] targeting VEGFR-2, Cetuximab [NCT00148109] targeting epidermal growth factor receptor (EGFR), Ganitumab (AMG 479) [NCT03041701], Teprotumumab [NCT00642941], Cixutumumab [NCT01016015] and Figitumumab [NCT00927966] targeting insulin-like growth factor 1 receptor (IGF-1R), Olaratumab [NCT03126591] targeting platelet derived growth factor α (PDGFRα), APX005M [NCT03719430] targeting cluster of differentiation 40 (CD40), Atezolizumab [NCT03474094], Avelumab [NCT04242238], Durvalumab [NCT03317457], and Envafolimab [NCT04480502] targeting programmed death-ligand 1 (PD-L1), ABBV-085 [NCT02565758] targeting leucine-rich repeat containing 15 (LRRC15), CAB-ROR2-ADC [NCT03504488] targeting receptor tyrosine kinase-like orphan receptor 2 (ROR2) and Ipilimumab [NCT04118166], and Tremelimumab [NCT03317457] targeting cytotoxic T-Lymphocyte-associated protein 4 (CTLA-4).

The PubMed search based on the cell surface-expressed biomarkers targeted by clinically available monoclonal antibodies identified 1856 articles (Figure 1). After screening the titles and abstracts, 1604 articles were excluded. Subsequently, 252 full-text articles were assessed for eligibility, of which 171 articles did not meet eligibility criteria; 107 articles did not study expression of the included biomarkers on human STS cells, for 19 articles data was not suitable for extraction, 16 articles had a sample size of less than 4 samples, 11 articles did not have full-text available, 10 articles had more than 5% of samples which were not primary STS and therefore their results were no longer a valid representation of STS samples, and 8 articles were reviews or letters to journals without an accompanying methods section. Data regarding internalization and previously imaged was not always described in STS. Therefore, a separate search was performed to obtain these data from other tissue types (Appendix B). This resulted in an additional 16 included articles. Ultimately, 97 articles were included for this review.

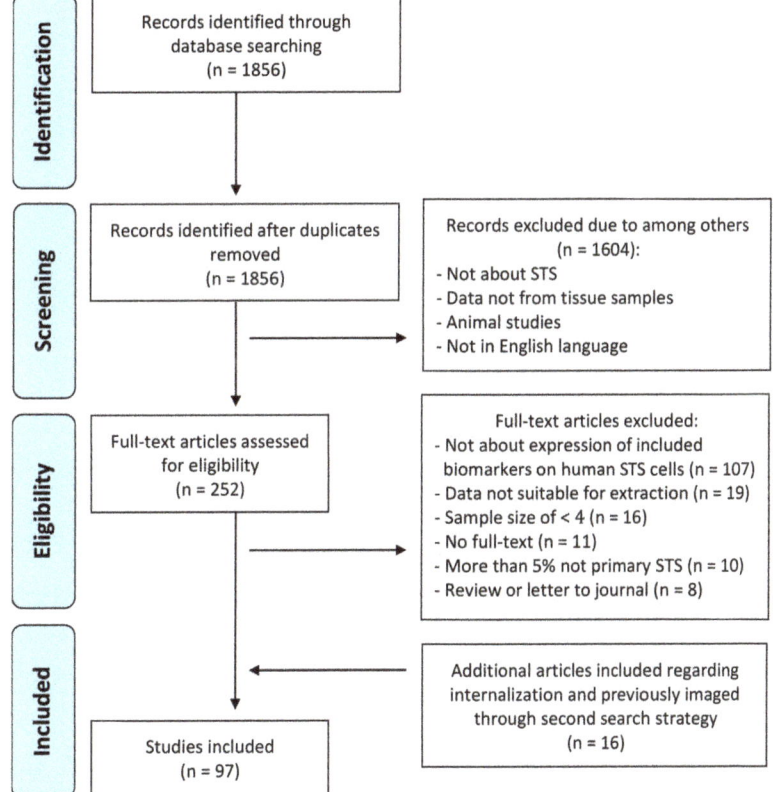

Figure 1. Flowchart of study selection process.

Table 2. Summarized data regarding eleven reviewed biomarkers (in descending order of the modified target selection criteria score).

Biomarker	Therapeutic Antibody	N	% Positive STS (Mean % + Range)	Pattern of Expression	Internalization	Previously Imaged	Score	Literature
Tumor endothelial marker 1 (TEM1/endosialin/CD248)	Ontuxizumab (MORAb-004)	768	77% (55–100)	Diffuse	Yes, [25]	NIRF imaging [26]	9	[26–29]
Vascular endothelial growth factor receptor-1 (VEGFR-1)	Aflibercept Bevacizumab	477	76% (22–100)	Diffuse	Yes, [30]	NIRF imaging [30,31]	8	[32–39]
Epidermal growth factor receptor (EGFR)	Cetuximab	1918	53% (0–100)	Diffuse	Yes, [40]	NIRF imaging [41]	8	[27,42–76]
Vascular endothelial growth factor receptor-2 (VEGFR-2)	Aflibercept Bevacizumab Ramucirumab	449	71% (11–100)	Diffuse	Yes, [77]	NIRF imaging [78]	7	[33–36,38,39,79–81]
Insulin-like growth factor 1 receptor (IGF-1R)	Ganitumab (AMG 479) Teprotumumab Cixutumumab Figitumumab	507	63% (25–100)	Diffuse	Yes, [82]	NIRF imaging [83]	7	[63,64,82,84–89]
Platelet derived growth factor receptor α (PDGFRα)	Olaratumab	1536	64% (0–100)	Diffuse	Yes, [84]	NIRF imaging [85]	7	[27,34,36,38,42–49,51,82,86–92]
Cluster of differentiation 40 (CD40)	APX005M	153	62% (17–86)	Diffuse	Yes, [93]	NIRF imaging [94]	7	[95–98]
Programmed death-ligand 1 (PD-L1/CD 274/B7-H1)	Atezolizumab Avelumab Durvalumab Envafolimab	1492	31% (0–76)	Heterogeneous (focal and diffuse)	Yes, [99]	NIRF imaging [100]	6	[101–118]
Leucine-rich repeat containing 15 (LRRC15)	ABBV-085	635	40%	Diffuse	Not described	Not described	4	[102]
Receptor tyrosine kinase-like orphan receptor 2 (ROR2) Cytotoxic	CAB-ROR2-ADC	237	72%	Not described	Not described	Not described	3	[119]
T-Lymphocyte-associated protein 4 (CTLA-4/CD152)	Ipilimumab Tremelimumab	10	30%	Not described	Yes, [120]	Not with NIRF imaging [120]	2	[59]

Note. Abbreviations: N, total number of samples; STS, soft tissue sarcoma; NIRF, near-infrared fluorescence.

3.2. Candidate Biomarkers

A modified Target Selection Criteria TASC)-scoring system was applied to eleven cell surface-expressed biomarkers (Table 1). Seven promising candidate targets for NIRF imaging emerged with a minimum score of 7 out of 9. The biomarkers arranged in descending order based on their scores were: TEM1 (9), VEGFR-1 (8), EGFR (8), VEGFR-2 (7), IGF-1R (7), PDGFRα (7) and CD40 (7). Further details of these biomarkers are described below and in Table 2, focusing on their physiological role, expression in STS, the availability of clinically used monoclonal antibodies targeting these biomarkers, and latest developments.

3.2.1. TEM1

Tumor Endothelial Marker 1, also referred to as Endosialin or CD248, is a highly glycosylated type I transmembrane protein classified among the C-type lectin-like domain superfamily 14. It has been suggested that TEM1 plays a critical role in wound healing and angiogenesis [121,122]. Moreover, while it is expressed minimally in normal conditions, it is markedly upregulated in the setting of injury and malignant tumor growth. In (soft tissue) sarcomas TEM1 was observed to be present on malignant cells [28]. Stromal TEM1 promotes spontaneous metastasis and TEM1-expressing pericytes were shown to facilitate distant site metastasis by stimulating tumor cell intravasation [123]. Furthermore, TEM1 expression is associated with enhanced tumor growth, presumably due to tumor-specific angiogenesis [124].

The presence of the biomarker in STS samples, regardless of the percentage of positive tumor cells, was determined on both tumor and stromal cells for TEM1. In STS, 77% (range 55–100%, n = 768) of the samples showed presence of TEM1 on average, reported in 4 different articles [26–29]. Staining was performed in 17 subtypes of STS (Appendix C). The expression pattern for TEM1 was diffuse. Corresponding to the expression in other cancer types, TEM1 expression is correlated with advanced tumor grade in STS [121,125].

In MFS it was demonstrated that TEM1 was present in all 34 investigated samples, with a diffuse pattern of expression [27]. Staining was negative or very limited in normal adjacent tissue such as muscular fascia and peripheral nerve bundles. For USTS an average of 81% (range 73–89%, n = 128) of the samples expressed TEM1, with a diffuse pattern of expression [28,29]. In SS, 71% (range 62–80%, n = 70) of the tissue samples stained positive for TEM1. The pattern of expression was heterogeneous with samples expressing TEM1 either focally or diffusely. Besides, Thway et al. [29] demonstrated in representative images that the spindle cell component of biphasic SS samples is positive, while the glandular epithelial areas are negative. Regarding monophasic SS, both positive and negative samples were reported [28,29]. Data are summarized in Table 3.

Exclusively Ontuxizumab has been clinically investigated as a therapeutic drug in STS [130]. However, it still needs to be modified into a NIRF imaging tracer. A high-affinity human single-chain variable fragment (scFv)-Fc fusion protein (78Fc) targeting TEM1 has been engineered and conjugated with the near-infrared fluorochrome VivoTag-S750, which proved to be an efficient tracer in preclinical osteosarcoma and lung cancer models [25,27,124,127].

In conclusion, TEM1 can be targeted in NIRF imaging by Ontuxizumab upon conjugation to a NIRF dye and small proteins have been produced pre-clinically for similar purposes. A major advantage of TEM1 is that it has minimal to no expression on adjacent normal tissue and therefore it is characterized by a high tumor-to-background ratio. Additional benefits are its diffuse pattern of expression, the high frequency of positivity (STS 77%, MFS 100%, USTS 81% and SS 71%), and its correlation with advanced tumor grades. A disadvantage is its heterogeneous pattern of expression in the SS subtype with samples illustrating focal expression of TEM1.

Table 3. Summarized data regarding biomarkers in myxofibrosarcoma, undifferentiated soft tissue sarcoma, and synovial sarcoma.

Biomarker	N	Positive Tumors Mean% (Range)	Expression Pattern	Present after RTx	Literature
Myxofibrosarcoma					
TEM1	34	100 (100)	Diffuse	Yes, [27]	[27]
EGFR	97	38 (0–89)	Heterogeneous	Yes, [27]	[26,53,65]
PDGFRα	34	77 (77)	Not described	Yes, [27]	[27]
Undifferentiated soft tissue sarcoma					
TEM1	128	81 (73–89)	Diffuse	N.D.	[28,29]
VEGFR-1	81	68 (68)	Not described	N.D.	[36]
EGFR	287	62 (5–95)	Heterogeneous	N.D.	[50,57,65,70]
VEGFR-2	81	6 (6)	Not described	N.D.	[36]
IGF-1R	120	25 (25)	Not described	N.D.	[90]
PDGFRα	432	79 (63–99)	Diffuse	N.D.	[35,50,126]
Synovial sarcoma					
TEM1	70	71 (62–80)	Heterogeneous	N.D.	[28,29]
VEGFR-1	27	70 (70)	Not described	N.D.	[27]
EGFR	160	86 (71–100)	Heterogeneous	Yes, [127]	[52,58,66,69–71]
VEGFR-2	27	4 (4)	Not described	N.D.	[27]
IGF-1R	195	57 (35–80)	Not described	N.D.	[81,82,128,129]
PDGFRα	136	69 (44–84)	Not described	N.D.	[35,81,88,91]

Abbreviations: N, total number of samples and/or cell lines; STS, soft tissue sarcoma; RTx, radiotherapy; N.D. not described. No distinction was made between monophasic and biphasic synovial sarcoma.

3.2.2. VEGFR

The VEGFR family consists of the 3 members VEGFR-1, -2 and -3 which are receptors for ligands VEGF-A, -B, -C, -D, and Placenta Growth Factor [22]. The receptors contain a split tyrosine kinase domain and a ligand-binding part. The individual VEGFR members have separate roles in various signaling pathways, but as a family they collectively function as the principal driver of angiogenesis and lymph angiogenesis. Hence, VEGFRs are mainly expressed on vascular and lymphatic endothelial cells in healthy tissue [21,130,131]. In various tumor types, including STS, they are expressed by both endothelial cells and tumor cells [131]. Here they stimulate tumor growth [132]. VEGFR-1 and VEGFR-2 have been clinically targeted by antibodies in STS, in contrast to VEGFR-3. Therefore, only VEGFR-1 and VEGFR-2 will be evaluated.

VEGFR-1 presence was found in an average of 76% (range 22–100%, n = 477) of the STS patients in 8 different studies [32–39]. Staining was performed in 15 STS subtypes (Appendix C). The VEGFR-1 expression pattern was demonstrated to be diffuse. Expression was found in the cytoplasm, and on the nuclear and cell membrane [32,35]. VEGFR-2 expression was present in 71% (range 11–100%, n = 449) on average in 9 different studies, and 16 STS subtypes were evaluated [33–36,38,39,79–81]. The pattern of expression was heterogeneous, and expression was found in the cytoplasm, and on the nuclear and cell membrane [35,81]. Interestingly, Kilvaer et al. [131] states that VEGFR overexpression is correlated with an increased tumor grade.

No data were found for VEGFR immunohistochemical staining in MFS. One paper reported on the presence of VEGFR-1 and VEGFR-2 in USTS and SS [36]. VEGFR-1 and VEGFR-2 expression was found in 68% and 6% of 81 USTS samples, respectively. In SS, this was 70% and 4% for respectively VEGFR-1 and VEGFR-2 in 27 samples (Table 3). Moreover, the pattern of expression was described for neither USTS nor SS [36]. Additionally, no distinction was made between monophasic and biphasic SS in the published data.

Ramucirumab binds to VEGFR-2 and is currently in its recruitment phase for clinical testing in SS [133]. Besides, VEGFR-1 and VEGFR-2 may be targeted indirectly using Bevacizumab-IRDye800CW or Aflibercept upon conjugation to a NIRF dye [29,30,134,135]. Recently published study results showed visualization of all 15 included STS patients with

Bevacizumab-IRDye800CW targeting VEGF-A. In this paper, in vivo tumor-to-background ratios of 2.0-2.5 were found with doses of 10-25mg tracer and no tracer-related adverse events occurred within 2 weeks after surgery [136]. Additionally, targeting tumors with Bevacizumab-IRDye800CW has been investigated extensively in clinical trials for several tumor types [134–137]. Here, its tolerable safety profile was confirmed in primary breast cancer patients [138].

In conclusion, VEGFR-1 and VEGFR-2 are receptors that may be targeted indirectly with a tracer, Bevacizumab-IRDye800CW, that has already widely proven its benefit in multiple cancer types. The direct targeting of VEGFR-2, however, may additionally be performed with Ramucirumab. Major advantages of VEGFR-1 are the high frequency of positivity in STS (76%), the diffuse pattern of expression in tumors and increasing expression associated with enhanced tumor grade. However, while VEGFR-1 is commonly present in USTS and SS, there is no data concerning its pattern of expression in these STS subtypes. Furthermore, advantages of VEGFR-2 are its high presence of 71% in STS samples and increasing expression associated with enhanced tumor grade. Disadvantages are a heterogeneous, and therefore unpredictable, pattern of expression in the evaluated tissue samples and the fact that only 6% of USTS and 4% of SS are positive. Additionally, both VEGFRs are commonly expressed in healthy tissue, potentially resulting in a low tumor-to-background ratio.

3.2.3. EGFR

Epidermal Growth Factor Receptor is a transmembrane glycoprotein belonging to the ErbB/HER family together with 3 additional distinct receptor tyrosine kinases: ErbB2/HER2, ErbB3/HER3, and ErbB4/HER4 [139]. Seven different ligands trigger intracellular signals for fundamental cellular functions including proliferation, differentiation, migration and survival of tumor cells [140,141]. EGFR is mainly expressed in proliferating keratinocytes [142,143]. In tumors, EGFR overexpression can trigger tumor invasion and metastasis. Furthermore, it is a central regulator of autophagy, which is strongly involved in resistance to cancer therapies [144,145].

EGFR expression in STS was described in 36 scientific papers [27,42–76]. The presence of EGFR on STS tissue was observed in an average of 53% of the samples (range 0–100%, n = 1918). Expression was evaluated in 29 different subtypes of STS (Appendix C). The pattern of expression was diffuse. Importantly, EGFR expression in STS was strongly correlated to higher histological grade [46,48,70].

In MFS, EGFR presence was observed in an average of 38% (range 0–89%, n = 97) of the samples in 3 articles (Table 3) [26,53,65]. This wide range might be explained by the fact that 1 article included 10 low-grade MFS samples of which none expressed EGFR. The remaining 2 articles had a higher percentage of positive samples with a diffuse pattern of expression. This confirms the positive correlation of EGFR expression with increased histological grade STS [26,53,65]. For USTS, EGFR expression was detected in an average of 62% (range 5–95%, n = 287) of the samples with a heterogeneous pattern of expression. Similar to MFS, a wide range was observed with 1 article reporting 5% of 200 samples to be positive for EGFR staining, 1 article reporting 58% in 24 samples, and 2 articles reporting 91% and 95% positive samples in 44 and 19 samples, respectively. Here, the correlation to increased histological grade could not explain the variable expression [50,57,65,70]. Lastly, EGFR presence was seen in an average of 86% (range 71–100%, n = 160) of the SS samples. The pattern of expression was noticeably heterogeneous, extending from focal to diffuse expression [52,58,66,69–71]. Furthermore, Gusterson et al. [58] and Sato et al. [66] compared the spindle cell and epithelial components of biphasic SS samples. They described that the former is strongly positive, whereas the latter is mainly negative for EGFR expression. Regarding monophasic SS, both positive and negative samples were reported.

Currently, Cetuximab is the only clinically investigated EGFR-targeting monoclonal antibody for STS [146]. It has been conjugated to IRDye800 and examined in several clinical trials in other tumor types. To appraise its utility in the detection of metastatic lymph nodes in pancreatic cancer, a total of 144 human lymph nodes were evaluated *ex-vivo*. The Cetuximab-IRDye800 conjugate demonstrated a sensitivity and specificity of 100% and 78% [147]. Additionally, no grade 2 or higher adverse events were observed with Cetuximab-IRDye800 in glioblastoma and head and neck squamous cell carcinoma [148,149].

A clinical trial investigating the use of ABY-029, an affibody conjugated to IRDye800CW targeting EGFR, is in the recruitment phase for targeting STS [150]. Based on pre-clinical research it is a promising tracer for STS and is safe for human use [41,151]. Other clinical trials in their recruitment phase explore the use of Panitumumab-IRDye800 in imaging of head and neck cancer, lung cancer, and metastatic lymph nodes [152–154].

In summary, there are multiple promising tracers available which can be applied for NIR fluorescence-guided surgery in STS. Main advantages of EGFR, apart from the readily available tracers, are its diffuse pattern of expression in STS in general, the increased expression in STS of higher histological grade, and the high frequency of expression (88%) among SS samples. Yet, some drawbacks are the mediocre percentage (54%) of positive tumor samples in STS in general and the highly heterogeneous expression pattern in SS.

3.2.4. IGF-1R

Insulin-like Growth Factor 1 Receptor is a receptor tyrosine kinase that is activated upon binding with IGF-1 or IGF-2. Under normal physiological circumstances, this provokes a chain of signaling events that induce cellular transformations such as hypertrophy in skeletal muscle. IGF-1R is upregulated in multiple malignancies, including prostate, breast and lung cancer, where it is involved in tumor growth. Besides, it enables cancer cells to resist the cytotoxic properties of radiotherapy and chemotherapeutic drugs by inducing an anti-apoptotic effect [24].

IGF-1R presence was detected in 63% (range 25–100%, n = 507) of STS samples on average in 9 different studies [63,64,82,90,126,128,129,155,156]. Staining was performed in 15 subtypes of STS (Appendix C). The receptor was dispersed diffusely in the cytoplasm, and on the nuclear and cell membrane [62,82,128]. No correlation between histological grade and IGF-1R expression was observed [64,128].

No data are available on IGF-1R presence in MFS. Presence of IGF-1R in USTS and SS was evaluated in 1 and 4 articles respectively [81,82,126,128,129]. IGF-1R presence was found in 25% of the USTS samples (n = 120), while in SS an average of 57% (range 35–100%, n = 195) of the samples stained positive. The pattern of expression was described for neither (Table 3). However, Friedrichs et al. [155] reported that vast areas of tumorous tissue showed membranous staining in monophasic (comprising spindle cells) SS. In contrast, biphasic SS samples displayed predominantly positive staining in the epithelial component. Regarding monophasic SS, both positive and negative samples were reported [81,126,128,129].

Clinical trials targeting IGF-1R in STS have been conducted with Teprotumumab, Cixutumumab, Figitumumab, and Ganitumab [157–161]. Nevertheless, these monoclonal antibodies have not been evaluated for their potential in NIRF imaging.

AVE-1642, a humanized anti-IGF-1R antibody, labelled with Alexa 680 has been pre-clinically investigated in in vivo breast cancer models and adequately identified receptor expression [162].

Overall, IGF-1R may be targeted in NIRF imaging by several potential antibodies after conjugation to a NIRF dye. In addition, pre-clinical advances have resulted in promising tracers that may find future clinical use. An advantage of IGF-1R is its relatively common (63%) presence in all STS samples. However, its expression has no correlation with tumor grade, and data on pattern of expression in MFS, USTS and SS is limited.

3.2.5. PDGFR

Platelet-Derived Growth Factor is a receptor tyrosine kinase characterized by two isoforms, PDGFRα and PDGFRβ [163]. The receptors can be activated after binding by ligands from the PDGF-family. Upon activation, PDGFR is known to control angiogenesis in endothelial cells, and cell migration and growth in mesenchymal cells. Moreover, in healthy tissue both PDGFRs are mainly expressed in mesenchymal cells during inflammation, whereas during non-inflammatory conditions the expression is minimal [164,165]. In tumor biology, PDGFR activation stimulates cell growth and enhances metastatic behavior by attracting fibroblasts, which secrete factors that promote proliferation and migration of tumor cells. Both PDGFRα and -β are expressed by tumor cells of STS, yet expression of specifically PDGFRα is evaluated in this review as a monoclonal antibody against this receptor has been clinically tested in STS, while not against PDGFRβ [42,46,166,167].

Based on the literature search, PDGFRα was present in 64% of STS samples on average (range 0–100%, n = 1536) in 21 different articles [27,34,36,38,42–49,51,82,86–92]. Expression was evaluated in 22 different subtypes of STS (Appendix C). The pattern of expression was diffuse, and expression was identified in the cytoplasm, and on the nuclear and cell membrane of the tumor cells [45,86,168].

PDGFRα expression in the specific STS subtypes of interest, MFS, USTS, and SS, were evaluated separately in 1, 4, and 5 articles, respectively. In MFS PDGFRα was present in 77% of 34 tissue samples [27]. In USTS, 78% of the tumors (range 63–99%, n = 475) were positive for PDGFRα, while for SS 69% (range 44–84%, n = 136) stained positive. Moreover, expression was reported to be diffuse in USTS. No data regarding the pattern of expression of MFS and SS were reported [35,50,88,91,126,155]. However, opposing data was published regarding differences in expression of either spindle cell or epithelial components in biphasic SS. While Fleuren et al. [89] displayed images where exclusively the spindle cell component expressed PDGFRα, Lopez-Guerrero et al. [92] reported that membranous staining was more prominent in the epithelial component. Regarding monophasic SS, both positive and negative samples were reported. Data are summarized in Table 3.

Multiple drugs targeting PDGFRα are currently FDA approved or subject to clinical trials. However, Olaratumab is the only monoclonal antibody that has been clinically investigated for STS. It binds specifically PDGFRα [169]. No clinical NIRF imaging studies have been performed using Olaratumab conjugated with a fluorophore in any cancer type.

In summary, PDGFRα may be targeted in NIRF imaging by Olaratumab after conjugation to a NIRF dye. The advantages of PDGFRα are its relatively regular (65%) presence in STS samples and its diffuse pattern of expression in specifically USTS with 78% of samples expressing PDGFRα. The disadvantages are the non-reported patterns of expression for MFS and SS, and no article addressed a correlation between enhanced PDGFRα expression and histological grade.

3.2.6. CD40

Cluster of Differentiation 40 is a member of the tumor necrosis factor family and can be ligated by CD40 Ligand (CD40L). CD40 is detected on dendritic cells, B-cells and myeloid cells that can mediate cytotoxic T-cell priming upon CD40L ligation [170]. Moreover, it is constitutively expressed on platelets, smooth muscle cells, and endothelial cells [166]. In cancer, CD40 has been found in nearly all B-cell malignancies and many solid tumors, where it induces a direct cytotoxic effect in the absence of immune accessory cells [167]. It is hypothesized that it confers a growth and survival stimulus via signaling pathways such as PI3Kinase/Akt and NFκB and/or that it modulates anti-tumor immune responses [168].

CD40 was present in 62% of STS samples (range 17–86%, n = 153) on average in 4 different scientific papers [95–98]. The pattern of expression was diffuse, when assessed in 7 subtypes (Appendix C). Expression was observed on the membrane and in the cytoplasm of tumor cells [95–98]. No association between enhanced CD40 expression and histological grade was found after comparing low-grade to high-grade STS samples [97]. Furthermore, no articles published data regarding CD40 expression on MFS, USTS and SS separately.

A phase II clinical trial applying APX005M, a second-generation agonistic CD40 monoclonal antibody, combined with Doxorubicin in STS is currently recruiting participants [171]. Nonetheless, the antibody has not yet been evaluated for NIRF imaging and no other CD40-targeting drug has thus far been clinically examined for CD40.

Apart from 2 articles focusing on respectively B-cell activation by targeting CD40 with nanoparticles and cerebral ischemia by targeting CD40 with an anti-CD40 antibody conjugated to Cy5.5, no pre-clinical advances in the field of NIRF imaging can be addressed using CD40 as a target [94,172].

In conclusion, APX005M may be utilized as tracer after conjugation to a NIRF dye for imaging in STS. Pre-clinical studies have developed tracers targeting CD40, yet these have not been tested in STS models thus far. Advantages of CD40 are a diffuse pattern of expression and the fact that expression is relatively common (62%) in STS samples in general. Disadvantages are the small number of evaluated STS samples and the lack of data regarding CD40 expression in MFS, USTS and SS.

3.3. Potential NIRF Imaging Tracers Safety Profile

In this review, 7 potential targets for fluorescence-guided surgery of STS (TEM1, VEGFR-1, EGFR, VEGFR-2, IGF-1R, PDGFRα, and CD40) were selected based on antibodies that are clinically available and mostly used in the antibody-based therapy of STS. Several tracers have already proven to be well suitable for NIRF imaging. Among these tracers, Bevacizumab-IRDye800CW targeting VEGF-A (indirectly VEGFR-1 and VEGFR-2) has already shown promising results in STS [136]. Besides, Cetuximab-IRDye800 targeting EGFR is an adequate tracer in several tumor types [147–149]. This section elaborates on clinically available monoclonal antibodies which can be modified into tracers: Ontuxizumab targeting TEM1, Teprotumumab, Cixutumumab and Figitumumab targeting IGF-1R, and Olaratumab targeting PDGFRα [130,159–161,173–176]. APX005M targeting CD40 is currently under investigation and therefore its efficacy and safety profile in STS are yet to be determined. In contrast to therapy, a single dose of tracer is injected for imaging and an increase in adverse effects compared to therapy is not expected. Further, no increase in adverse effects is expected after conjugation of a fluorophore and antibody [136,177–179]. This paragraph summarizes the safety profiles of each clinically available monoclonal antibody extracted from advanced clinical trials conducted with STS-patients to evaluate their potential for translation towards NIRF imaging. Only high grade (grade $\geq$ 3) Adverse Events (AE) are displayed.

Ontuxizumab was compared to a placebo when both were combined with Gemcitabine and Docetaxel. While the total of grade $\geq$3 AEs was not reported, the incidence of Serious Adverse Events (SAE) was comparable between Ontuxizumab and placebo (50% vs. 48%). The most frequent treatment related SAEs were pyrexia (4% vs. 0%) and anemia (1% vs. 3%) (Appendix A). No substantial differences were observed in laboratory values or electrocardiogram parameters [130].

Targeting IGF-1R, Teprotumumab, Cixutumumab, and Figitumumab were investigated as a monotherapy. These trials have reported a minor incidence of high-grade AEs. AEs such as hyperglycemia, pain, thrombocytopenia, and vomiting were the most common high-grade AEs with incidences ranging from 3–5%. Of all included study subjects, 10% and 17% of patients acquired grade $\geq$3 AEs for Teprotumumab and Figitumumab, respectively. Among these 3 antibodies, Teprotumumab was demonstrated to have the most tolerable and Cixutumumab the most toxic safety profile in STS [159–161].

Two studies on Olaratumab reported grade $\geq$3 Adverse Events (AE) in 58–67% of the patients when combined with Doxorubicin alone [174,180]. In addition, 2 studies observed contrasting AEs when Olaratumab plus Doxorubicin was compared to Doxorubicin. A phase 2 trial observed an increased incidence of high-grade AEs for the combination therapy while a phase 3 trial found no significant differences and therefore concluded no additional adverse events to be attributed to Olaratumab [179–181]. Hematologic grade $\geq$3 AEs were most common in these trials with incidences reaching 40–50% (Appendix A).

4. Discussion

4.1. Research Aim

The success of surgical treatment for localized STS highly depends on complete tumor resection as positive margins are associated with LR and decreased overall survival. Determining the surgical margin is a major challenge for STS surgeons as they generally try to balance the aim of a functional limb against the risk of LR. Real-time tumor-specific imaging can improve surgical margins by visualizing tumor tissue during resection. This review selected TEM1 (score 9), VEGFR-1 (score 8), EGFR (score 8), VEGFR-2 (score 7), IGF-1R (score 7), PDGFRα (score 7), and CD40 (score 7) as the most promising cell surface-expressed biomarkers for tumor-specific NIRF imaging in STS, for which clinically available monoclonal antibodies are already present. Additionally, these potential future NIRF tracers, which are antibodies that have already been clinically tested in STS but not yet conjugated to a NIRF-dye for imaging practices, are expected to be safe for their use in NIRF guided surgery.

4.2. Comparing the Selected Biomarkers

All the suitable biomarkers have already been evaluated for NIRF imaging preclinically, demonstrating their potential [25,29,30,77,82,84,93]. Furthermore, all the selected cell surface-expressed biomarkers internalize after binding with an antibody (derivative) [24,29,39,76,81,92,156]. This causes a better tumor-to-background ratio and a long-lasting signal important for fluorescence-guided surgery [19,20]. However, the indirect targeting of VEGFR-1 and VEGFR-2 by targeting VEGF-A with, for instance, Bevacizumab-IRDye800CW, has not been proven to result in internalization of tracers.

TEM1 and VEGFR-1 were most frequently present in STS samples, 77% and 76% respectively. VEGFR-2 was third most frequently expressed (71%), followed by PDGFRα (64%), IGF-1R (63%), CD40 (62%), and EGFR (53%). Furthermore, apart from CD40 (n = 153), presence of every biomarker of the top 7 has been studied in a large number of STS samples. Therefore, the summarized data in this review are a good representation of biomarker presence in STS patients: EGFR (n = 1918), PDGFRα (n = 1536), TEM1 (n = 768), IGF-1R (n = 507), VEGFR-1 (n = 477), and VEGFR-2 (n = 449).

A particularly important parameter for successful NIRF imaging, which is not included in the TASC score, is the tumor-to-background ratio of a biomarker. With the currently available literature it is impossible to address the expression of each biomarker in healthy tissue, and thus the tumor-to-background ratio, because data on the expression of the biomarkers in normal tissue is very limited. Nevertheless, VEGFR-1 and VEGFR-2 are highly expressed in healthy tissue, while TEM1 and PDGFRα are biomarkers with low expression in healthy tissue. TEM1 has already shown high tumor-to-background ratios with immunohistochemistry [27]. However, both biomarkers are expressed in inflammatory tissue as well as in tumors [28,182]. As STS can be surrounded by inflammation during their growth, it is possible that no clear distinction can be made between tumor and surrounding inflammatory tissue [183]. Unfortunately, none of the selected studies reported on inflammation status of surrounding tissue. In addition, neoadjuvant therapy is frequently used in STS treatment. Successful fluorescence guided surgery is only possible if the overexpression of cell surface-expressed biomarkers is preserved after neoadjuvant therapy. It was demonstrated that EGFR, TEM1, and PDGFRα expression is preserved after neoadjuvant radiotherapy of MFS [27]. This has also been confirmed for EGFR in SS [127]. No other data is available on the expression of these or the remaining evaluated biomarkers after neoadjuvant therapy in STS. Therefore, further research is needed to assess if surrounding inflammatory tissue or neoadjuvant therapy interferes with tumor border identification in STS.

4.3. MFS, USTS and SS

We chose to focus on MFS, USTS, and SS because of their aggressive and infiltrative growth pattern. TEM1 was present in 100% of the MFS samples (Table 3). Besides, its pattern of expression was diffuse in all tested MFS samples [27]. This indicates that TEM1 is likely to be extensively expressed in tumors of every individual MFS patient. Besides, a sharp contrast between tumor and adjacent normal tissue, such as fascia, muscle, and fat, was seen on microscopic pictures of stained MFS samples. This clearly identifies the tumor border and therefore TEM1 seems the most promising biomarker to facilitate complete MFS resections using NIRF imaging [27].

For USTS the average presence of TEM1 and PDGFRα was 81 and 79% of the tumor samples. Apart from being expressed in a substantial percentage of USTS samples, TEM1 and PDGFRα were primarily expressed diffusely [27,28,35,50,126]. However, there is no data published regarding contrast between expression on tumor and normal tissue in USTS. According to the human protein atlas TEM1 and PDGFRα expression is not detected in skeletal muscle tissue and adipose tissue. For smooth muscle tissue, TEM1 displays low expression, while PDGFRα is not detected [184,185]. These characteristics suggest that TEM1 and PDGFRα are promising biomarkers for NIRF imaging in USTS patients.

In SS, the presence of TEM1 and EGFR was demonstrated in 71% and 86% of the assessed samples, respectively. EGFR and TEM1 are both characterized by a variable expression pattern in SS [28,29,52,58,66,69–71]. Moreover, both targets are reported to be not or minimally expressed in the epithelial components of biphasic SS tumors, while it was expressed in the spindle cell components. This might complicate NIRF imaging of biphasic SS tumors when solely targeting either of these biomarkers. Interestingly, EGFR remains present on SS after neoadjuvant radiotherapy. This has not been researched for TEM1, therefore providing EGFR a further advantage over TEM1 [127].

Lastly, most biomarkers are not present in 100% of the evaluated STS (subtype) tumor samples. The disadvantage of not knowing expression in advance to surgery can be overcome by evaluating the expression of each biomarker in preoperative biopsies to assess which biomarker would be most appropriate to target for NIRF imaging during surgery.

4.4. Comparison of Potential NIRF Imaging Tracers

Several monoclonal antibodies targeting STS have already been adjusted to tracers suitable for NIRF imaging and additional monoclonal antibodies used in therapy may be applicable for future NIRF imaging in STS after conjugation to a fluorescent dye/fluorophore. Five distinct antibodies have been assessed for their toxicity profile in STS (Appendix A). Nevertheless, comparing the results of these drugs is complicated, since Olaratumab and Ontuxizumab have solely been investigated combined with chemotherapeutic agents. Still, no evident increase in high-grade toxicity was detected for either antibodies when compared to placebo suggesting a tolerable safety profile. These results are confirmed in trials investigating Olaratumab in metastatic gastrointestinal stromal tumor (GIST) and Ontuxizumab in metastatic colorectal cancer where respectively 10 and 11% grade of ≥ 3 treatment-related adverse events were reported [175,186]. These data are similar to the percentages of patients acquiring grade ≥ 3 AE after treatment with IGF-1R targeting antibodies (Teprotomumab, Figitumumab and Cixutumumab) and therefore all antibodies studied here can be safely modified into NIRF imaging tracers.

It should, however, be emphasized that data on toxicity in antibody-based therapy are presumably an overestimation for imaging, because doses of antibodies injected for NIRF imaging are substantially lower compared to therapeutic doses. For instance, a single dose of 10mg Bevacizumab-IRDye800CW was found to be optimal for NIRF imaging in STS, whereas therapeutic doses comprise of 5–15mg/kg Bevacizumab every 2–3 weeks [134,185,186]. Consequently, the serum concentration of the antibody (conjugated to a fluorophore) is lower when used for NIRF imaging and less toxicity of these monoclonal antibodies is expected [181]. Preferably, dose-finding studies, where single and low doses of the five evaluated compounds have been given to STS patients, should be reviewed to predict toxicity when used for NIRF imaging, yet such articles have not been published.

4.5. Strengths and Limitations

The first limitation is that the heterogeneity of the included studies complicates ranking of the biomarkers. Studies have used various antibodies for immunohistochemistry. The percentage of positive tumors may be variable depending on type of antibodies, dilutions, epitope, and clone used [187]. Also, immunohistochemistry protocols differ between labs which may cause variable results while the same type of antibodies is used. This creates discrepancy in immunohistochemical results published by different researchers. Secondly, the heterogeneity of STS complicates selecting the optimal biomarkers. There are over 50 subtypes of STS, and different subtypes have different biomarker expression patterns [71]. Therefore, finding one optimal biomarker for each subtype is challenging.

A strength of this study is our focus on MFS, USTS, and SS as they are STS subtypes which show an infiltrative growth pattern, and consequently have high percentages of positive margins and high percentages of LR. Patients with these subtypes might benefit the most from implementation of NIRF imaging. Nevertheless, published data regarding some biomarkers in MFS is scarce. Another strength is that clinically available monoclonal antibodies were the starting point of this systematic review. This was because primary development of a NIRF tumor-specific tracer for a rare disease such as STS is time consuming and costly which hampers rapid clinical implementation. However, alternative antigens that might be interesting for tumor-specific imaging in STS can be missed because no clinically available antibodies (or antibody derivatives) are available. Nevertheless, clinical implementation is of utmost importance to prove feasibility of NIRF imaging for STS surgery and subsequently stimulate primary development of STS specific tracers. This progression is enabled by this review as each evaluated biomarker is accompanied by a clinically available antibody (derivative) that can be transformed into a NIRF tracer.

5. Conclusions

In STS, TEM1, VEGFR-1, EGFR, VEGFR-2, IGF-1R, PDGFRα, and CD40 were identified in descending order as the most suitable biomarkers for NIRF imaging according to the modified TASC-scoring system. However, as the category of STS comprises an extensive and heterogenous group of tumors, it was chosen to specify the most optimal target for three common subtypes with infiltrative growth that are characterized by high rates of local recurrence: MFS, USTS and SS. While TEM1 was the optimal target for MFS, both TEM1 and PDGFRα were concluded to be most promising for USTS. In SS EGFR was considered most promising, yet closely followed by TEM1, VEGFR-1, and PDGFRα. However, as the expression of biomarkers and its extent is often not certain, an evaluation of the expression of biomarkers in preoperative biopsies could assist in designating the appropriate tracer for every patient. More importantly, for their potential use in NIRF imaging, data on contrast of expression on malignant and adjacent normal tissue is needed. Altogether, this systematic review paves the way for implementing fluorescence-guided surgery to optimize STS treatment.

Author Contributions: Conceptualization, Z.R., A.N.S., S.E.B., P.J.K.K., A.L.V., S.K., J.V.M.G.B., M.A.J.v.d.S., C.F.M.S. and P.B.A.A.v.D.; methodology, Z.R., A.N.S., C.F.M.S. and P.B.A.A.v.D.; software, Z.R.; validation, Z.R., A.N.S., C.F.M.S. and P.B.A.A.v.D.; formal analysis, not applicable; investigation, Z.R., A.N.S., S.E.B., C.F.M.S. and P.B.A.A.v.D.; resources, Z.R. and A.N.S.; data curation, Z.R. and A.N.S.; writing—original draft preparation, Z.R. and A.N.S.; writing—review and editing, Z.R., A.N.S., S.E.B., P.J.K.K., A.L.V., S.K., J.V.M.G.B., M.A.J.v.d.S., C.F.M.S. and P.B.A.A.v.D.; visualization, Z.R., A.N.S. and C.F.M.S.; supervision, M.A.J.v.d.S., C.F.M.S. and P.B.A.A.v.D.; project administration, Z.R. All authors have read and agreed to the published version of the manuscript.

Funding: This research received no external funding. CS was in part funded by the European Commission under two Marie Skłodowska-Curie Action awards: H2020-MSCA-RISE-2019 (Project number: 872860-PRISAR2) and H2020-MSCA-ITN-2019 (Project number: 857894-CAST).

Institutional Review Board Statement: Not applicable.

Informed Consent Statement: Not applicable.

Data Availability Statement: No new data were created or analyzed in this study. Data sharing is not applicable to this article.

Acknowledgments: The authors would like to acknowledge J.W.M. Plevier, MA (medical librarian, LUMC) for her assistance with the PubMed search.

Conflicts of Interest: The authors declare no conflict of interest.

Appendix A. Search Strategy

("Sarcoma"[Mesh] OR "soft tissue sarcoma*"[tw]) AND ("Receptors, Vascular Endothelial Growth Factor"[Mesh] OR "VEGF"[tw] OR "vascular endothelial growth factor receptor"[tw] OR "EGFR"[tw] OR "epithelial growth factor receptor"[tw] OR "Endosialin"[tw] OR "TEM1"[tw] OR "CD248"[tw] OR "Receptors, Platelet-Derived Growth Factor"[Mesh] OR "Platelet-Derived Growth Factor Receptor*"[tw] OR "PDGFR"[tw] OR "programmed death ligand 1"[tw] OR "PD-L1"[tw] OR "Insulin-Like Growth Factor I"[Mesh] OR "Insulin-Like Growth Factor I"[tw] OR "IGF-1R"[tw] OR "TRAIL-R2"[tw] OR "CTLA-4 Antigen" [Mesh] OR "CTLA-4"[tw] OR "CD40 Antigens"[Mesh] OR "CD40"[tw] OR "Receptor Tyrosine Kinase-like Orphan Receptors"[Mesh] OR "Receptor Tyrosine Kinase-like Orphan Receptor*"[tw] OR "ROR2"[tw] OR "LRRC15"[tw]) NOT ("Animals" [Mesh] NOT "Humans"[Mesh])

Appendix B. Search Previously Imaged and Search Internalization

("Spectroscopy, Near-Infrared"[Mesh] OR "Near-Infrared"[tw] OR "Near infrared"[tw] OR "NIR"[tw] OR "fluorescence"[MeSH] OR "fluorescence"[tw] OR "fluorescent"[tw] OR "imaging"[tw] OR "Positron Emission Tomography Computed Tomography"[tw] OR "PET-CT"[tw] OR "PET"[tw] OR "immune-pet"[tw] OR "tomography, emission-computed, single-photon"[MeSH] OR "spect"[tw] OR "radiolabelled"[tw] OR "radio-labelled"[tw] AND ("Receptors, Vascular Endothelial Growth Factor"[Mesh] OR "VEGF"[tw] OR "vascular endothelial growth factor receptor"[tw] OR "EGFR"[tw] OR "epithelial growth factor receptor"[tw] OR "Endosialin"[tw] OR "TEM1"[tw] OR "CD248"[tw] OR "Receptors, Platelet-Derived Growth Factor"[Mesh] OR "Platelet-Derived Growth Factor Receptor*"[tw] OR "PDGFR"[tw] OR "programmed death ligand 1"[tw] OR "PD-L1"[tw] OR "Insulin-Like Growth Factor I"[Mesh] OR "Insulin-Like Growth Factor I"[tw] OR "IGF-1R"[tw] OR "TRAIL-R2"[tw] OR "CTLA-4 Antigen" [Mesh] OR "CTLA-4"[tw] OR "CD40 Antigens"[Mesh] OR "CD40"[tw] OR "Receptor Tyrosine Kinase-like Orphan Receptors"[Mesh] OR "Receptor Tyrosine Kinase-like Orphan Receptor*"[tw] OR "ROR2"[tw] OR "LRRC15"[tw])

("Internalization"[tw] OR "Internalize"[tw] OR "Internalisation"[tw] OR "Internalise" [tw] OR "Endocytosis"[Mesh] OR "Endocytosis"[tw] OR "Endocyte"[tw]) AND ("Receptors, Vascular Endothelial Growth Factor"[Mesh] OR "VEGF"[tw] OR "vascular endothelial growth factor receptor"[tw] OR "EGFR"[tw] OR "epithelial growth factor receptor"[tw] OR "Endosialin"[tw] OR "TEM1"[tw] OR "CD248"[tw] OR "Receptors, Platelet-Derived Growth Factor"[Mesh] OR "Platelet-Derived Growth Factor Receptor*"[tw] OR "PDGFR"[tw] OR "programmed death ligand 1"[tw] OR "PD-L1"[tw] OR "Insulin-Like Growth Factor I"[Mesh] OR "Insulin-Like Growth Factor I"[tw] OR "IGF-1R"[tw] OR "TRAIL-R2"[tw] OR "CTLA-4 Antigen" [Mesh] OR "CTLA-4"[tw] OR "CD40 Antigens" [Mesh] OR "CD40"[tw] OR "Receptor Tyrosine Kinase-like Orphan Receptors"[Mesh] OR "Receptor Tyrosine Kinase-like Orphan Receptor*"[tw] OR "ROR2"[tw] OR "LRRC15"[tw])

Appendix C. STS Subtypes Examined for Each of the Top 7 Biomarkers

Table A1. Overview of the studied STS subtypes for each of the top 7 biomarkers.

Biomarker	STS Subtypes
TEM1	Angiosarcoma, desmoplastic small round cell, epithelioid haemangioendothelioma, epithelioid sarcoma, fibrosarcoma, inflammatory myofibroblastic sarcoma, kaposi sarcoma, LMS, liposarcoma, MPNST, malignant solitary fibrous tumor, myxofibrosarcoma, RMS, spindle cell sarcoma NOS, synovial sarcoma, USTS, and uterine sarcoma
VEGFR-1	Alveolar STS, angiosarcoma, endometrial stromal sarcoma, Kaposi sarcoma, LMS, liposarcoma, MPNST, malignant solitary fibrous tumor, myxofibrosarcoma, myxoid liposarcoma, pulmonary artery sarcoma, RMS, sarcoma NOS, synovial sarcoma, and USTS
VEGFR-2	Alveolar STS, angiosarcoma, endometrial stromal sarcoma, epithelioid hemangioendotheliomas, fibrosarcoma, LMS, liposarcoma, MPNST, malignant solitary fibrous tumor, myxofibrosarcoma, pulmonary artery sarcoma, RMS, sarcoma NOS, synovial sarcoma, and USTS
EGFR	Acral myxoinflammatory fibroblastic sarcoma, alveolar soft part sarcoma, atypical fibroxanthoma, desmoplastic tumor, endometrial stromal sarcoma, epithelioid sarcoma, fibromatosis, fibromyxoid sarcoma, fibrosarcoma, follicular dendritic cell sarcoma, intimal sarcoma, liposarcoma, LMS, MPNST, myofibroblastic sarcoma, myoxyoinflammatory fibroblastic sarcoma, myxofibrosarcoma, myxoid lipsarcoma, myxoid sarcoma, pleomorphic dermal sarcoma, RMS, sarcoma NOS, synovial sarcoma, endifferentiated endometrial sarcoma, USTS, and undifferentiated stromal sarcoma
IGF-1R	Alveolar STS, angiosarcoma, desmoplastic tumor, fibrosarcoma, LMS, liposarcoma, MPNST, mesenchyoma, myxofibrosarcoma, RMS, sarcoma NOS, spindle cell sarcoma, synovial sarcoma, and USTS
PDGFRα	Alveolar soft part sarcoma, Angiosarcoma, dermatofibrosarcoma protuberans, endometrial stromal sarcoma, fibromyxoid sarcoma, fibrosarcoma, liposarcoma, LMS, MPNST, myofibroblastic sarcoma, myoxyoinflammatory fibroblastic sarcoma, myxofibrosarcoma, myxoid liposarcoma, pulmonary artery sarcoma, RMS, sarcoma NOS, solitary fibrous tumor, synovial sarcoma, undifferentiated endometrial sarcoma, undifferentiated uterine sarcoma, undifferentiated stromal sarcoma, and USTS
CD40	Kaposi sarcoma, liposarcoma, LMS, MPNST, RMS, and USTS

A. Toxicity of Clinically Available Monoclonal Antibodies in Patients with STS

Table A2. Overview of the Toxicity of Clinically Available Monoclonal Antibodies in STS Patients.

Clinical Trial	Phase	Tumor Type	Evaluable for Toxicity	Median [a,*] Age (Years)	Treatment	Most Common Adverse Events	Percentage Patients with ≥3 Adverse Events (vs. Placebo)	Most Common Grade ≥ 3 Adverse Events
TEM1 (Ontuxizumab)								
Jones et al., 2019	2	STS	209	55	Ontuxizumab 8mg/kg + G/D vs. placebo + G/D [b]	Fatigue (74% vs. 66%), anemia (61% vs. 60%), nausea (56% vs. 52%), diarrhea (44% vs. 36%), and peripheral edema (42% vs. 45%)	Not reported	Pyrexia (4% vs. 0%) and anemia (1% vs. 3%) [c]
IGF-1R (Teprotomumab, Figitumumab and Cixutumumab)								
Pappo et al., 2014	2	STS + osteosarcoma	163	31	Teprotumumab 9 mg/kg; 1 dose per week	Fatigue (20.2%), nausea (14.1%), hyperglycemia (9.2%), and muscle spasms (8.6%)	10.4%	Hyperglycemia (2.5%), dehydration (1.8%), fatigue (1.8%), and hyponatremia (1.2%)
Olmos et al., 2010	1	STS + Ewing sarcoma + myxoid chondrosarcoma	29	30	Figitumumab 20 mg/kg; 1 dose per 3–4 weeks	Hyperglycemia (17%), skin reactions (rash, urticaria, infection, eczema) (13.8%), increased GGT (10.3%), headache (10.3%), and fatigue (10.3%)	17.2%	Vomiting (3.4%), back pain (3.4%), DVT (3.4%), increased uric acid concentration (3.4%), and increased AST, ALT or GGT (3.4%)
Wagner et al., 2015	2	STS + Ewing sarcoma + osteosarcoma	44	14–181	Cixutumumab 6 mg/kg and Temsirolimus 8 mg/m²; 1 dose per week	Mucositis, electrolyte disturbances and myelosuppression	Not reported	Neutropenia (13.6%), thrombocytopenia (11.4%), hypokalemia (11.4%), oral mucositis (9.1%), and hypophosphatemia (9.1%)
Schöffski et al., 2013	2	STS + Ewing family of tumors	113	27.5–33.1	Cixutumumab 10 mg/kg; 1 dose per 2 weeks	Nausea (26.1%), fatigue (23.4%), diarrhea (22.5%), hyperglycemia (19.8%), and anorexia (17.1%)	Not reported	Hyperglycemia (5.4%), pain (5.4%), thrombocytopenia (4.5%), asthenia (4.5%), and Anemia (3.6%)
Schwartz et al., 2013	2	STS + sarcoma of bone	174	Mean: 48.1	Cixutumumab 6 mg/kg and Temsirolimus 25 mg; 1 dose per week	Oral mucositis (71.3%), hypercalcemia (68.4%), fatigue (65.5%), thrombocytopenia (63.8%), and anemia (62.6%)	Not reported	Anemia (9%), hyperglycemia (10%), hypophosphatemia (9%), lymphopenia (14%), oral mucositis (11%), and thrombocytopenia (11%)

Table A2. *Cont.*

Clinical Trial	Phase	Tumor Type	Evaluable for Toxicity	Median [a],* Age (Years)	Treatment	Most Common Adverse Events	Percentage Patients with ≥3 Adverse Events (vs. Placebo)	Most Common Grade ≥ 3 Adverse Events
PDGFR (Olaratumab)								
Tap et al., 2020	3	STS	506	Mean: 56.9	Olaratumab 15 mg/kg + Doxorubicin 75 mg/m² vs. Placebo + Doxorubicin 75 mg/m² [d]	Nausea (59.5% vs. 66.7%), neutropenia (55.3% vs. 57.8%), fatigue (54.1% vs. 59%), alopecia (43.6% vs. 49.8%), and anemia (42.8% vs. 45.4%)	Not reported	Neutropenia (46.3% vs. 49%), leukopenia (23.3% vs. 23.7%), febrile neutropenia (17.5% vs. 16.5%), anemia (13.6% vs. 12.4%), and thrombocytopenia (9.3% vs. 8.4%)
Yonemori et al., 2018	1	STS	19	41.5–52 [a]	Olaratumab 15 mg/kg + Doxorubicin 25–75 mg/m² [e]	ALT increased (52.6%), neutrophil count decreased (52.6%), WBC count decreased (47.4%), anemia (36.8%), and GGT increased (31.6%)	57.9%	Decreased neutrophil count (42.1%), decreased WBC count (42.1%), increased ALT (15.8%), anemia (10.5%), and febrile neutropenia (10.5%)
Tap et al., 2016	2	STS	133	58.5	Olaratumab 15 mg/kg + Doxorubicin 75 mg/m² vs. Doxorubicin [f]	Nausea (73.4% vs. 52.3%), fatigue (68.8% vs. 69.2%), neutropenia (57.8% vs. 35.4%), mucositis (53.1% vs. 35.4%), and alopecia (51.6% vs. 40%)	67% vs. 55%	Neutropenia (53.2% vs. 32.3%), leukopenia (36% vs. 16.9%), febrile neutropenia (12.5% vs. 13.8%), anemia (12.5% vs. 9.2%), and fatigue (9.4% vs. 3.1%)

Note. Abbreviations: STS, soft tissue sarcoma; ALT, alanine aminotransferase; WBC, white blood cell; GGT, gamma-glutamyl transferase; DVT, deep venous thrombosis; AST, aspartate aminotransferase. * Unless reported differently as some articles published mean data instead of median. [a] These trials had several cohorts with each a separate median age. Reported in the table is the range of median ages. [b] Full treatment schedule was: Ontuxizumab 8mg/kg (day 1 and 8) of a 21-day cycle or a placebo with G/D (G/D: 900 mg/m² gemcitabine (day 1 and 8) and 75 mg/m² docetaxel (day 8)). [c] These are the serious adverse events instead of all grade ≥3 adverse events, as the latter was not reported. [d] Full treatment schedule was: Olaratumab 20 mg/kg in cycle 1 and 15 mg/kg in subsequent cycles or placebo (days 1 and 8) combined with Doxorubicin 75 mg/m² (day 1) for up to 8 21-day cycles, followed by Olaratumab/placebo monotherapy. [e] Full treatment schedule was: Olaratumab 15 mg/kg (day 1 and 8) of each 21-day cycle until progressive disease (PD) or other discontinuation criteria were met. Patients in Cohort 3 received a 20 mg/kg loading dose of Olaratumab (Day 1 and 8) in Cycle 1. Doxorubicin was administered for up to 6 cycles (or a cumulative dose of 500 mg/m², whichever came later) until PD or other discontinuation criteria were met. Patients in Cohort 1 received doxorubicin 25mg/m² (day 1, 2, and 3) in each cycle, Cohorts 2 and 3 received doxorubicin 75 mg/m² (day 1) in each cycle. [f] Full treatment schedule was: Olaratumab 15 mg/kg (day 1 and 8) combined with doxorubicin 75mg/m2 or doxorubicin alone 75 mg/m² (day 1) of each 21-day cycle for up to eight cycles.

References

1. Vos, M.; Blaauwgeers, H.G.T.; Ho, V.K.Y.; van Houdt, W.J.; van der Hage, J.A.; Been, L.B.; Bonenkamp, J.J.; Bemelmans, M.H.A.; van Dalen, T.; Haas, R.L.; et al. Increased survival of non low-grade and deep-seated soft tissue sarcoma after surgical management in high-volume hospitals: A nationwide study from the Netherlands. *Eur. J. Cancer* **2019**, *110*, 98–106. [CrossRef] [PubMed]
2. ESMO/European Sarcoma Network Working Group. Soft tissue and visceral sarcomas: ESMO Clinical Practice Guidelines for diagnosis, treatment and follow-up. *Ann. Oncol.* **2014**, *25* (Suppl. 3), iii102–iii112. [CrossRef]
3. Stiller, C.A.; Trama, A.; Serraino, D.; Rossi, S.; Navarro, C.; Chirlaque, M.D.; Casali, P.G. Descriptive epidemiology of sarcomas in Europe: Report from the RARECARE project. *Eur. J. Cancer* **2013**, *49*, 684–695. [CrossRef] [PubMed]
4. Lawrence, W., Jr.; Donegan, W.L.; Natarajan, N.; Mettlin, C.; Beart, R.; Winchester, D. Adult soft tissue sarcomas. A pattern of care survey of the American College of Surgeons. *Ann. Surg.* **1987**, *205*, 349–359. [CrossRef] [PubMed]
5. WHO Classification of Tumours. *Tissue and Bone Tumours: WHO Classification of Tumours*, 5th ed.; IARC Publications: Lyon, France, 2020; Volume 3.
6. Enneking, W.F.; Spanier, S.S.; Goodman, M.A. A system for the surgical staging of musculoskeletal sarcoma. *Clin. Orthop. Relat. Res.* **1980**. [CrossRef]
7. Pasquali, S.; Colombo, C.; Pizzamiglio, S.; Verderio, P.; Callegaro, D.; Stacchiotti, S.; Martin Broto, J.; Lopez-Pousa, A.; Ferrari, S.; Poveda, A.; et al. High-risk soft tissue sarcomas treated with perioperative chemotherapy: Improving prognostic classification in a randomised clinical trial. *Eur. J. Cancer* **2018**, *93*, 28–36. [CrossRef]
8. Smolle, M.A.; Sande, M.V.; Callegaro, D.; Wunder, J.; Hayes, A.; Leitner, L.; Bergovec, M.; Tunn, P.U.; van Praag, V.; Fiocco, M.; et al. Individualizing Follow-Up Strategies in High-Grade Soft Tissue Sarcoma with Flexible Parametric Competing Risk Regression Models. *Cancers* **2019**, *12*, 47. [CrossRef]
9. Willeumier, J.; Fiocco, M.; Nout, R.; Dijkstra, S.; Aston, W.; Pollock, R.; Hartgrink, H.; Bovee, J.; van de Sande, M. High-grade soft tissue sarcomas of the extremities: Surgical margins influence only local recurrence not overall survival. *Int. Orthop.* **2015**, *39*, 935–941. [CrossRef]
10. Zagars, G.K.; Ballo, M.T.; Pisters, P.W.; Pollock, R.E.; Patel, S.R.; Benjamin, R.S.; Evans, H.L. Prognostic factors for patients with localized soft-tissue sarcoma treated with conservation surgery and radiation therapy: An analysis of 1225 patients. *Cancer* **2003**, *97*, 2530–2543. [CrossRef]
11. Kandel, R.; Coakley, N.; Werier, J.; Engel, J.; Ghert, M.; Verma, S. Surgical margins and handling of soft-tissue sarcoma in extremities: A clinical practice guideline. *Curr. Oncol.* **2013**, *20*, e247–e254. [CrossRef]
12. O'Sullivan, B.; Davis, A.M.; Turcotte, R.; Bell, R.; Catton, C.; Chabot, P.; Wunder, J.; Kandel, R.; Goddard, K.; Sadura, A.; et al. Preoperative versus postoperative radiotherapy in soft-tissue sarcoma of the limbs: A randomised trial. *Lancet* **2002**, *359*, 2235–2241. [CrossRef]
13. Yoo, H.J.; Hong, S.H.; Kang, Y.; Choi, J.Y.; Moon, K.C.; Kim, H.S.; Han, I.; Yi, M.; Kang, H.S. MR imaging of myxofibrosarcoma and undifferentiated sarcoma with emphasis on tail sign; diagnostic and prognostic value. *Eur. Radiol.* **2014**, *24*, 1749–1757. [CrossRef] [PubMed]
14. Bhangu, A.A.; Beard, J.A.S.; Grimer, R.J. Should Soft Tissue Sarcomas be Treated at a Specialist Centre? *Sarcoma* **2004**, *8*, 1–6. [CrossRef] [PubMed]
15. Chen, S.; Huang, W.; Luo, P.; Cai, W.; Yang, L.; Sun, Z.; Zheng, B.; Yan, W.; Wang, C. Undifferentiated Pleomorphic Sarcoma: Long-Term Follow-Up from a Large Institution. *Cancer Manag. Res.* **2019**, *11*, 10001–10009. [CrossRef] [PubMed]
16. Lewis, J.J.; Antonescu, C.R.; Leung, D.H.; Blumberg, D.; Healey, J.H.; Woodruff, J.M.; Brennan, M.F. Synovial sarcoma: A multivariate analysis of prognostic factors in 112 patients with primary localized tumors of the extremity. *J. Clin. Oncol.* **2000**, *18*, 2087–2094. [CrossRef] [PubMed]
17. Look Hong, N.J.; Hornicek, F.J.; Raskin, K.A.; Yoon, S.S.; Szymonifka, J.; Yeap, B.; Chen, Y.L.; DeLaney, T.F.; Nielsen, G.P.; Mullen, J.T. Prognostic factors and outcomes of patients with myxofibrosarcoma. *Ann. Surg. Oncol.* **2013**, *20*, 80–86. [CrossRef]
18. Odei, B.; Rwigema, J.C.; Eilber, F.R.; Eilber, F.C.; Selch, M.; Singh, A.; Chmielowski, B.; Nelson, S.D.; Wang, P.C.; Steinberg, M.; et al. Predictors of Local Recurrence in Patients With Myxofibrosarcoma. *Am. J. Clin. Oncol.* **2018**, *41*, 827–831. [CrossRef]
19. Hernot, S.; van Manen, L.; Debie, P.; Mieog, J.S.D.; Vahrmeijer, A.L. Latest developments in molecular tracers for fluorescence image-guided cancer surgery. *Lancet. Oncol.* **2019**, *20*, e354–e367. [CrossRef]
20. Keereweer, S.; Van Driel, P.B.; Snoeks, T.J.; Kerrebijn, J.D.; Baatenburg de Jong, R.J.; Vahrmeijer, A.L.; Sterenborg, H.J.; Lowik, C.W. Optical image-guided cancer surgery: Challenges and limitations. *Clin. Cancer Res.* **2013**, *19*, 3745–3754. [CrossRef]
21. Barth, C.; Gibbs, S.L. Fluorescence Image-Guided Surgery—A Perspective on Contrast Agent Development. *Proc. Spie. Int. Soc. Opt. Eng.* **2020**, *11222*. [CrossRef]
22. Karaman, S.; Leppanen, V.M.; Alitalo, K. Vascular endothelial growth factor signaling in development and disease. *Development* **2018**, *145*. [CrossRef] [PubMed]
23. Moher, D.; Liberati, A.; Tetzlaff, J.; Altman, D.G. Preferred reporting items for systematic reviews and meta-analyses: The PRISMA statement. *PLoS Med.* **2009**, *6*, e1000097. [CrossRef] [PubMed]
24. Bosma, S.E.; van Driel, P.B.; Hogendoorn, P.C.; Dijkstra, P.S.; Sier, C.F. Introducing fluorescence guided surgery into orthopedic oncology: A systematic review of candidate protein targets for Ewing sarcoma. *J. Surg. Oncol.* **2018**, *118*, 906–914. [CrossRef] [PubMed]

25. Lange, S.E.; Zheleznyak, A.; Studer, M.; O'Shannessy, D.J.; Lapi, S.E.; Van Tine, B.A. Development of 89Zr-Ontuxizumab for in vivo TEM-1/endosialin PET applications. *Oncotarget* **2016**, *7*, 13082–13092. [CrossRef]
26. Guo, Y.; Hu, J.; Wang, Y.; Peng, X.; Min, J.; Wang, J.; Matthaiou, E.; Cheng, Y.; Sun, K.; Tong, X.; et al. Tumour endothelial marker 1/endosialin-mediated targeting of human sarcoma. *Eur. J. Cancer* **2018**, *90*, 111–121. [CrossRef]
27. De Gooyer, J.M.; Versleijen-Jonkers, Y.M.H.; Hillebrandt-Roeffen, M.H.S.; Frielink, C.; Desar, I.M.E.; de Wilt, J.H.W.; Flucke, U.; Rijpkema, M. Immunohistochemical selection of biomarkers for tumor-targeted image-guided surgery of myxofibrosarcoma. *Sci. Rep.* **2020**, *10*, 2915. [CrossRef]
28. Rouleau, C.; Curiel, M.; Weber, W.; Smale, R.; Kurtzberg, L.; Mascarello, J.; Berger, C.; Wallar, G.; Bagley, R.; Honma, N.; et al. Endosialin protein expression and therapeutic target potential in human solid tumors: Sarcoma versus carcinoma. *Clin. Cancer Res.* **2008**, *14*, 7223–7236. [CrossRef]
29. Thway, K.; Robertson, D.; Jones, R.L.; Selfe, J.; Shipley, J.; Fisher, C.; Isacke, C.M. Endosialin expression in soft tissue sarcoma as a potential marker of undifferentiated mesenchymal cells. *Br. J. Cancer* **2016**, *115*, 473–479. [CrossRef]
30. Zhang, J.; Razavian, M.; Tavakoli, S.; Nie, L.; Tellides, G.; Backer, J.M.; Backer, M.V.; Bender, J.R.; Sadeghi, M.M. Molecular imaging of vascular endothelial growth factor receptors in graft arteriosclerosis. *Arter. Thromb. Vasc. Biol.* **2012**, *32*, 1849–1855. [CrossRef]
31. Saban, M.R.; Backer, J.M.; Backer, M.V.; Maier, J.; Fowler, B.; Davis, C.A.; Simpson, C.; Wu, X.R.; Birder, L.; Freeman, M.R.; et al. VEGF receptors and neuropilins are expressed in the urothelial and neuronal cells in normal mouse urinary bladder and are upregulated in inflammation. *Am. J. Physiol. Ren. Physiol.* **2008**, *295*, F60–F72. [CrossRef]
32. Andersson, M.K.; Goransson, M.; Olofsson, A.; Andersson, C.; Aman, P. Nuclear expression of FLT1 and its ligand PGF in FUS-DDIT3 carrying myxoid liposarcomas suggests the existence of an intracrine signaling loop. *BMC Cancer* **2010**, *10*, 249. [CrossRef] [PubMed]
33. Arita, S.; Kikkawa, F.; Kajiyama, H.; Shibata, K.; Kawai, M.; Mizuno, K.; Nagasaka, T.; Ino, K.; Nomura, S. Prognostic importance of vascular endothelial growth factor and its receptors in the uterine sarcoma. *Int. J. Gynecol. Cancer Off. J. Int. Gynecol. Cancer Soc.* **2005**, *15*, 329–336. [CrossRef]
34. Gaumann, A.; Strubel, G.; Bode-Lesniewska, B.; Schmidtmann, I.; Kriegsmann, J.; Kirkpatrick, C.J. The role of tumor vascularisation in benign and malignant cardiovascular neoplasms: A comparison of cardiac myxoma and sarcomas of the pulmonary artery. *Oncol. Rep.* **2008**, *20*, 309–318. [CrossRef] [PubMed]
35. Itakura, E.; Yamamoto, H.; Oda, Y.; Tsuneyoshi, M. Detection and characterization of vascular endothelial growth factors and their receptors in a series of angiosarcomas. *J. Surg. Oncol.* **2008**, *97*, 74–81. [CrossRef]
36. Kampmann, E.; Altendorf-Hofmann, A.; Gibis, S.; Lindner, L.H.; Issels, R.; Kirchner, T.; Knosel, T. VEGFR2 predicts decreased patients survival in soft tissue sarcomas. *Pathol. Res. Pract.* **2015**, *211*, 726–730. [CrossRef]
37. Lee, Y.J.; Chung, J.G.; Chien, Y.T.; Lin, S.S.; Hsu, F.T. Suppression of ERK/NF-κB Activation Is Associated With Amentoflavone-Inhibited Osteosarcoma Progression In Vivo. *Anticancer Res.* **2019**, *39*, 3669–3675. [CrossRef]
38. Yonemori, K.; Tsuta, K.; Ando, M.; Hirakawa, A.; Hatanaka, Y.; Matsuno, Y.; Chuman, H.; Yamazaki, N.; Fujiwara, Y.; Hasegawa, T. Contrasting prognostic implications of platelet-derived growth factor receptor-beta and vascular endothelial growth factor receptor-2 in patients with angiosarcoma. *Ann. Surg. Oncol.* **2011**, *18*, 2841–2850. [CrossRef]
39. Young, R.J.; Woll, P.J.; Staton, C.A.; Reed, M.W.; Brown, N.J. Vascular-targeted agents for the treatment of angiosarcoma. *Cancer Chemother. Pharmacol.* **2014**, *73*, 259–270. [CrossRef]
40. Harding, J.; Burtness, B. Cetuximab: An epidermal growth factor receptor chemeric human-murine monoclonal antibody. *Drugs Today* **2005**, *41*, 107–127. [CrossRef]
41. Samkoe, K.S.; Sardar, H.S.; Bates, B.D.; Tselepidakis, N.N.; Gunn, J.R.; Hoffer-Hawlik, K.A.; Feldwisch, J.; Pogue, B.W.; Paulsen, K.D.; Henderson, E.R. Preclinical imaging of epidermal growth factor receptor with ABY-029 in soft-tissue sarcoma for fluorescence-guided surgery and tumor detection. *J. Surg. Oncol.* **2019**, *119*, 1077–1086. [CrossRef]
42. Anderson, S.E.; Nonaka, D.; Chuai, S.; Olshen, A.B.; Chi, D.; Sabbatini, P.; Soslow, R.A. p53, epidermal growth factor, and platelet-derived growth factor in uterine leiomyosarcoma and leiomyomas. *Int. J. Gynecol. Cancer Off. J. Int. Gynecol. Cancer Soc.* **2006**, *16*, 849–853. [CrossRef] [PubMed]
43. Armistead, P.M.; Salganick, J.; Roh, J.S.; Steinert, D.M.; Patel, S.; Munsell, M.; El-Naggar, A.K.; Benjamin, R.S.; Zhang, W.; Trent, J.C. Expression of receptor tyrosine kinases and apoptotic molecules in rhabdomyosarcoma: Correlation with overall survival in 105 patients. *Cancer* **2007**, *110*, 2293–2303. [CrossRef] [PubMed]
44. Baek, M.H.; Park, J.Y.; Rhim, C.C.; Kim, J.H.; Park, Y.; Kim, K.R.; Nam, J.H. Investigation of New Therapeutic Targets in Undifferentiated Endometrial Sarcoma. *Gynecol. Obstet. Investig.* **2017**, *82*, 329–339. [CrossRef] [PubMed]
45. Cheng, X.; Yang, G.; Schmeler, K.M.; Coleman, R.L.; Tu, X.; Liu, J.; Kavanagh, J.J. Recurrence patterns and prognosis of endometrial stromal sarcoma and the potential of tyrosine kinase-inhibiting therapy. *Gynecol. Oncol.* **2011**, *121*, 323–327. [CrossRef] [PubMed]
46. Cossu-Rocca, P.; Contini, M.; Uras, M.G.; Muroni, M.R.; Pili, F.; Carru, C.; Bosincu, L.; Massarelli, G.; Nogales, F.F.; De Miglio, M.R. Tyrosine kinase receptor status in endometrial stromal sarcoma: An immunohistochemical and genetic-molecular analysis. *Int. J. Gynecol. Pathol.* **2012**, *31*, 570–579. [CrossRef]
47. Cuppens, T.; Annibali, D.; Coosemans, A.; Trovik, J.; Ter Haar, N.; Colas, E.; Garcia-Jimenez, A.; Van de Vijver, K.; Kruitwagen, R.P.; Brinkhuis, M.; et al. Potential Targets' Analysis Reveals Dual PI3K/mTOR Pathway Inhibition as a Promising Therapeutic Strategy for Uterine Leiomyosarcomas-an ENITEC Group Initiative. *Clin. Cancer. Res.* **2017**, *23*, 1274–1285. [CrossRef]

48. Hoffman, A.; Ghadimi, M.P.; Demicco, E.G.; Creighton, C.J.; Torres, K.; Colombo, C.; Peng, T.; Lusby, K.; Ingram, D.; Hornick, J.L.; et al. Localized and metastatic myxoid/round cell liposarcoma: Clinical and molecular observations. *Cancer* 2013, *119*, 1868–1877. [CrossRef]
49. Iwasaki, S.; Sudo, T.; Miwa, M.; Ukita, M.; Morimoto, A.; Tamada, M.; Ueno, S.; Wakahashi, S.; Yamaguchi, S.; Fujiwara, K.; et al. Endometrial stromal sarcoma: Clinicopathological and immunophenotypic study of 16 cases. *Arch. Gynecol. Obs.* 2013, *288*, 385–391. [CrossRef]
50. Park, J.Y.; Kim, K.R.; Nam, J.H. Immunohistochemical analysis for therapeutic targets and prognostic markers in low-grade endometrial stromal sarcoma. *Int. J. Gynecol. Cancer Off. J. Int. Gynecol. Cancer Soc.* 2013, *23*, 81–89. [CrossRef]
51. Ruping, K.; Altendorf-Hofmann, A.; Chen, Y.; Kampmann, E.; Gibis, S.; Lindner, L.; Katenkamp, D.; Petersen, I.; Knosel, T. High IGF2 and FGFR3 are associated with tumour progression in undifferentiated pleomorphic sarcomas, but EGFR and FGFR3 mutations are a rare event. *J. Cancer Res. Clin. Oncol* 2014, *140*, 1315–1322. [CrossRef]
52. Barbashina, V.; Benevenia, J.; Aviv, H.; Tsai, J.; Patterson, F.; Aisner, S.; Cohen, S.; Fernandes, H.; Skurnick, J.; Hameed, M. Oncoproteins and proliferation markers in synovial sarcomas: A clinicopathologic study of 19 cases. *J. Cancer Res. Clin. Oncol.* 2002, *128*, 610–616. [CrossRef] [PubMed]
53. Cascio, M.J.; O'Donnell, R.J.; Horvai, A.E. Epithelioid sarcoma expresses epidermal growth factor receptor but gene amplification and kinase domain mutations are rare. *Mod. Pathol.* 2010, *23*, 574–580. [CrossRef] [PubMed]
54. Cates, J.M.; Memoli, V.A.; Gonzalez, R.S. Cell cycle and apoptosis regulatory proteins, proliferative markers, cell signaling molecules, CD209, and decorin immunoreactivity in low-grade myxofibrosarcoma and myxoma. *Virchows Arch.* 2015, *467*, 211–216. [CrossRef] [PubMed]
55. Dewaele, B.; Floris, G.; Finalet-Ferreiro, J.; Fletcher, C.D.; Coindre, J.M.; Guillou, L.; Hogendoorn, P.C.; Wozniak, A.; Vanspauwen, V.; Schoffski, P.; et al. Coactivated platelet-derived growth factor receptor {alpha} and epidermal growth factor receptor are potential therapeutic targets in intimal sarcoma. *Cancer Res.* 2010, *70*, 7304–7314. [CrossRef]
56. Ganti, R.; Skapek, S.X.; Zhang, J.; Fuller, C.E.; Wu, J.; Billups, C.A.; Breitfeld, P.P.; Dalton, J.D.; Meyer, W.H.; Khoury, J.D. Expression and genomic status of EGFR and ErbB-2 in alveolar and embryonal rhabdomyosarcoma. *Mod. Pathol.* 2006, *19*, 1213–1220. [CrossRef]
57. Garcia, C.; Kubat, J.S.; Fulton, R.S.; Anthony, A.T.; Combs, M.; Powell, C.B.; Littell, R.D. Clinical outcomes and prognostic markers in uterine leiomyosarcoma: A population-based cohort. *Int. J. Gynecol. Cancer Off. J. Int. Gynecol. Cancer Soc.* 2015, *25*, 622–628. [CrossRef]
58. Gusterson, B.; Cowley, G.; McIlhinney, J.; Ozanne, B.; Fisher, C.; Reeves, B. Evidence for increased epidermal growth factor receptors in human sarcomas. *Int. J. Cancer* 1985, *36*, 689–693. [CrossRef]
59. Helbig, D.; Ihle, M.A.; Putz, K.; Tantcheva-Poor, I.; Mauch, C.; Buttner, R.; Quaas, A. Oncogene and therapeutic target analyses in atypical fibroxanthomas and pleomorphic dermal sarcomas. *Oncotarget* 2016, *7*, 21763–21774. [CrossRef]
60. Kovarik, C.L.; Barrett, T.; Auerbach, A.; Cassarino, D.S. Acral myxoinflammatory fibroblastic sarcoma: Case series and immunohistochemical analysis. *J. Cutan. Pathol.* 2008, *35*, 192–196. [CrossRef]
61. Leibl, S.; Moinfar, F. Mammary NOS-type sarcoma with CD10 expression: A rare entity with features of myoepithelial differentiation. *Am. J. Surg. Pathol.* 2006, *30*, 450–456. [CrossRef]
62. Moinfar, F.; Gogg-Kamerer, M.; Sommersacher, A.; Regitnig, P.; Man, Y.G.; Zatloukal, K.; Denk, H.; Tavassoli, F.A. Endometrial stromal sarcomas frequently express epidermal growth factor receptor (EGFR, HER-1): Potential basis for a new therapeutic approach. *Am. J. Surg. Pathol.* 2005, *29*, 485–489. [CrossRef] [PubMed]
63. Asmane, I.; Watkin, E.; Alberti, L.; Duc, A.; Marec-Berard, P.; Ray-Coquard, I.; Cassier, P.; Decouvelaere, A.V.; Ranchere, D.; Kurtz, J.E.; et al. Insulin-like growth factor type 1 receptor (IGF-1R) exclusive nuclear staining: A predictive biomarker for IGF-1R monoclonal antibody (Ab) therapy in sarcomas. *Eur. J. Cancer* 2012, *48*, 3027–3035. [CrossRef] [PubMed]
64. Conti, A.; Espina, V.; Chiechi, A.; Magagnoli, G.; Novello, C.; Pazzaglia, L.; Quattrini, I.; Picci, P.; Liotta, L.A.; Benassi, M.S. Mapping protein signal pathway interaction in sarcoma bone metastasis: Linkage between rank, metalloproteinases turnover and growth factor signaling pathways. *Clin. Exp. Metastasis* 2014, *31*, 15–24. [CrossRef] [PubMed]
65. Lazar, A.J.; Lahat, G.; Myers, S.E.; Smith, K.D.; Zou, C.; Wang, W.L.; Lopez-Terrada, D.; Lev, D. Validation of potential therapeutic targets in alveolar soft part sarcoma: An immunohistochemical study utilizing tissue microarray. *Histopathology* 2009, *55*, 750–755. [CrossRef] [PubMed]
66. Sato, O.; Wada, T.; Kawai, A.; Yamaguchi, U.; Makimoto, A.; Kokai, Y.; Yamashita, T.; Chuman, H.; Beppu, Y.; Tani, Y.; et al. Expression of epidermal growth factor receptor, ERBB2 and KIT in adult soft tissue sarcomas: A clinicopathologic study of 281 cases. *Cancer* 2005, *103*, 1881–1890. [CrossRef]
67. Sun, X.; Chang, K.C.; Abruzzo, L.V.; Lai, R.; Younes, A.; Jones, D. Epidermal growth factor receptor expression in follicular dendritic cells: A shared feature of follicular dendritic cell sarcoma and Castleman's disease. *Hum. Pathol.* 2003, *34*, 835–840. [CrossRef]
68. Tamborini, E.; Casieri, P.; Miselli, F.; Orsenigo, M.; Negri, T.; Piacenza, C.; Stacchiotti, S.; Gronchi, A.; Pastorino, U.; Pierotti, M.A.; et al. Analysis of potential receptor tyrosine kinase targets in intimal and mural sarcomas. *J. Pathol.* 2007, *212*, 227–235. [CrossRef]
69. Tawbi, H.; Thomas, D.; Lucas, D.R.; Biermann, J.S.; Schuetze, S.M.; Hart, A.L.; Chugh, R.; Baker, L.H. Epidermal growth factor receptor expression and mutational analysis in synovial sarcomas and malignant peripheral nerve sheath tumors. *Oncologist* 2008, *13*, 459–466. [CrossRef]

70. Teng, H.W.; Wang, H.W.; Chen, W.M.; Chao, T.C.; Hsieh, Y.Y.; Hsih, C.H.; Tzeng, C.H.; Chen, P.C.; Yen, C.C. Prevalence and prognostic influence of genomic changes of EGFR pathway markers in synovial sarcoma. *J. Surg. Oncol.* **2011**, *103*, 773–781. [CrossRef]
71. Vesely, K.; Jurajda, M.; Nenutil, R.; Vesela, M. Expression of p53, cyclin D1 and EGFR correlates with histological grade of adult soft tissue sarcomas: A study on tissue microarrays. *Neoplasma* **2009**, *56*, 239–244. [CrossRef]
72. Xie, X.; Ghadimi, M.P.; Young, E.D.; Belousov, R.; Zhu, Q.S.; Liu, J.; Lopez, G.; Colombo, C.; Peng, T.; Reynoso, D.; et al. Combining EGFR and mTOR blockade for the treatment of epithelioid sarcoma. *Clin. Cancer Res.* **2011**, *17*, 5901–5912. [CrossRef] [PubMed]
73. Yang, J.L.; Gupta, R.D.; Goldstein, D.; Crowe, P.J. Significance of Phosphorylated Epidermal Growth Factor Receptor and Its Signal Transducers in Human Soft Tissue Sarcoma. *Int. J. Mol. Sci.* **2017**, *18*, 1159. [CrossRef] [PubMed]
74. Yang, J.L.; Hannan, M.T.; Russell, P.J.; Crowe, P.J. Expression of HER1/EGFR protein in human soft tissue sarcomas. *Eur. J. Surg. Oncol.* **2006**, *32*, 466–468. [CrossRef] [PubMed]
75. Alves, P.M.; de Arruda, J.A.A.; Arantes, D.A.C.; Costa, S.F.S.; Souza, L.L.; Pontes, H.A.R.; Fonseca, F.P.; Mesquita, R.A.; Nonaka, C.F.W.; Mendonça, E.F.; et al. Evaluation of tumor-infiltrating lymphocytes in osteosarcomas of the jaws: A multicenter study. *Virchows Arch.* **2019**, *474*, 201–207. [CrossRef] [PubMed]
76. Capobianco, G.; Pili, F.; Contini, M.; De Miglio, M.R.; Marras, V.; Santeufemia, D.A.; Cherchi, C.; Dessole, M.; Cherchi, P.L.; Cossu-Rocca, P. Analysis of epidermal growth factor receptor (EGFR) status in endometrial stromal sarcoma. *Eur. J. Gynaecol. Oncol.* **2012**, *33*, 629–632.
77. Backer, M.V.; Levashova, Z.; Patel, V.; Jehning, B.T.; Claffey, K.; Blankenberg, F.G.; Backer, J.M. Molecular imaging of VEGF receptors in angiogenic vasculature with single-chain VEGF-based probes. *Nat. Med.* **2007**, *13*, 504–509. [CrossRef]
78. Winkler, A.M.; Rice, P.F.; Weichsel, J.; Watson, J.M.; Backer, M.V.; Backer, J.M.; Barton, J.K. In vivo, dual-modality OCT/LIF imaging using a novel VEGF receptor-targeted NIR fluorescent probe in the AOM-treated mouse model. *Mol. Imaging Biol.* **2011**, *13*, 1173–1182. [CrossRef]
79. Liu, L.; Kakiuchi-Kiyota, S.; Arnold, L.L.; Johansson, S.L.; Wert, D.; Cohen, S.M. Pathogenesis of human hemangiosarcomas and hemangiomas. *Hum. Pathol.* **2013**, *44*, 2302–2311. [CrossRef]
80. Pakos, E.E.; Goussia, A.C.; Tsekeris, P.G.; Papachristou, D.J.; Stefanou, D.; Agnantis, N.J. Expression of vascular endothelial growth factor and its receptor, KDR/Flk-1, in soft tissue sarcomas. *Anticancer Res.* **2005**, *25*, 3591–3596.
81. Stacher, E.; Gruber-Mosenbacher, U.; Halbwedl, I.; Dei Tos, A.P.; Cavazza, A.; Papotti, M.; Carvalho, L.; Huber, M.; Ermert, L.; Popper, H.H. The VEGF-system in primary pulmonary angiosarcomas and haemangioendotheliomas: New potential therapeutic targets? *Lung Cancer* **2009**, *65*, 49–55. [CrossRef]
82. Ho, A.L.; Vasudeva, S.D.; Lae, M.; Saito, T.; Barbashina, V.; Antonescu, C.R.; Ladanyi, M.; Schwartz, G.K. PDGF receptor alpha is an alternative mediator of rapamycin-induced Akt activation: Implications for combination targeted therapy of synovial sarcoma. *Cancer Res.* **2012**, *72*, 4515–4525. [CrossRef] [PubMed]
83. Zhou, H.; Qian, W.; Uckun, F.M.; Zhou, Z.; Wang, L.; Wang, A.; Mao, H.; Yang, L. IGF-1 receptor targeted nanoparticles for image-guided therapy of stroma-rich and drug resistant human cancer. *Proc. SPIE Int. Soc. Opt. Eng.* **2016**, *9836*. [CrossRef]
84. Moroncini, G.; Maccaroni, E.; Fiordoliva, I.; Pellei, C.; Gabrielli, A.; Berardi, R. Developments in the management of advanced soft-tissue sarcoma—Olaratumab in context. *Onco. Targets* **2018**, *11*, 833–842. [CrossRef] [PubMed]
85. Camorani, S.; Hill, B.S.; Collina, F.; Gargiulo, S.; Napolitano, M.; Cantile, M.; Di Bonito, M.; Botti, G.; Fedele, M.; Zannetti, A.; et al. Targeted imaging and inhibition of triple-negative breast cancer metastases by a PDGFRbeta aptamer. *Theranostics* **2018**, *8*, 5178–5199. [CrossRef]
86. Adams, S.F.; Hickson, J.A.; Hutto, J.Y.; Montag, A.G.; Lengyel, E.; Yamada, S.D. PDGFR-alpha as a potential therapeutic target in uterine sarcomas. *Gynecol. Oncol.* **2007**, *104*, 524–528. [CrossRef]
87. Liegl, B.; Gully, C.; Reich, O.; Nogales, F.F.; Beham, A.; Regauer, S. Expression of platelet-derived growth factor receptor in low-grade endometrial stromal sarcomas in the absence of activating mutations. *Histopathology* **2007**, *50*, 448–452. [CrossRef]
88. Rossi, G.; Valli, R.; Bertolini, F.; Marchioni, A.; Cavazza, A.; Mucciarini, C.; Migaldi, M.; Federico, M.; Trentini, G.P.; Sgambato, A. PDGFR expression in differential diagnosis between KIT-negative gastrointestinal stromal tumours and other primary soft-tissue tumours of the gastrointestinal tract. *Histopathology* **2005**, *46*, 522–531. [CrossRef]
89. Fleuren, E.D.G.; Vlenterie, M.; van der Graaf, W.T.A.; Hillebrandt-Roeffen, M.H.S.; Blackburn, J.; Ma, X.; Chan, H.; Magias, M.C.; van Erp, A.; van Houdt, L.; et al. Phosphoproteomic Profiling Reveals ALK and MET as Novel Actionable Targets across Synovial Sarcoma Subtypes. *Cancer Res.* **2017**, *77*, 4279–4292. [CrossRef]
90. Roland, C.L.; May, C.D.; Watson, K.L.; Al Sannaa, G.A.; Dineen, S.P.; Feig, R.; Landers, S.; Ingram, D.R.; Wang, W.L.; Guadagnolo, B.A.; et al. Analysis of Clinical and Molecular Factors Impacting Oncologic Outcomes in Undifferentiated Pleomorphic Sarcoma. *Ann. Surg. Oncol.* **2016**, *23*, 2220–2228. [CrossRef]
91. Hiraki-Hotokebuchi, Y.; Yamada, Y.; Kohashi, K.; Yamamoto, H.; Endo, M.; Setsu, N.; Yuki, K.; Ito, T.; Iwamoto, Y.; Furue, M.; et al. Alteration of PDGFRbeta-Akt-mTOR pathway signaling in fibrosarcomatous transformation of dermatofibrosarcoma protuberans. *Hum. Pathol.* **2017**, *67*, 60–68. [CrossRef]
92. Lopez-Guerrero, J.A.; Navarro, S.; Noguera, R.; Carda, C.; Farinas, S.C.; Pellin, A.; Llombart-Bosch, A. Mutational analysis of the c-KIT AND PDGFRalpha in a series of molecularly well-characterized synovial sarcomas. *Diagn. Mol. Pathol. Am. J. Surg. Pathol. Part B* **2005**, *14*, 134–139. [CrossRef] [PubMed]

93. Sieber, T.; Schoeler, D.; Ringel, F.; Pascu, M.; Schriever, F. Selective internalization of monoclonal antibodies by B-cell chronic lymphocytic leukaemia cells. *Br. J. Haematol.* **2003**, *121*, 458–461. [CrossRef]
94. Klohs, J.; Grafe, M.; Graf, K.; Steinbrink, J.; Dietrich, T.; Stibenz, D.; Bahmani, P.; Kronenberg, G.; Harms, C.; Endres, M.; et al. In vivo imaging of the inflammatory receptor CD40 after cerebral ischemia using a fluorescent antibody. *Stroke* **2008**, *39*, 2845–2852. [CrossRef] [PubMed]
95. Kennedy, M.M.; Biddolph, S.; Lucas, S.B.; Howells, D.D.; Picton, S.; McGee, J.O.; O'Leary, J.J. CD40 upregulation is independent of HHV-8 in the pathogenesis of Kaposi's sarcoma. *Mol. Pathol.* **1999**, *52*, 32–36. [CrossRef] [PubMed]
96. Mechtersheimer, G.; Barth, T.; Ludwig, R.; Staudter, M.; Moller, P. Differential expression of leukocyte differentiation antigens in small round blue cell sarcomas. *Cancer* **1993**, *71*, 237–248. [CrossRef]
97. Ottaiano, A.; De Chiara, A.; Perrone, F.; Botti, G.; Fazioli, F.; De Rosa, V.; Mozzillo, N.; Ravo, V.; Morrica, B.; Gallo, C.; et al. Prognostic value of CD40 in adult soft tissue sarcomas. *Clin. Cancer Res.* **2004**, *10*, 2824–2831. [CrossRef] [PubMed]
98. Pammer, J.; Plettenberg, A.; Weninger, W.; Diller, B.; Mildner, M.; Uthman, A.; Issing, W.; Sturzl, M.; Tschachler, E. CD40 antigen is expressed by endothelial cells and tumor cells in Kaposi's sarcoma. *Am. J. Pathol.* **1996**, *148*, 1387–1396.
99. Kalim, M.; Wang, S.; Liang, K.; Khan, M.S.I.; Zhan, J. Engineered scPDL1-DM1 drug conjugate with improved in vitro analysis to target PD-L1 positive cancer cells and intracellular trafficking studies in cancer therapy. *Genet. Mol. Biol.* **2020**, *42*, e20180391. [CrossRef]
100. Zhang, M.; Jiang, H.; Zhang, R.; Jiang, H.; Xu, H.; Pan, W.; Gao, X.; Sun, Z. Near-infrared fluorescence-labeled anti-PD-L1-mAb for tumor imaging in human colorectal cancer xenografted mice. *J. Cell. Biochem.* **2019**, *120*, 10239–10247. [CrossRef]
101. Asanuma, K.; Nakamura, T.; Hayashi, A.; Okamoto, T.; Iino, T.; Asanuma, Y.; Hagi, T.; Kita, K.; Nakamura, K.; Sudo, A. Soluble programmed death-ligand 1 rather than PD-L1 on tumor cells effectively predicts metastasis and prognosis in soft tissue sarcomas. *Sci. Rep.* **2020**, *10*, 9077. [CrossRef]
102. Ben-Ami, E.; Barysauskas, C.M.; Solomon, S.; Tahlil, K.; Malley, R.; Hohos, M.; Polson, K.; Loucks, M.; Severgnini, M.; Patel, T.; et al. Immunotherapy with single agent nivolumab for advanced leiomyosarcoma of the uterus: Results of a phase 2 study. *Cancer* **2017**, *123*, 3285–3290. [CrossRef]
103. D'Angelo, S.P.; Shoushtari, A.N.; Agaram, N.P.; Kuk, D.; Qin, L.X.; Carvajal, R.D.; Dickson, M.A.; Gounder, M.; Keohan, M.L.; Schwartz, G.K.; et al. Prevalence of tumor-infiltrating lymphocytes and PD-L1 expression in the soft tissue sarcoma microenvironment. *Hum. Pathol.* **2015**, *46*, 357–365. [CrossRef] [PubMed]
104. Gabrych, A.; Pęksa, R.; Kunc, M.; Krawczyk, M.; Izycka-Swieszewska, E.; Biernat, W.; Bień, E. The PD-L1/PD-1 axis expression on tumor-infiltrating immune cells and tumor cells in pediatric rhabdomyosarcoma. *Pathol. Res. Pract.* **2019**, *215*, 152700. [CrossRef] [PubMed]
105. Kawamura, A.; Kawamura, T.; Riddell, M.; Hikita, T.; Yanagi, T.; Umemura, H.; Nakayama, M. Regulation of programmed cell death ligand 1 expression by atypical protein kinase C lambda/iota in cutaneous angiosarcoma. *Cancer Sci.* **2019**, *110*, 1780–1789. [CrossRef] [PubMed]
106. Kim, C.; Kim, E.K.; Jung, H.; Chon, H.J.; Han, J.W.; Shin, K.H.; Hu, H.; Kim, K.S.; Choi, Y.D.; Kim, S.; et al. Prognostic implications of PD-L1 expression in patients with soft tissue sarcoma. *BMC Cancer* **2016**, *16*, 434. [CrossRef] [PubMed]
107. Kim, J.S.; Kim, M.W.; Park, D.Y. Indirect ultrasound guidance increased accuracy of the glenohumeral injection using the superior approach: A cadaveric study of injection accuracy. *Ann. Rehabil. Med.* **2013**, *37*, 202–207. [CrossRef]
108. Klein, S.; Mauch, C.; Wagener-Ryczek, S.; Schoemmel, M.; Buettner, R.; Quaas, A.; Helbig, D. Immune-phenotyping of pleomorphic dermal sarcomas suggests this entity as a potential candidate for immunotherapy. *Cancer Immunol. Immunother.* **2019**, *68*, 973–982. [CrossRef]
109. Kosemehmetoglu, K.; Ozogul, E.; Babaoglu, B.; Tezel, G.G.; Gedikoglu, G. Programmed Death Ligand 1 (PD-L1) Expression in Malignant Mesenchymal Tumors. *Turk. Patoloji. Derg.* **2017**, *1*, 192–197. [CrossRef]
110. Orth, M.F.; Buecklein, V.L.; Kampmann, E.; Subklewe, M.; Noessner, E.; Cidre-Aranaz, F.; Romero-Pérez, L.; Wehweck, F.S.; Lindner, L.; Issels, R.; et al. A comparative view on the expression patterns of PD-L1 and PD-1 in soft tissue sarcomas. *Cancer Immunol. Immunother.* **2020**, *69*, 1353–1362. [CrossRef]
111. Park, H.K.; Kim, M.; Sung, M.; Lee, S.E.; Kim, Y.J.; Choi, Y.L. Status of programmed death-ligand 1 expression in sarcomas. *J. Transl. Med.* **2018**, *16*, 303. [CrossRef]
112. Paydas, S.; Bagir, E.K.; Deveci, M.A.; Gonlusen, G. Clinical and prognostic significance of PD-1 and PD-L1 expression in sarcomas. *Med Oncol.* **2016**, *33*, 93. [CrossRef] [PubMed]
113. Pollack, S.M.; He, Q.; Yearley, J.H.; Emerson, R.; Vignali, M.; Zhang, Y.; Redman, M.W.; Baker, K.K.; Cooper, S.; Donahue, B.; et al. T-cell infiltration and clonality correlate with programmed cell death protein 1 and programmed death-ligand 1 expression in patients with soft tissue sarcomas. *Cancer* **2017**, *123*, 3291–3304. [CrossRef] [PubMed]
114. Shanes, E.D.; Friedman, L.A.; Mills, A.M. PD-L1 Expression and Tumor-infiltrating Lymphocytes in Uterine Smooth Muscle Tumors: Implications for Immunotherapy. *Am. J. Surg. Pathol.* **2019**, *43*, 792–801. [CrossRef] [PubMed]
115. Torabi, A.; Amaya, C.N.; Wians, F.H., Jr.; Bryan, B.A. PD-1 and PD-L1 expression in bone and soft tissue sarcomas. *Pathology* **2017**, *49*, 506–513. [CrossRef] [PubMed]
116. Vargas, A.C.; Maclean, F.M.; Sioson, L.; Tran, D.; Bonar, F.; Mahar, A.; Cheah, A.L.; Russell, P.; Grimison, P.; Richardson, L.; et al. Prevalence of PD-L1 expression in matched recurrent and/or metastatic sarcoma samples and in a range of selected sarcomas subtypes. *PLoS ONE* **2020**, *15*, e0222551. [CrossRef]

117. Yan, L.; Wang, Z.; Cui, C.; Guan, X.; Dong, B.; Zhao, M.; Wu, J.; Tian, X.; Hao, C. Comprehensive immune characterization and T-cell receptor repertoire heterogeneity of retroperitoneal liposarcoma. *Cancer Sci.* **2019**, *110*, 3038–3048. [CrossRef]
118. Zheng, B.; Wang, J.; Cai, W.; Lao, I.; Shi, Y.; Luo, X.; Yan, W. Changes in the tumor immune microenvironment in resected recurrent soft tissue sarcomas. *Ann. Transl. Med.* **2019**, *7*, 387. [CrossRef]
119. Edris, B.; Espinosa, I.; Muhlenberg, T.; Mikels, A.; Lee, C.H.; Steigen, S.E.; Zhu, S.; Montgomery, K.D.; Lazar, A.J.; Lev, D.; et al. ROR2 is a novel prognostic biomarker and a potential therapeutic target in leiomyosarcoma and gastrointestinal stromal tumour. *J. Pathol.* **2012**, *227*, 223–233. [CrossRef]
120. Ehlerding, E.B.; England, C.G.; Majewski, R.L.; Valdovinos, H.F.; Jiang, D.; Liu, G.; McNeel, D.G.; Nickles, R.J.; Cai, W. ImmunoPET Imaging of CTLA-4 Expression in Mouse Models of Non-small Cell Lung Cancer. *Mol. Pharm.* **2017**, *14*, 1782–1789. [CrossRef]
121. Hong, Y.K.; Lee, Y.C.; Cheng, T.L.; Lai, C.H.; Hsu, C.K.; Kuo, C.H.; Hsu, Y.Y.; Li, J.T.; Chang, B.I.; Ma, C.Y.; et al. Tumor Endothelial Marker 1 (TEM1/Endosialin/CD248) Enhances Wound Healing by Interacting with Platelet-Derived Growth Factor Receptors. *J. Investig. Derm.* **2019**, *139*, 2204–2214.e7. [CrossRef]
122. Naylor, A.J.; McGettrick, H.M.; Maynard, W.D.; May, P.; Barone, F.; Croft, A.P.; Egginton, S.; Buckley, C.D. A differential role for CD248 (Endosialin) in PDGF-mediated skeletal muscle angiogenesis. *PLoS ONE* **2014**, *9*, e107146. [CrossRef] [PubMed]
123. Teicher, B.A. CD248: A therapeutic target in cancer and fibrotic diseases. *Oncotarget* **2019**, *10*, 993–1009. [CrossRef] [PubMed]
124. Pietrzyk, Ł. Biomarkers Discovery for Colorectal Cancer: A Review on Tumor Endothelial Markers as Perspective Candidates. *Dis. Markers* **2016**, *2016*, 4912405. [CrossRef] [PubMed]
125. Rouleau, C.; Smale, R.; Fu, Y.S.; Hui, G.; Wang, F.; Hutto, E.; Fogle, R.; Jones, C.M.; Krumbholz, R.; Roth, S.; et al. Endosialin is expressed in high grade and advanced sarcomas: Evidence from clinical specimens and preclinical modeling. *Int. J. Oncol.* **2011**, *39*, 73–89. [CrossRef]
126. Palmerini, E.; Benassi, M.S.; Quattrini, I.; Pazzaglia, L.; Donati, D.; Benini, S.; Gamberi, G.; Gambarotti, M.; Picci, P.; Ferrari, S. Prognostic and predictive role of CXCR4, IGF-1R and Ezrin expression in localized synovial sarcoma: Is chemotaxis important to tumor response? *Orphanet. J. Rare. Dis.* **2015**, *10*, 6. [CrossRef]
127. Ptaszyński, K.; Szumera-Ciećkiewicz, A.; Zakrzewska, K.; Tuziak, T.; Mrozkowiak, A.; Rutkowski, P. Her2, EGFR and TOPIIA gene amplification and protein expression in synovial sarcoma before and after combined treatment. *Pol. J. Pathol.* **2009**, *60*, 10–18.
128. Ahlen, J.; Wejde, J.; Brosjo, O.; von Rosen, A.; Weng, W.H.; Girnita, L.; Larsson, O.; Larsson, C. Insulin-like growth factor type 1 receptor expression correlates to good prognosis in highly malignant soft tissue sarcoma. *Clin. Cancer Res.* **2005**, *11*, 206–216.
129. Van der Ven, L.T.; Roholl, P.J.; Gloudemans, T.; Van Buul-Offers, S.C.; Welters, M.J.; Bladergroen, B.A.; Faber, J.A.; Sussenbach, J.S.; Den Otter, W. Expression of insulin-like growth factors (IGFs), their receptors and IGF binding protein-3 in normal, benign and malignant smooth muscle tissues. *Br. J. Cancer* **1997**, *75*, 1631–1640. [CrossRef]
130. Jones, R.L.; Chawla, S.P.; Attia, S.; Schöffski, P.; Gelderblom, H.; Chmielowski, B.; Le Cesne, A.; Van Tine, B.A.; Trent, J.C.; Patel, S.; et al. A phase 1 and randomized controlled phase 2 trial of the safety and efficacy of the combination of gemcitabine and docetaxel with ontuxizumab (MORAb-004) in metastatic soft-tissue sarcomas. *Cancer* **2019**, *125*, 2445–2454. [CrossRef]
131. Kilvaer, T.K.; Valkov, A.; Sorbye, S.; Smeland, E.; Bremnes, R.M.; Busund, L.T.; Donnem, T. Profiling of VEGFs and VEGFRs as prognostic factors in soft tissue sarcoma: VEGFR-3 is an independent predictor of poor prognosis. *PLoS ONE* **2010**, *5*, e15368. [CrossRef]
132. Patwardhan, P.P.; Musi, E.; Schwartz, G.K. Preclinical Evaluation of Nintedanib, a Triple Angiokinase Inhibitor, in Soft-tissue Sarcoma: Potential Therapeutic Implication for Synovial Sarcoma. *Mol. Cancer* **2018**, *17*, 2329–2340. [CrossRef] [PubMed]
133. Clinicaltrials.gov Ramucirumab. Available online: https://clinicaltrials.gov/ct2/show/NCT04145700?term=ramucirumab&cond=Soft+Tissue+Sarcoma&draw=2&rank=1 (accessed on 22 June 2020).
134. Harlaar, N.J.; Koller, M.; de Jongh, S.J.; van Leeuwen, B.L.; Hemmer, P.H.; Kruijff, S.; van Ginkel, R.J.; Been, L.B.; de Jong, J.S.; Kats-Ugurlu, G.; et al. Molecular fluorescence-guided surgery of peritoneal carcinomatosis of colorectal origin: A single-centre feasibility study. *Lancet. Gastroenterol. Hepatol.* **2016**, *1*, 283–290. [CrossRef]
135. Mitsiades, N.; Yu, W.H.; Poulaki, V.; Tsokos, M.; Stamenkovic, I. Matrix metalloproteinase-7-mediated cleavage of Fas ligand protects tumor cells from chemotherapeutic drug cytotoxicity. *Cancer Res.* **2001**, *61*, 577–581. [PubMed]
136. Steinkamp, P.J.; Pranger, B.K.; Li, M.; Linssen, M.D.; Voskuil, F.J.; Been, L.B.; van Leeuwen, B.L.; Suurmeijer, A.J.H.; Nagengast, W.B.; Kruijff, S.K.; et al. Fluorescence-guided visualization of soft tissue sarcomas by targeting vascular endothelial growth factor-A: A phase 1 single-center clinical trial. *J. Nucl. Med.* **2020**. [CrossRef] [PubMed]
137. De Jongh, S.J.; Tjalma, J.J.J.; Koller, M.; Linssen, M.D.; Vonk, J.; Dobosz, M.; Jorritsma-Smit, A.; Kleibeuker, J.H.; Hospers, G.A.P.; Havenga, K.; et al. Back-Table Fluorescence-Guided Imaging for Circumferential Resection Margin Evaluation Using Bevacizumab-800CW in Patients with Locally Advanced Rectal Cancer. *J. Nucl. Med.* **2020**, *61*, 655–661. [CrossRef] [PubMed]
138. Lamberts, L.E.; Koch, M.; de Jong, J.S.; Adams, A.L.L.; Glatz, J.; Kranendonk, M.E.G.; Terwisscha van Scheltinga, A.G.T.; Jansen, L.; de Vries, J.; Lub-de Hooge, M.N.; et al. Tumor-Specific Uptake of Fluorescent Bevacizumab-IRDye800CW Microdosing in Patients with Primary Breast Cancer: A Phase I Feasibility Study. *Clin. Cancer Res.* **2017**, *23*, 2730–2741. [CrossRef]
139. Wang, Z. ErbB Receptors and Cancer. *Methods Mol. Biol.* **2017**, *1652*, 3–35. [CrossRef]
140. Pellat, A.; Vaquero, J.; Fouassier, L. Role of ErbB/HER family of receptor tyrosine kinases in cholangiocyte biology. *Hepatology* **2018**, *67*, 762–773. [CrossRef]
141. Singh, B.; Carpenter, G.; Coffey, R.J. EGF receptor ligands: Recent advances. *F1000Research* **2016**, *5*. [CrossRef]

142. Duan, C.; Li, C.W.; Zhao, L.; Subramaniam, S.; Yu, X.M.; Li, Y.Y.; de Chen, H.; Li, T.Y.; Shen, L.; Shi, L.; et al. Differential Expression Patterns of EGF, EGFR, and ERBB4 in Nasal Polyp Epithelium. *PLoS ONE* **2016**, *11*, e0156949. [CrossRef]
143. Huisman, B.W.; Burggraaf, J.; Vahrmeijer, A.L.; Schoones, J.W.; Rissmann, R.A.; Sier, C.F.M.; van Poelgeest, M.I.E. Potential targets for tumor-specific imaging of vulvar squamous cell carcinoma: A systematic review of candidate biomarkers. *Gynecol. Oncol.* **2020**, *156*, 734–743. [CrossRef] [PubMed]
144. Sasaki, T.; Hiroki, K.; Yamashita, Y. The role of epidermal growth factor receptor in cancer metastasis and microenvironment. *Biomed. Res. Int.* **2013**, *2013*, 546318. [CrossRef] [PubMed]
145. Sigismund, S.; Avanzato, D.; Lanzetti, L. Emerging functions of the EGFR in cancer. *Mol. Oncol.* **2018**, *12*, 3–20. [CrossRef] [PubMed]
146. Clinicaltrials.gov Cetuximab. Available online: https://clinicaltrials.gov/ct2/show/NCT00148109?term=cetuximab&cond=Soft+Tissue+Sarcoma&draw=3&rank=1 (accessed on 22 June 2020).
147. Tummers, W.S.; Miller, S.E.; Teraphongphom, N.T.; Gomez, A.; Steinberg, I.; Huland, D.M.; Hong, S.; Kothapalli, S.R.; Hasan, A.; Ertsey, R.; et al. Intraoperative Pancreatic Cancer Detection using Tumor-Specific Multimodality Molecular Imaging. *Ann. Surg. Oncol.* **2018**, *25*, 1880–1888. [CrossRef] [PubMed]
148. Miller, S.E.; Tummers, W.S.; Teraphongphom, N.; van den Berg, N.S.; Hasan, A.; Ertsey, R.D.; Nagpal, S.; Recht, L.D.; Plowey, E.D.; Vogel, H.; et al. First-in-human intraoperative near-infrared fluorescence imaging of glioblastoma using cetuximab-IRDye800. *J. Neurooncol.* **2018**, *139*, 135–143. [CrossRef] [PubMed]
149. Rosenthal, E.L.; Warram, J.M.; de Boer, E.; Chung, T.K.; Korb, M.L.; Brandwein-Gensler, M.; Strong, T.V.; Schmalbach, C.E.; Morlandt, A.B.; Agarwal, G.; et al. Safety and Tumor Specificity of Cetuximab-IRDye800 for Surgical Navigation in Head and Neck Cancer. *Clin. Cancer. Res.* **2015**, *21*, 3658–3666. [CrossRef]
150. Colman, R.W.; Pixley, R.A.; Sainz, I.M.; Song, J.S.; Isordia-Salas, I.; Muhamed, S.N.; Powell, J.A., Jr.; Mousa, S.A. Inhibition of angiogenesis by antibody blocking the action of proangiogenic high-molecular-weight kininogen. *J. Thromb. Haemost.* **2003**, *1*, 164–170. [CrossRef]
151. Samkoe, K.S.; Gunn, J.R.; Marra, K.; Hull, S.M.; Moodie, K.L.; Feldwisch, J.; Strong, T.V.; Draney, D.R.; Hoopes, P.J.; Roberts, D.W.; et al. Toxicity and Pharmacokinetic Profile for Single-Dose Injection of ABY-029: A Fluorescent Anti-EGFR Synthetic Affibody Molecule for Human Use. *Mol. Imaging Biol.* **2017**, *19*, 512–521. [CrossRef]
152. Clinicaltrials.gov Panitumumab (Head&Neck Cancer). Available online: https://clinicaltrials.gov/ct2/show/NCT03405142?term=Panitumumab-IRDye800&draw=2&rank=4 (accessed on 22 June 2020).
153. Clinicaltrials.gov Panitumumab (Lung Cancer). Available online: https://clinicaltrials.gov/ct2/show/NCT03582124?term=Panitumumab-IRDye800&draw=2&rank=3 (accessed on 22 June 2020).
154. Clinicaltrials.gov Panitumumab. Available online: https://clinicaltrials.gov/ct2/show/NCT02415881?term=Panitumumab-IRDye800&draw=2&rank=2 (accessed on 22 June 2020).
155. Friedrichs, N.; Kuchler, J.; Endl, E.; Koch, A.; Czerwitzki, J.; Wurst, P.; Metzger, D.; Schulte, J.H.; Holst, M.I.; Heukamp, L.C.; et al. Insulin-like growth factor-1 receptor acts as a growth regulator in synovial sarcoma. *J. Pathol.* **2008**, *216*, 428–439. [CrossRef]
156. Xie, Y.; Skytting, B.; Nilsson, G.; Brodin, B.; Larsson, O. Expression of insulin-like growth factor-1 receptor in synovial sarcoma: Association with an aggressive phenotype. *Cancer Res.* **1999**, *59*, 3588–3591.
157. Clinicaltrials.gov Ganitumab. Available online: https://clinicaltrials.gov/ct2/show/NCT00819169?term=Ganitumab&cond=Soft+Tissue+Sarcoma&draw=2&rank=8 (accessed on 22 June 2020).
158. Clinicaltrials.gov AMG-479. Available online: https://clinicaltrials.gov/ct2/show/NCT00562380?term=Ganitumab&cond=Soft+Tissue+Sarcoma&draw=2&rank=6 (accessed on 22 June 2020).
159. Olmos, D.; Postel-Vinay, S.; Molife, L.R.; Okuno, S.H.; Schuetze, S.M.; Paccagnella, M.L.; Batzel, G.N.; Yin, D.; Pritchard-Jones, K.; Judson, I.; et al. Safety, pharmacokinetics, and preliminary activity of the anti-IGF-1R antibody figitumumab (CP-751,871) in patients with sarcoma and Ewing's sarcoma: A phase 1 expansion cohort study. *Lancet. Oncol.* **2010**, *11*, 129–135. [CrossRef]
160. Pappo, A.S.; Vassal, G.; Crowley, J.J.; Bolejack, V.; Hogendoorn, P.C.; Chugh, R.; Ladanyi, M.; Grippo, J.F.; Dall, G.; Staddon, A.P.; et al. A phase 2 trial of R1507, a monoclonal antibody to the insulin-like growth factor-1 receptor (IGF-1R), in patients with recurrent or refractory rhabdomyosarcoma, osteosarcoma, synovial sarcoma, and other soft tissue sarcomas: Results of a Sarcoma Alliance for Research Through Collaboration study. *Cancer* **2014**, *120*, 2448–2456. [CrossRef] [PubMed]
161. Schoffski, P.; Adkins, D.; Blay, J.Y.; Gil, T.; Elias, A.D.; Rutkowski, P.; Pennock, G.K.; Youssoufian, H.; Gelderblom, H.; Willey, R.; et al. An open-label, phase 2 study evaluating the efficacy and safety of the anti-IGF-1R antibody cixutumumab in patients with previously treated advanced or metastatic soft-tissue sarcoma or Ewing family of tumours. *Eur. J. Cancer* **2013**, *49*, 3219–3228. [CrossRef] [PubMed]
162. Zhang, H.; Zeng, X.; Li, Q.; Gaillard-Kelly, M.; Wagner, C.R.; Yee, D. Fluorescent tumour imaging of type I IGF receptor in vivo: Comparison of antibody-conjugated quantum dots and small-molecule fluorophore. *Br. J. Cancer* **2009**, *101*, 71–79. [CrossRef]
163. Lai, Y.T.; Chao, H.W.; Lai, A.C.; Lin, S.H.; Chang, Y.J.; Huang, Y.S. CPEB2-activated PDGFRalpha mRNA translation contributes to myofibroblast proliferation and pulmonary alveologenesis. *J. Biomed. Sci.* **2020**, *27*, 52. [CrossRef] [PubMed]
164. Andrae, J.; Gallini, R.; Betsholtz, C. Role of platelet-derived growth factors in physiology and medicine. *Genes Dev.* **2008**, *22*, 1276–1312. [CrossRef] [PubMed]

165. Lin, L.H.; Lin, J.S.; Yang, C.C.; Cheng, H.W.; Chang, K.W.; Liu, C.J. Overexpression of Platelet-Derived Growth Factor and Its Receptor Are Correlated with Oral Tumorigenesis and Poor Prognosis in Oral Squamous Cell Carcinoma. *Int. J. Mol. Sci.* **2020**, *21*, 2360. [CrossRef]
166. Santilli, F.; Basili, S.; Ferroni, P.; Davi, G. CD40/CD40L system and vascular disease. *Intern. Emerg. Med.* **2007**, *2*, 256–268. [CrossRef]
167. Vonderheide, R.H. Prospect of targeting the CD40 pathway for cancer therapy. *Clin. Cancer Res.* **2007**, *13*, 1083–1088. [CrossRef]
168. Elmetwali, T.; Young, L.S.; Palmer, D.H. Fas-associated factor (Faf1) is a novel CD40 interactor that regulates CD40-induced NF-kappaB activation via a negative feedback loop. *Cell Death Dis.* **2014**, *5*, e1213. [CrossRef]
169. Gennatas, S.; Chamberlain, F.; Carter, T.; Slater, S.; Cojocaru, E.; Lambourn, B.; Stansfeld, A.; Todd, R.; Verrill, M.; Ali, N.; et al. Real-world experience with doxorubicin and olaratumab in soft tissue sarcomas in England and Northern Ireland. *Clin. Sarcoma Res.* **2020**, *10*, 9. [CrossRef] [PubMed]
170. Piechutta, M.; Berghoff, A.S. New emerging targets in cancer immunotherapy: The role of Cluster of Differentiation 40 (CD40/TNFR5). *Esmo Open* **2019**, *4*, e000510. [CrossRef] [PubMed]
171. Clinicaltrials.gov APX005M. Available online: https://clinicaltrials.gov/ct2/show/NCT03719430?term=APX005M&cond=Soft+Tissue+Sarcoma&draw=2&rank=1 (accessed on 22 June 2020).
172. Gu, L.; Ruff, L.E.; Qin, Z.; Corr, M.; Hedrick, S.M.; Sailor, M.J. Multivalent porous silicon nanoparticles enhance the immune activation potency of agonistic CD40 antibody. *Adv. Mater.* **2012**, *24*, 3981–3987. [CrossRef]
173. Tap, W.D.; Wagner, A.J.; Schöffski, P.; Martin-Broto, J.; Krarup-Hansen, A.; Ganjoo, K.N.; Yen, C.C.; Abdul Razak, A.R.; Spira, A.; Kawai, A.; et al. Effect of Doxorubicin Plus Olaratumab vs Doxorubicin Plus Placebo on Survival in Patients With Advanced Soft Tissue Sarcomas: The ANNOUNCE Randomized Clinical Trial. *JAMA* **2020**, *323*, 1266–1276. [CrossRef] [PubMed]
174. Yonemori, K.; Kodaira, M.; Satoh, T.; Kudo, T.; Takahashi, S.; Nakano, K.; Ando, Y.; Shimokata, T.; Mori, J.; Inoue, K.; et al. Phase 1 study of olaratumab plus doxorubicin in Japanese patients with advanced soft-tissue sarcoma. *Cancer Sci.* **2018**, *109*, 3962–3970. [CrossRef]
175. Wagner, A.J.; Kindler, H.; Gelderblom, H.; Schoffski, P.; Bauer, S.; Hohenberger, P.; Kopp, H.G.; Lopez-Martin, J.A.; Peeters, M.; Reichardt, P.; et al. A phase II study of a human anti-PDGFRalpha monoclonal antibody (olaratumab, IMC-3G3) in previously treated patients with metastatic gastrointestinal stromal tumors. *Ann. Oncol.* **2017**, *28*, 541–546. [CrossRef]
176. Schwartz, G.K.; Tap, W.D.; Qin, L.X.; Livingston, M.B.; Undevia, S.D.; Chmielowski, B.; Agulnik, M.; Schuetze, S.M.; Reed, D.R.; Okuno, S.H.; et al. Cixutumumab and temsirolimus for patients with bone and soft-tissue sarcoma: A multicentre, open-label, phase 2 trial. *Lancet. Oncol.* **2013**, *14*, 371–382. [CrossRef]
177. Chisholm, K.M.; Chang, K.W.; Truong, M.T.; Kwok, S.; West, R.B.; Heerema-McKenney, A.E. β-Adrenergic receptor expression in vascular tumors. *Mod. Pathol.* **2012**, *25*, 1446–1451. [CrossRef]
178. Federico, S.M.; Caldwell, K.J.; McCarville, M.B.; Daryani, V.M.; Stewart, C.F.; Mao, S.; Wu, J.; Davidoff, A.M.; Santana, V.M.; Furman, W.L.; et al. Phase I expansion cohort to evaluate the combination of bevacizumab, sorafenib and low-dose cyclophosphamide in children and young adults with refractory or recurrent solid tumours. *Eur. J. Cancer* **2020**, *132*, 35–42. [CrossRef]
179. Hong, D.S.; Garrido-Laguna, I.; Ekmekcioglu, S.; Falchook, G.S.; Naing, A.; Wheler, J.J.; Fu, S.; Moulder, S.L.; Piha-Paul, S.; Tsimberidou, A.M.; et al. Dual inhibition of the vascular endothelial growth factor pathway: A phase 1 trial evaluating bevacizumab and AZD2171 (cediranib) in patients with advanced solid tumors. *Cancer* **2014**, *120*, 2164–2173. [CrossRef]
180. Tap, W.D.; Federman, N.; Eilber, F.C. Targeted therapies for soft-tissue sarcomas. *Expert Rev. Anticancer* **2007**, *7*, 725–733. [CrossRef] [PubMed]
181. Coats, S.; Williams, M.; Kebble, B.; Dixit, R.; Tseng, L.; Yao, N.S.; Tice, D.A.; Soria, J.C. Antibody-Drug Conjugates: Future Directions in Clinical and Translational Strategies to Improve the Therapeutic Index. *Clin. Cancer Res.* **2019**, *25*, 5441–5448. [CrossRef] [PubMed]
182. Petrus, P.; Fernandez, T.L.; Kwon, M.M.; Huang, J.L.; Lei, V.; Safikhan, N.S.; Karunakaran, S.; O'Shannessy, D.J.; Zheng, X.; Catrina, S.B.; et al. Specific loss of adipocyte CD248 improves metabolic health via reduced white adipose tissue hypoxia, fibrosis and inflammation. *EBioMedicine* **2019**, *44*, 489–501. [CrossRef] [PubMed]
183. Vodanovich, D.A.; Choong, P.F.M. Soft-tissue Sarcomas. *Indian J. Orthop.* **2018**, *52*, 35–44. [CrossRef] [PubMed]
184. Uhlén, M.; Fagerberg, L.; Hallström, B.M.; Lindskog, C.; Oksvold, P.; Mardinoglu, A.; Sivertsson, Å.; Kampf, C.; Sjöstedt, E.; Asplund, A.; et al. Proteomics. Tissue-based map of the human proteome. *Science* **2015**, *347*, 1260419. [CrossRef]
185. Human Protein Atlas. Available online: http://www.proteinatlas.org (accessed on 13 December 2020).
186. Grothey, A.; Strosberg, J.R.; Renfro, L.A.; Hurwitz, H.I.; Marshall, J.L.; Safran, H.; Guarino, M.J.; Kim, G.P.; Hecht, J.R.; Weil, S.C.; et al. A Randomized, Double-Blind, Placebo-Controlled Phase II Study of the Efficacy and Safety of Monotherapy Ontuxizumab (MORAb-004) Plus Best Supportive Care in Patients with Chemorefractory Metastatic Colorectal Cancer. *Clin. Cancer Res.* **2018**, *24*, 316–325. [CrossRef]
187. Kersting, C.; Packeisen, J.; Leidinger, B.; Brandt, B.; von Wasielewski, R.; Winkelmann, W.; van Diest, P.J.; Gosheger, G.; Buerger, H. Pitfalls in immunohistochemical assessment of EGFR expression in soft tissue sarcomas. *J. Clin. Pathol.* **2006**, *59*, 585–590. [CrossRef]

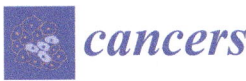

Article

The Feasibility Study of Hypofractionated Radiotherapy with Regional Hyperthermia in Soft Tissue Sarcomas

Mateusz Jacek Spałek [1,*], Aneta Maria Borkowska [1], Maria Telejko [2], Michał Wągrodzki [3], Daria Niebyłowska [2], Aldona Uzar [2], Magdalena Białobrzeska [2] and Piotr Rutkowski [1]

[1] Department of Soft Tissue/Bone Sarcoma and Melanoma, Maria Sklodowska-Curie National Research Institute of Oncology, 02-781 Warsaw, Poland; aneta.borkowska@pib-nio.pl (A.M.B.); piotr.rutkowski@pib-nio.pl (P.R.)
[2] Department of Radiotherapy, Maria Sklodowska-Curie National Research Institute of Oncology, 02-781 Warsaw, Poland; maria.telejko@pib-nio.pl (M.T.); daria.niebylowska@pib-nio.pl (D.N.); aldona.lesniewska-mazur@pib-nio.pl (A.U.); magdalena.bialobrzeska@pib-nio.pl (M.B.)
[3] Department of Pathology and Laboratory Medicine, Maria Sklodowska-Curie National Research Institute of Oncology, 02-781 Warsaw, Poland; michal.wagrodzki@pathologist.cc
* Correspondence: mateusz@spalek.co; Tel.: +48-22-546-24-55

Simple Summary: The recommended management of marginally resectable or unresectable soft tissue sarcomas is an attempt of neoadjuvant therapy. The use of neoadjuvant chemotherapy is limited in low-grade tumors, sarcomas with chemoresistant pathology or in unfit patients. There is a growing evidence on hypofractionated radiotherapy in soft tissue sarcomas, but its efficacy may be limited by radioresistance that is frequently associated with chemoresistance. Regional hyperthermia is a potent and minimally invasive radiosensitizer. We aimed to investigate the feasibility of moderately hypofractionated radiotherapy combined with regional hyperthermia in aforementioned clinical situations. Our findings indicate that proposed combination is feasible while maintaining good short-term local efficacy and tolerance. It could serve as a basis for further studies on radiotherapy with hyperthermia in soft tissue sarcomas.

Abstract: Introduction: Management of marginally resectable or unresectable soft tissue sarcomas (STS) in patients who are not candidates for neoadjuvant chemotherapy due to chemoresistant pathology or contraindications remains a challenge. Therefore, in these indications, we aimed to investigate a feasibility of 10x 3.25 Gy radiotherapy combined with regional hyperthermia (HT) that could be followed by surgery or 4x 4 Gy radiotherapy with HT. Materials and methods: We recruited patients with locally advanced marginally resectable or unresectable STS who (1) presented chemoresistant STS subtype, or (2) progressed after neoadjuvant chemotherapy, or (3) were unfit for chemotherapy. The primary endpoint was the feasibility of the proposed regimen. Results: Thirty patients were enrolled. All patients received the first part of the treatment, namely radiotherapy with HT. Among them, 14 received the second part of radiotherapy with HT whereas 13 patients underwent surgery. Three patients did not complete the treatment protocol. The feasibility criteria were fulfilled in 90% of patients. Two patients developed distant metastases. One patient died due to distant progression. One patient developed rapid local recurrence after surgery. Conclusions: Hypofractionated radiotherapy with HT is a feasible treatment for marginally resectable or unresectable STS in patients who are not candidates for chemotherapy. Results of this clinical trial support the further validation of RT and HT combinations in STS.

Keywords: sarcoma; radiotherapy; neoadjuvant therapy; hypofractionated radiotherapy; thermotherapy; hyperthermia

Citation: Spałek, M.J.; Borkowska, A.M.; Telejko, M.; Wągrodzki, M.; Niebyłowska, D.; Uzar, A.; Białobrzeska, M.; Rutkowski, P. The Feasibility Study of Hypofractionated Radiotherapy with Regional Hyperthermia in Soft Tissue Sarcomas. *Cancers* 2021, 13, 1332. https://doi.org/10.3390/cancers 13061332

Academic Editors: Joanna Szkandera and Dimosthenis Andreou

Received: 1 February 2021
Accepted: 12 March 2021
Published: 16 March 2021

Publisher's Note: MDPI stays neutral with regard to jurisdictional claims in published maps and institutional affiliations.

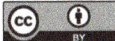

Copyright: © 2021 by the authors. Licensee MDPI, Basel, Switzerland. This article is an open access article distributed under the terms and conditions of the Creative Commons Attribution (CC BY) license (https://creativecommons.org/licenses/by/4.0/).

1. Introduction

The recommended management of marginally resectable or unresectable soft tissue sarcomas (STS) is an attempt of neoadjuvant therapy, namely radiotherapy (RT) and chemotherapy [1–3]. Neoadjuvant chemotherapy was a preferred approach in the vast majority of European sarcoma tertiary centers as per the expert survey performed by the European Organization for Research and Treatment of Cancer [4]. However, the most effective but toxic chemotherapy regimens used in STS may be not suitable for elderly patients or those with significant comorbidities [5]. Moreover, low-grade STS and selected histopathological STS subtypes are considered chemoresistant [6–12]. Another approach could be the use of high-dose definitive RT. In a large cohort analysis on RT for unresectable STS, total dose and tumor size influenced on local control, disease-free survival and overall survival [13]. This study identified a threshold dose of 63 Gy. However, delivery of such doses to large volume with extensive margins may lead to increase of RT-related toxicity as per results of the aforementioned analysis.

The solution may be the introduction of hypofractionated regimens. Alpha/beta ratio of STS, especially low-grade, is presumably low or very low [14,15]. Therefore, a higher dose per fraction may enable better tumor control with lower total equivalent dose in 2-Gy fractions (EQD2) and the similar toxicity profile [16]. This hypothesis was validated in several early-phase clinical trials with hypofractionation for STS [17–24]. Unfortunately, chemoresistance is frequently associated with radioresistance; thus, hypofractionated RT alone may not provide satisfactory local control [25,26]. The efficacy of RT could be additionally increased by using various methods that may overcome radioresistance. Hyperthermia (HT) is known as a potent radiosensitizer that enhance the cell-killing effect of RT and chemotherapy [27,28]. Focused heat directly damages tumor cells that are more heat-sensitive than surrounding tissues. It also indirectly intensifies RT damage by increasing oxygenation and inducing apoptosis, instability of the cell membrane, and dysregulation of proteins, including DNA repair enzymes [29]. Despite supporting evidence from preclinical studies, the addition of HT to standard neoadjuvant therapy was rarely a matter of prospective clinical trials [30–32]. The only randomized phase 3 clinical trial showed increased survival, as well as local progression-free survival among patients with locally advanced STS who received regional HT additionally to neoadjuvant chemotherapy [33,34]. Such an evidence for RT with HT does not exist. However, this combination provided encouraging results in management of melanomas that are also considered as chemo- and radioresistant tumors [35].

Therefore, we hypothesized that hypofractionated RT combined with regional HT is a feasible method of treatment of patients with STS who are not candidates for chemotherapy. We aimed to design feasible and flexible regimen that provides benefits from both hypofractionation and HT, as well as it can be applied for marginally resectable and unresectable tumors. Thus, we proposed two-week regimen of 32.5 Gy in 10 fractions with four HT sessions that could be followed by surgery or the second part of RT with HT.

Hence, we report the results of the clinical trial hypofractionated RT with regional HT for STS.

2. Materials and Methods

We conducted a prospective proof-of-concept phase II, open-label, single-arm clinical trial (NCT03989596). Ethical approval for this study was obtained from the Institutional Ethics committee of Maria Sklodowska-Curie National Research Institute of Oncology in June 2018, approval number 35/2018.

2.1. Inclusion Criteria

We recruited adult patients with locally advanced marginally resectable or unresectable STS localized to the extremities, trunk wall and pelvis who were not candidates for neoadjuvant chemotherapy. Resectability, chemoresistance, and/or non-eligibility for chemotherapy (for example, due to patient's comorbidities) were discussed individually in each case during the sarcoma multidisciplinary tumor board (MTB).

The major institutional criteria of marginal resectability and unresectability included extracompartmental extension of the tumor, involvement of the bone or major vessels that may require vascular reconstruction, an extension of the tumor through natural foramina, or technical difficulties with resectability due to the tumor volume or its anatomical localization.

Patients who were not appropriate candidates for chemotherapy included those with chemoresistant STS or unfit to tolerate such a treatment as per MTB decision. Chemoresistance was defined as clinical or radiological local progression of primary tumor on neoadjuvant chemotherapy or the diagnosis of potentially chemoresistant STS (low-grade STS, epithelioid sarcoma, clear cell sarcoma, alveolar soft part tissue sarcoma, solitary fibrous tumor).

All patients were 18 or older and had Eastern Cooperative Oncology Group (ECOG) performance status 0 to 2. All patients provided written informed consent as approved by the Institutional Ethics Committee.

2.2. Exclusion Criteria

Patients with distant metastases, lymph node involvement or contraindications to RT or HT were excluded. Excluded pathological diagnoses were Ewing sarcoma, osteogenic sarcoma, embryonal, or alveolar rhabdomyosarcoma, and aggressive fibromatosis. Neither prior RT within or close to the currently planned target volume (PTV) nor second active malignancy were permitted.

2.3. Treatment Schedule

After a screening, which consists of local assessment of primary tumor in magnetic resonance imaging (MRI) or computed tomography (CT), biopsy or central pathological assessment of previously taken tumor sample, physical examination, exclusion of distant metastases in staging imaging, and case analysis at the MTB meeting, a patient received 32.5 Gy in ten fractions with regional HT twice a week within two weeks. The response analysis in CT or MRI and toxicity assessment were performed after at least six weeks.

During the second MDT meeting, final decisions about resectability and operability were made. In the case of resectability, operability, or consent for amputation if required, a patient was referred to surgery. Otherwise, the patient received a second part of local treatment which consisted of 16 Gy in four fractions with regional HT twice a week within one week. The treatment schedule was presented in Figure 1.

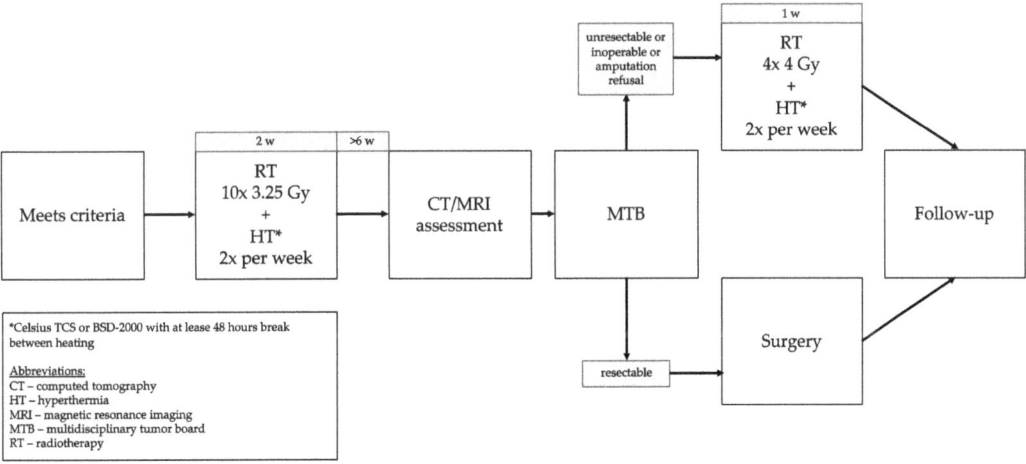

Figure 1. Treatment schedule.

2.4. Radiotherapy

Previous clinical trials with moderate hypofractionation combined with chemotherapy showed good local efficacy and favorable toxicity profile of such treatment. The most common fractionation regimens comprised of 28–35 Gy in eight to ten fractions combined with anthracycline-based chemotherapy. We used the alpha/beta ratio for STS of 4 Gy, in alignment with other studies. Then, we decided to use 32.5 Gy in ten fractions. That translated into equivalent dose in 2-Gy fractions (EQD2) of 39.3 Gy. The addition of four HT sessions should compensate the lack of chemotherapy and lower EQD2 than in conventionally fractionated regimens; thus, we expected high local control. Moreover, there is theoretical dependence between higher total dose and a risk of RT-related toxicity, mostly wound complications. Thus, investigated regimen with lower EQD2 should provide a substantial benefit for the patients with locally advanced STS who are not candidates for chemotherapy.

In the case of unresectability, inoperability or refusal to amputation if limb-sparing surgery was not possible, the patient received the second part of RT with HT. It consisted of 16 Gy in four fractions combined with two HT sessions. That translated into higher dose intensity and EQD2 of 21.3 Gy. Then, the total EQD2 from the whole RT with HT was 60.6 Gy.

Delineation and treatment planning was performed by a team experienced in STS. The immobilization and the application of bolus was selected on a case-by-case basis. The gross tumor volume (GTV) was contoured on planning CT fused with contrast-enhanced MRI or diagnostic contrast-enhanced CT. The general rule was to create clinical target volume (CTV) by expanding GTV at least 2 cm in each direction, and, in extremity STS, at least 4 cm longitudinally. Nevertheless, due to the variety of clinical situations, the final choice of CTV was based on the benefit-risk assessment and opinion of at least two other radiation oncologists. In the case of second part RT with HT, it was allowed to reduce CTV to 1.5 cm in each direction. Then, CTV was adapted to anatomical borders of tumor spread (i.e., bones, fascias, or vital organs). All delineated target volumes and organs at risk were reviewed by another radiation oncologist. Planning target volume (PTV) was created by expanding CTV, adding safety margins (0.5–1.0 cm).

We used three-dimensional RT techniques with daily image guidance (cone beam computed tomography or planar kilovoltage) to deliver the prescribed dose. Techniques with dose intensity modulation were preferred over static RT. The dose was prescribed on mean PTV.

2.5. Hyperthermia

We used two regional HT systems, Celsius TCS and BSD-2000. The choice of the equipment for heat delivery in each case was based on tumor and patient-related factors, such as tumor localization or weight and height. BSD-2000 was preferred in the case of deeply seated abdominal and pelvic tumors or tumors localized to lower limbs; however, due to the properties of the Sigma-Eye applicator, it was not possible to use it in the majority of obese and overweight patients. Celsius TCS system was used in the other situations. The final decision was made by a radiation oncologist after discussion with radiation therapists specialized in HT.

Celsius TCS system uses the changeable two-electrode and water bolus system that allow homogeneous temperature development within the heated volume. The heat energy is generated by electromagnetic waves of 13.56 MHz to transfer energy based on the principle of capacitive coupling. More detailed data are provided in the manufacturer's site [36]. The disadvantage of the Celsius TCS system include lack of tumor temperature control; however, we used pre-defined treatment protocols tailored to anatomical site and patient's parameters to ensure proper delivery of necessary heat energy. The choice of treatment protocol was discussed within the HT team, taking into account tumor site, volume, and comorbidities.

BSD-2000 3D system uses 24 antennas surrounding patient's body that generate electromagnetic waves at the frequency range of 75 to 140 MHz to deliver heat energy. The energy is focused on heated volume using dedicated software. More detailed data are provided in the manufacturer's site [37]. We aimed to reach temperature within the treated volume between 39 and 42 Celsius degree. The indirect temperature control was performed using intraluminal or skin sensors.

Institutional contraindications to HT included implanted medical devices or objects (for example pacemakers, stabilizers, prostheses), significant tumor-related pain that cannot be controlled with medications, severe cardiac or pulmonary diseases, uncontrolled hypertension, myocardial infarction or cerebrovascular incident <6 months ago, pregnancy or breastfeeding.

HT was performed by a dedicated team of radiation therapists. Thermotolerance and all protocols deviations were strictly monitored and reported. The treatment was applied twice a week, with a minimum 48-h gap between sessions. The patient received RT fraction within one hour after each HT session.

2.6. Assessment of Response and Toxicity

Radiological response was assessed according to the Response Evaluation Criteria in Solid Tumors (RECIST), version 1.1. RT and HT toxicities were assessed according to the Common Terminology Criteria for Adverse Events v 5.0 (CTCAE). Acute toxicity was defined as from start of the RT with HT to 90 days after treatment completion. Late toxicity was defined as at any time after 90 days.

2.7. Follow-Up

The patients are followed-up according to the national and international guidelines. The minimum is a first visit 30 days after treatment completion to assess RT toxicity or wound healing and then every three months in the first two years, then twice a year up to the fifth year, and once a year thereafter. All patients are followed for evidence of local recurrence or distant metastases using CT or X-ray of the chest, and MRI or CT of the treated site.

2.8. Primary Endpoint

In this proof-of-concept study, the primary endpoint was the protocol feasibility that comprised treatment tolerance and compliance. The study would be terminated earlier in the case of unacceptable toxicity of treatment defined as the frequency of occurrence of grade 3 or higher acute toxicity according to CTCAE in over 40% of the treated patients.

The intervention would be deemed feasible if it meets safety rule and at least 80% of participants fulfil all the criteria:
- Able to finish all planned treatment according to the protocol (intention-to-treat principle); a permanent treatment termination regardless of the reason, including consent withdrawal, lost to follow-up or disease progression, was treated as the protocol failure.
- Able to tolerate HT; reduction of delivered heat energy or temporary breaks were allowed, but permanent discontinuation was treated as the protocol failure.
- Able to tolerate hypofractionated RT without unplanned breaks.

Using the Wilson method for calculating confidence intervals for proportions, the exact 95% confidence interval for an estimated feasibility proportion of 80% (23 of 30 patients) does not include (60–80%) a value of 50%. Thus, for a sample size of 30 patients, a feasibility of 80% is above chance level performance (50%).

2.9. Secondary Endpoints

The secondary endpoints were one-year local control, one-year sarcoma-specific survival (SSS), one-year progression-free survival (PFS) and rate of late toxicities. Local control was assessed by calculating time to local progression (TTLP) and local progression-free survival (LPFS).

2.10. Statistical Considerations

Statistical analyses were performed using R version 3.6.3 software (R Foundation for Statistical Computing, Vienna, Austria) and jamovi version 1.2 software (The jamovi project, Sydney, Australia).

The one-sample proportions test and the one-sided alternative were used to assess whether the feasibility proportion is larger than 50%. Median follow-up was estimated by Kaplan–Meier analysis with the reversed meaning of the status indicator. TTLP was calculated from the day of surgery or start of the last part of RT with HT to the last follow-up (censored), death without local progression (censored) or confirmed local progression. LPFS was calculated from the day of surgery or start of the last part of RT with HT to the last follow-up (censored), confirmed local progression, or death. SSS was calculated from the enrollment to the last follow-up (censored), death from STS, or death from other reasons (censored). PFS was calculated from the enrollment to the last follow-up (censored), disease progression or death. The Kaplan–Meier method was used to estimate survival. All p-values < 0.05 were considered significant.

3. Results

3.1. Patient and Tumor Data

Between June 2018 and September 2020, 30 patients were enrolled. The most frequent pathological diagnosis was solitary fibrous tumor (23%). The vast majority of STS were low grade tumors (73%). Over one third of the treated tumors developed in the pelvic area (37%). The median largest tumor dimension was 9.8 cm. At the MTB, 17 tumors were classified as marginally resectable, eight as locally unresectable but with possible amputation of the extremity and five as unresectable regardless of the extent of surgery. The patient and tumor characteristics are presented in Table 1. Detailed patient, tumor and treatment data are available in Table S1.

Table 1. Patient and tumor characteristics.

Characteristic		Value
Age at the enrollment	Median	69.5
	Interquartile range	52–74.8
Largest tumor dimension	Median	9.8 cm
	Interquartile range	7.7–13.5 cm
		Number of patients (%)
Sex	Female	17 (56.7)
	Male	13 (43.3)
Tumor grade	1	22 (73.3)
	2	3 (10)
	3	4 (13.3)
	Not assessed *	1 (3.3)
Pathological diagnosis (biopsy)	Solitary fibrous tumor	7 (23.3)
	Leiomyosarcoma	5 (16.7)
	Sarcoma not otherwise specified	4 (13.3)
	Undifferentiated pleomorphic sarcoma	3 (10)
	Myxoid liposarcoma	2 (6.7)
	Myogenic sarcoma	1 (3.3)
	Pleomorphic rhabdomyosarcoma	1 (3.3)

Table 1. *Cont.*

Characteristic		Value
	Sclerosing epithelioid fibrosarcoma	1 (3.3)
	Alveolar soft part tissue sarcoma	1 (3.3)
	Myxoinflammatory fibroblastic sarcoma	1 (3.3)
	Low grade fibromyxoid sarcoma	1 (3.3)
	Myxofibrosarcoma	1 (3.3)
	Well-differentiated liposarcoma	1 (3.3)
	Dedifferentiated liposarcoma	1 (3.3)
Primary tumor site	Pelvis	11 (36.7)
	Thigh	9 (30)
	Calf	4 (13.3)
	Forearm	2 (6.7)
	Arm	1 (3.3)
	Thorax	1 (3.3)
	Lumbar area	1 (3.3)
	Foot	1 (3.3)

* Alveolar soft part tissue sarcoma.

3.2. Feasibility and Applied Treatment

Using intention-to-treat principle, all patients received the first part of RT with HT (BSD-2000, $n = 7$; Celsius-TCS, $n = 23$), whereas all but three received the second part of treatment, namely surgery or the second part of RT with HT (BSD-2000, $n = 3$; Celsius-TCS, $n = 11$). One patient received three out of four planned HT sessions due to HT equipment breakdown; however, this event was not considered as treatment failure. Thus, the feasibility proportion was 90% (27/30), with a 95% confidence interval (CI) equal to 76–100%. The feasibility proportion was greater than 50% with a *p*-value < 0.001.

The first patient who did not complete the protocol refused further cancer treatment due to the deterioration of performance status caused by comorbidities. The second one developed multiple lung metastases after RT with HT and was referred to palliative treatment. The third patient was lost to follow-up after the first RT with HT and did not answer phone calls.

Among patients who completed the whole protocol, 13 underwent surgery while 14 were referred to the second part of RT with HT. The median GTV, CTV, and PTV during the first part of RT with HT were 299 cm^3, 1586 cm^3, and 2153 cm^3, respectively. The corresponding median values of target volumes in the second part of the local treatment were 228 cm^3, 638 cm^3, and 1041 cm^3, respectively. Among patients who underwent surgery, microscopically negative margins were achieved in 13/15 patients (87%). The summary is presented in Table 2. Interestingly, complete or almost complete pathological responses according to the European Organization for Research and Treatment of Cancer-Soft Tissue and Bone Sarcoma Group recommendations were found in three and one postoperative specimens, respectively (Figure 2).

RT was well-tolerated. The analysis of RT-related toxicities is presented in Table 3. The full analysis of late toxicities will be possible after longer follow-up.

The tolerance of HT was acceptable. The most common adverse event during heating was an unpleasant sensation of high heat (43.3% of patients). HT-related adverse events were presented in Table 4. We did not observe any HT-related toxicity after heating. Full data regarding used electrodes, applicators sensors and protocols, temperature range, delivered energies, heating times, detailed description of adverse events and thermotolerance are available in Table S2.

Table 2. Outcomes of treatment among patients who completed the protocol.

Parameter		Second Part of Radiotherapy with Hyperthermia: Best Local Response		Surgery: Surgical Margins	
		Stable Disease	Partial Response	R0	R1
Grade	1	5	6	8	1
	2	1	0	1	0
	3	0	1	2	1
	NA	0	1	0	0
Reason for inclusion	Chemoresistant subtype	5	6	9	1
	Progression after neoadjuvant CHT	0	1	1	0
	Unfit for CHT	1	1	1	1
Resectability	Marginally resectable	1	1	11	2
	Amputation only	4	4	0	0
	Unresectable	1	3	0	0

CHT—chemotherapy; R0—microscopically negative surgical margin; R1—microscopically positive surgical margin.

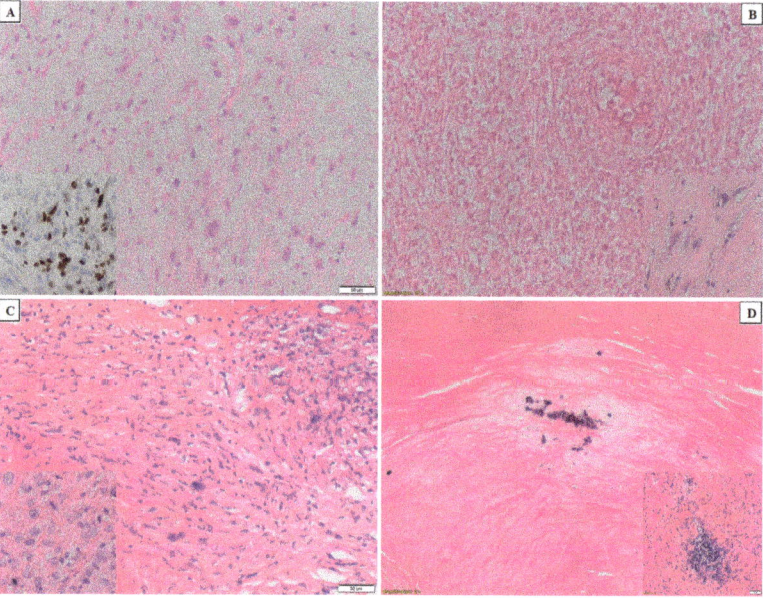

Figure 2. Histological response to the treatment: (**A**) A pleomorphic rhabdomyosarcoma before treatment confirmed by the myogenin expression (clone F5D, Daco, inlet); (**B**) diffuse necrotic changes in the pleomorphic rhabdomyosarcoma after treatment with only single, degenerated neoplastic cells present (less than 1% of tumoral tissue, inlet); (**C**) biopsy of a high-grade, undifferentiated spindle cell and focally pleomorphic sarcoma with brisk mitotic activity (inlet); (**D**) diffuse sclerosis with focal calcifications and scattered lymphocytic infiltrates in more fibrotic areas (inlet) in the undifferentiated sarcoma after treatment.

Table 3. Toxicity of radiotherapy.

Toxicity	Grade	Part of treatment	
		I	II
Early			
Radiation dermatitis	1	7	3
	2	4	
Edema	1	3	
Diarrhea	2	3	
Pain	1	1	
Hematuria	1	1	
Wound complications	1	1	NA
	2	2	NA
	3	2	NA
Late			
Recurrent hematuria	1		1
Superficial soft tissue fibrosis	1		4
Deep connective tissue fibrosis	2		1
Lymphedema	1		1
	2		2
Colonic bleeding	3		1

NA—not applicable.

Table 4. The summary of hyperthermia-related adverse events.

Adverse Events	Equipment	Grade *	Number of Patients (%)	Number of Hyperthermia Sessions (%)
			n = 30	n = 148
Sensation of high heat	Celsius TCS	1	5 (16.7)	10 (6.8)
		2	8 (26.7)	10 (6.8)
Pain	Celsius TCS	2	2 (6.7)	7 (4.7)
	BSD-2000	1	1 (3.3)	2 (1.4)
Inability to keep position	Celsius TCS	not applicable	4 (13.3)	4 (2.7)
Frequent breaks	Celsius TCS	not applicable	2 (6.7)	2 (1.4)
Electrode translocation	Celsius TCS	not applicable	2 (6.7)	2 (1.4)
Power reduction	Celsius TCS	not applicable	3 (10)	7 (4.7)
Heating time reduction	Celsius TCS	not applicable	9 (30)	15 (10.1)
	BSD-2000	not applicable	1 (3.3)	1 (0.7)
Temporary electrode breakdown	Celsius TCS	not applicable	1 (3.3)	1 (0.7)
Device breakdown	Celsius TCS	not applicable	1 (3.3)	1 (0.7)

* grade 1—sensation only, grade 2—required intervention, grade 3—hospitalization or medically significant, grade 4—life-threatening or urgent intervention indicated (prepared on the basis of the Common Terminology Criteria for Adverse Events).

3.3. Local Control and Survival

Median follow-up time was 13 months (interquartile range: 10–17 months). At the moment of analysis, 29 patients were alive (97%). Rapid local recurrence treated with extremity amputation was observed in one patient who underwent RT with HT followed by R1 surgery. Distant metastases were diagnosed in two patients, being the cause of death in one of them. One-year TTLP and LPFS were 97% and 93%, respectively. One-year SSS and PFS were 97% and 88%, respectively. Survival curves are available in Figure S1.

4. Discussion

Our study prospectively examined the feasibility of moderately hypofractionated RT combined with regional HT that was performed using two HT-dedicated devices. Despite large volumes of treated tumors (median 9.8 cm) and anatomically challenging localizations, such as pelvis (37%), the feasibility criteria were fulfilled by 90% of enrolled patients. There is lack of other clinical trials that investigate the combination of RT with HT in STS, thus, the comparison of results is not possible.

Preliminary results for local efficacy, occurrence of acute toxicity and ratio of wound complications are similar to those achieved in other series with hypofractionated RT [17,20]. Despite relatively low EQD2 of the proposed regimen, we observed four very good pathological responses among patients who underwent surgery (31%) and partial radiological responses among patients who received the second part of RT with HT (57%). It indicates vast radiosensitizing effect of HT. Any grade HT-related adverse events occurred in 19/30 patients (63%), leading to decrease of HT intensity (power reduction or shortened heating time) in 11 cases (Table S2). In turn, we did not observe any serious adverse event after heating or toxicity that could be detected in physical examination, such as blisters or burns. Mild and moderate HT-related adverse events were also reported in the largest study on neoadjuvant chemotherapy with HT for STS that was published by Issels et al. [34]. Then we can assume that HT is well-tolerated treatment in comparison to other modalities used in STS management.

Until the moment of the analysis, we observed few late toxicities (Table S1). All but one of the late toxicities affected patients who underwent the second part of RT with HT. Only one patient who underwent RT for pelvic STS experience serious late toxicity, namely grade 3 colonic bleeding due to massive telangiectasia that required blood transfusion and laser treatment. Nevertheless, the full impact of investigated regimen on long-term local efficacy and occurrence of late toxicities will be assessed after longer follow-up.

The study has several limitations. The first weakness is the lack of clear definitions of marginal resectability and unresectability in STS. In our study, resectability was assessed by surgical oncologists experienced in STS who used institutional and international criteria during MTB meeting [38].

Second, one may ask whether the definitive RT is appropriate method for patients with low-grade STS localized to extremities that can be removed with amputation. However, after amputation refusal, RT seems to be a better treatment option than chemotherapy or observation only. The risk of distant metastases in this group remains low [39,40]. In the case of local progression after RT, amputation still remains an option. Importantly, in our group none of the patients locally progressed after two parts of RT with HT in short-term follow-up.

Third, our study group is heterogenous. The patients were diagnosed with numerous STS subtypes and presented different clinical situations. Nevertheless, we aimed to design a flexible regimen that covers challenges related to STS treatment and could be used in various indications.

Finally, data regarding proper application of HT in STS are greatly limited. The choice of HT equipment, protocols, energies, and other aspects of heating was based upon HT team decision rather than on objective criteria. However, such recommendations do not exist. Moreover, we were only able to estimate the real intratumoral temperature during HT. To maintain feasibility and tolerability we did not use risky invasive intratumoral temperature monitoring. We used pre-defined protocols for Celsius TCS without temperature control due to unavailability of dedicated temperature sensors. In the case of BSD-200, skin and intraluminal sensors enable only indirect measurements. The solution could be the introduction of magnetic resonance thermometry or other methods of temperature measurement in further investigations [41].

The study does not provide a new standard of treatment, neither confirms long-term efficacy of the proposed regimen. This trial rather suggests that moderately hypofractionated RT could be combined with regional HT while maintaining treatment compliance, short-term local efficacy and favorable toxicity profile in challenging clinical situations with locally advanced STS. The results could serve as the basis for the development of new studies on RT with HT in STS.

5. Conclusions

Moderately hypofractionated RT with regional HT seems to be feasible method of neoadjuvant or definitive treatment for marginally resectable or unresectable locally advanced STS in patients who are not candidates for chemotherapy due to chemoresistance or contraindications. Preliminary observations suggest good tolerance and no decrease in local efficacy of such treatment; however, the optimal application of HT remains a challenge. Results of this clinical trial support the further validation of RT and HT combinations in STS.

Supplementary Materials: The following are available online at https://www.mdpi.com/2072-6694/13/6/1332/s1, Table S1: Patient Data, Table S2: Hyperthermia Data, Figure S1: Survival Curves.

Author Contributions: Conceptualization, M.J.S.; methodology, M.J.S.; software, M.J.S.; validation, P.R.; formal analysis, M.J.S.; investigation, M.J.S. and A.M.B.; resources, M.J.S., A.M.B., M.T., D.N., A.U., and M.B.; data curation, M.J.S.; writing—original draft preparation, M.J.S.; writing—review and editing, M.J.S., A.M.B., M.T., M.W., and P.R.; visualization, M.J.S. and M.W.; supervision, P.R.; project administration, M.J.S. All authors have read and agreed to the published version of the manuscript.

Funding: This research did not receive any specific grant from funding agencies in the public, commercial, or not-for-profit sectors. The processing charges cost was covered by the Maria Sklodowska-Curie National Research Institute of Oncology, Warsaw, Poland.

Institutional Review Board Statement: The study was conducted according to the guidelines of the Declaration of Helsinki, and approved by the Institutional Ethics Committee of the Maria Sklodowska-Curie National Research Institute of Oncology (SINDIR1, protocol code 35/2018, date of approval 7 June 2018).

Informed Consent Statement: Informed consent was obtained from all subjects involved in the study.

Data Availability Statement: All data generated and analyzed during this study are included in this published article (and its Supplementary Information Files).

Conflicts of Interest: The authors declare that the research was conducted in the absence of any commercial or financial relationships that could be construed as a potential conflict of interest.

References

1. Spałek, M.J.; Kozak, K.; Czarnecka, A.M.; Bartnik, E.; Borkowska, A.; Rutkowski, P. Neoadjuvant Treatment Options in Soft Tissue Sarcomas. *Cancers* **2020**, *12*, 2061. [CrossRef] [PubMed]
2. Von Mehren, M.; Randall, R.L.; Benjamin, R.S.; Boles, S.; Bui, M.M.; Ganjoo, K.N.; George, S.; Gonzalez, R.J.; Heslin, M.J.; Kane, J.M.; et al. Soft Tissue Sarcoma, Version 2.2018, NCCN Clinical Practice Guidelines in Oncology. *J. Natl. Compr. Cancer Netw.* **2018**, *16*, 536–563. [CrossRef]
3. Casali, P.G.; Abecassis, N.; Aro, H.T.; Bauer, S.; Biagini, R.; Bielack, S.; Bonvalot, S.; Boukovinas, I.; Bovee, J.V.M.G.; Brodowicz, T.; et al. Soft Tissue and Visceral Sarcomas: ESMO-EURACAN Clinical Practice Guidelines for Diagnosis, Treatment and Follow-Up. *Ann. Oncol.* **2018**, *29*, iv51–iv67. [CrossRef]
4. Rothermundt, C.; Fischer, G.F.; Bauer, S.; Blay, J.; Grünwald, V.; Italiano, A.; Kasper, B.; Kollár, A.; Lindner, L.H.; Miah, A.; et al. Pre- and Postoperative Chemotherapy in Localized Extremity Soft Tissue Sarcoma: A European Organization for Research and Treatment of Cancer Expert Survey. *Oncologist* **2018**, *23*, 461–467. [CrossRef]

5. Garbay, D.; Maki, R.G.; Blay, J.Y.; Isambert, N.; Piperno Neumann, S.; Blay, C.; Zanardi, E.; Boudou-Rouquette, P.; Bozec, L.; Duffaud, F.; et al. Advanced Soft-Tissue Sarcoma in Elderly Patients: Patterns of Care and Survival. *Ann. Oncol.* **2013**, *24*, 1924–1930. [CrossRef]
6. Levy, A.; Le Péchoux, C.; Terrier, P.; Bouaita, R.; Domont, J.; Mir, O.; Coppola, S.; Honoré, C.; Le Cesne, A.; Bonvalot, S. Epithelioid Sarcoma: Need for a Multimodal Approach to Maximize the Chances of Curative Conservative Treatment. *Ann. Surg. Oncol.* **2014**, *21*, 269–276. [CrossRef] [PubMed]
7. Touati, N.; Schöffski, P.; Litière, S.; Judson, I.; Sleijfer, S.; van der Graaf, W.T.; Italiano, A.; Isambert, N.; Gil, T.; Blay, J.Y.; et al. European Organisation for Research and Treatment of Cancer Soft Tissue and Bone Sarcoma Group Experience with Advanced/Metastatic Epithelioid Sarcoma Patients Treated in Prospective Trials: Clinical Profile and Response to Systemic Therapy. *Clin. Oncol.* **2018**, *30*, 448–454. [CrossRef] [PubMed]
8. Kawai, A.; Hosono, A.; Nakayama, R.; Matsumine, A.; Matsumoto, S.; Ueda, T.; Tsuchiya, H.; Beppu, Y.; Morioka, H.; Yabe, H.; et al. Clear Cell Sarcoma of Tendons and Aponeuroses: A Study of 75 Patients. *Cancer* **2007**, *109*, 109–116. [CrossRef] [PubMed]
9. Czarnecka, A.M.; Sobczuk, P.; Zdzienicki, M.; Spałek, M.; Dudzisz-Śledź, M.; Rutkowski, P. Clear cell sarcoma. *Oncol. Clin. Pract.* **2018**, *14*, 354–363. [CrossRef]
10. Jones, R.L.; Constantinidou, A.; Thway, K.; Ashley, S.; Scurr, M.; Al-Muderis, O.; Fisher, C.; Antonescu, C.R.; D'Adamo, D.R.; Keohan, M.L.; et al. Chemotherapy in Clear Cell Sarcoma. *Med. Oncol.* **2011**, *28*, 859–863. [CrossRef] [PubMed]
11. Orbach, D.; Brennan, B.; Casanova, M.; Bergeron, C.; Mosseri, V.; Francotte, N.; Van Noesel, M.; Rey, A.; Bisogno, G.; Pierron, G.; et al. Paediatric and Adolescent Alveolar Soft Part Sarcoma: A Joint Series from European Cooperative Groups. *Pediatr. Blood Cancer* **2013**, *60*, 1826–1832. [CrossRef]
12. Reichardt, P.; Lindner, T.; Pink, D.; Thuss-Patience, P.C.; Kretzschmar, A.; Dörken, B. Chemotherapy in Alveolar Soft Part Sarcomas. What Do We Know? *Eur. J. Cancer* **2003**, *39*, 1511–1516. [CrossRef]
13. Kepka, L.; DeLaney, T.F.; Suit, H.D.; Goldberg, S.I. Results of Radiation Therapy for Unresected Soft-Tissue Sarcomas. *Int. J. Radiat. Oncol. Biol. Phys.* **2005**, *63*, 852–859. [CrossRef] [PubMed]
14. Thames, H.D.; Suit, H.D. Tumor Radioresponsiveness versus Fractionation Sensitivity. *Int. J. Radiat. Oncol. Biol. Phys.* **1986**, *12*, 687–691. [CrossRef]
15. van Leeuwen, C.M.; Oei, A.L.; Crezee, J.; Bel, A.; Franken, N.a.P.; Stalpers, L.J.A.; Kok, H.P. The Alfa and Beta of Tumours: A Review of Parameters of the Linear-Quadratic Model, Derived from Clinical Radiotherapy Studies. *Radiat. Oncol.* **2018**, *13*, 96. [CrossRef] [PubMed]
16. Hegemann, N.-S.; Guckenberger, M.; Belka, C.; Ganswindt, U.; Manapov, F.; Li, M. Hypofractionated Radiotherapy for Prostate Cancer. *Radiat. Oncol.* **2014**, *9*, 275. [CrossRef]
17. Spałek, M.J.; Rutkowski, P. Coronavirus Disease (COVID-19) Outbreak: Hypofractionated Radiotherapy in Soft Tissue Sarcomas as a Valuable Option in the Environment of Limited Medical Resources and Demands for Increased Protection of Patients. *Front. Oncol.* **2020**, *10*. [CrossRef]
18. Koseła-Paterczyk, H.; Szacht, M.; Morysiński, T.; Ługowska, I.; Dziewirski, W.; Falkowski, S.; Zdzienicki, M.; Pieńkowski, A.; Szamotulska, K.; Świtaj, T.; et al. Preoperative Hypofractionated Radiotherapy in the Treatment of Localized Soft Tissue Sarcomas. *Eur. J. Surg. Oncol.* **2014**, *40*, 1641–1647. [CrossRef]
19. Koseła-Paterczyk, H.; Spałek, M.; Borkowska, A.; Teterycz, P.; Wągrodzki, M.; Szumera-Ciećkiewicz, A.; Morysiński, T.; Castaneda-Wysocka, P.; Cieszanowski, A.; Zdzienicki, M.; et al. Hypofractionated Radiotherapy in Locally Advanced Myxoid Liposarcomas of Extremities or Trunk Wall: Results of a Single-Arm Prospective Clinical Trial. *J. Clin. Med.* **2020**, *9*, 2471. [CrossRef] [PubMed]
20. Haas, R.L.M.; Miah, A.B.; LePechoux, C.; DeLaney, T.F.; Baldini, E.H.; Alektiar, K.; O'Sullivan, B. Preoperative Radiotherapy for Extremity Soft Tissue Sarcoma; Past, Present and Future Perspectives on Dose Fractionation Regimens and Combined Modality Strategies. *Radiother. Oncol.* **2016**, *119*, 14–21. [CrossRef]
21. Kalbasi, A.; Kamrava, M.; Chu, F.-I.; Telesca, D.; Dams, R.V.; Yang, Y.; Ruan, D.; Nelson, S.D.; Dry, S.; Hernandez, J.; et al. A Phase 2 Trial of Five-Day Neoadjuvant Radiation Therapy for Patients with High-Risk Primary Soft Tissue Sarcoma. *Clin. Cancer Res.* **2020**. [CrossRef] [PubMed]
22. Parsai, S.; Lawrenz, J.; Mesko, N.; Nystrom, L.; Kilpatrick, S.; Campbell, S.R.; Billings, S.; Goldblum, J.; Rubin, B.; Shah, C.S.; et al. Early Outcomes of Preoperative 5-Fraction Radiation Therapy for Soft Tissue Sarcoma with Immediate Resection. *Int. J. Radiat. Oncol. Biol. Phys.* **2019**, *105*, E809–E810. [CrossRef]
23. Temple, W.J.; Temple, C.L.; Arthur, K.; Schachar, N.S.; Paterson, A.H.; Crabtree, T.S. Prospective Cohort Study of Neoadjuvant Treatment in Conservative Surgery of Soft Tissue Sarcomas. *Ann. Surg. Oncol.* **1997**, *4*, 586–590. [CrossRef]
24. Spalek, M.; Koseła-Paterczyk, H.; Borkowska, A.; Wągrodzki, M.; Szumera-Ciećkiewicz, A.; Cieszanowski, A.; Castaneda-Wysocka, P.; Świtaj, T.; Dudzisz-Śledź, M.; Czarnecka, A.; et al. OC-0069 5 × 5 Gy with Chemotherapy in Borderline Resectable Soft Tissue Sarcomas: Early Results of a Trial. *Radiother. Oncol.* **2019**, *133*, S31–S32. [CrossRef]
25. Schulz, A.; Meyer, F.; Dubrovska, A.; Borgmann, K. Cancer Stem Cells and Radioresistance: DNA Repair and Beyond. *Cancers* **2019**, *11*, 862. [CrossRef]
26. Bergman, P.J.; Harris, D. Radioresistance, Chemoresistance, and Apoptosis Resistance. The Past, Present, and Future. *Vet. Clin. N. Am. Small Anim. Pract.* **1997**, *27*, 47–57. [CrossRef]

27. Elming, P.B.; Sørensen, B.S.; Oei, A.L.; Franken, N.A.P.; Crezee, J.; Overgaard, J.; Horsman, M.R. Hyperthermia: The Optimal Treatment to Overcome Radiation Resistant Hypoxia. *Cancers* **2019**, *11*, 60. [CrossRef] [PubMed]
28. Bull, J.M.C. An Update on the Anticancer Effects of a Combination of Chemotherapy and Hyperthermia. *Cancer Res.* **1984**, *44*, 4853s–4856s. [PubMed]
29. Pennacchioli, E.; Fiore, M.; Gronchi, A. Hyperthermia as an Adjunctive Treatment for Soft-Tissue Sarcoma. *Expert Rev. Anticancer* **2009**, *9*, 199–210. [CrossRef]
30. Dewey, W.C.; Hopwood, L.E.; Sapareto, S.A.; Gerweck, L.E. Cellular Responses to Combinations of Hyperthermia and Radiation. *Radiology* **1977**, *123*, 463–474. [CrossRef] [PubMed]
31. Yagawa, Y.; Tanigawa, K.; Kobayashi, Y.; Yamamoto, M. Cancer Immunity and Therapy Using Hyperthermia with Immunotherapy, Radiotherapy, Chemotherapy, and Surgery. *JCMT* **2017**, *3*, 218. [CrossRef]
32. Jha, S.; Sharma, P.K.; Malviya, R. Hyperthermia: Role and Risk Factor for Cancer Treatment. *Achiev. Life Sci.* **2016**, *10*, 161–167. [CrossRef]
33. Issels, R.D.; Lindner, L.H.; Verweij, J.; Wessalowski, R.; Reichardt, P.; Wust, P.; Ghadjar, P.; Hohenberger, P.; Angele, M.; Salat, C.; et al. Effect of Neoadjuvant Chemotherapy Plus Regional Hyperthermia on Long-Term Outcomes Among Patients With Localized High-Risk Soft Tissue Sarcoma: The EORTC 62961-ESHO 95 Randomized Clinical Trial. *JAMA Oncol.* **2018**, *4*, 483–492. [CrossRef] [PubMed]
34. Issels, R.D.; Lindner, L.H.; Verweij, J.; Wust, P.; Reichardt, P.; Schem, B.-C.; Abdel-Rahman, S.; Daugaard, S.; Salat, C.; Wendtner, C.-M.; et al. Neo-Adjuvant Chemotherapy Alone or with Regional Hyperthermia for Localised High-Risk Soft-Tissue Sarcoma: A Randomised Phase 3 Multicentre Study. *Lancet Oncol.* **2010**, *11*, 561–570. [CrossRef]
35. Overgaard, J.; Gonzalez Gonzalez, D.; Hulshof, M.C.; Arcangeli, G.; Dahl, O.; Mella, O.; Bentzen, S.M. Randomised Trial of Hyperthermia as Adjuvant to Radiotherapy for Recurrent or Metastatic Malignant Melanoma. European Society for Hyperthermic Oncology. *Lancet* **1995**, *345*, 540–543. [CrossRef]
36. Loco-Regional Hyperthermia Device. Available online: http://www.htsystems.com.pl/en/products/loco-regional-hyperthermia-celsius-tcs (accessed on 24 January 2021).
37. BSD-2000 3D Microwave Hyperthermia System. Available online: https://www.pyrexar.com/hyperthermia/bsd-2000-3d (accessed on 24 January 2021).
38. Dangoor, A.; Seddon, B.; Gerrand, C.; Grimer, R.; Whelan, J.; Judson, I. UK Guidelines for the Management of Soft Tissue Sarcomas. *Clin. Sarcoma Res.* **2016**, *6*, 20. [CrossRef] [PubMed]
39. Donohue, J.H.; Collin, C.; Friedrich, C.; Godbold, J.; Hajdu, S.I.; Brennan, M.F. Low-Grade Soft Tissue Sarcomas of the Extremities. Analysis of Risk Factors for Metastasis. *Cancer* **1988**, *62*, 184–193. [CrossRef]
40. Canter, R.J.; Qin, L.-X.; Ferrone, C.R.; Maki, R.G.; Singer, S.; Brennan, M.F. Why Do Patients with Low Grade Soft Tissue Sarcoma Die? *Ann. Surg. Oncol.* **2008**, *15*, 3550–3560. [CrossRef]
41. Curto, S.; Aklan, B.; Mulder, T.; Mils, O.; Schmidt, M.; Lamprecht, U.; Peller, M.; Wessalowski, R.; Lindner, L.H.; Fietkau, R.; et al. Quantitative, Multi-Institutional Evaluation of MR Thermometry Accuracy for Deep-Pelvic MR-Hyperthermia Systems Operating in Multi-Vendor MR-Systems Using a New Anthropomorphic Phantom. *Cancers* **2019**, *11*, 1709. [CrossRef]

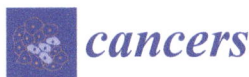

Article

Does the Duration of Primary and First Revision Surgery Influence the Probability of First and Subsequent Implant Failures after Extremity Sarcoma Resection and Megaprosthetic Reconstruction?

Christoph Theil [1,*], Kristian Nikolaus Schneider [1], Georg Gosheger [1], Ralf Dieckmann [1,2], Niklas Deventer [1], Jendrik Hardes [1,3], Tom Schmidt-Braekling [1] and Dimosthenis Andreou [1,4]

1. Department of General Orthopedics and Tumor Orthopedics, Muenster University Hospital, Albert-Schweitzer Campus 1, 48149 Muenster, Germany; kristian.schneider@ukmuenster.de (K.N.S.); georg.gosheger@ukmuenster.de (G.G.); r.dieckmann@bk-trier.de (R.D.); niklas.deventer@ukmuenster.de (N.D.); Jendrik.hardes@uk-essen.de (J.H.); tom.schmidt-braekling@ukmuenster.de (T.S.-B.); Dimosthenis.andreou@helios-gesundheit.de (D.A.)
2. Department of Orthopedics, Krankenhaus der Barmherzigen Brueder, Nordallee 1, 54292 Trier, Germany
3. Department of Musculoskeletal Oncology, Essen University Hospital, Hufelandstraße 55, 45147 Essen, Germany
4. Department of Orthopedic Oncology and Sarcoma Surgery, Sarcoma Centre Berlin-Brandenburg, Helios Klinikum Bad Saarow, 15526 Bad Saarow, Germany
* Correspondence: christoph.theil@ukmuenster.de; Tel.: +49-2514-4278

Citation: Theil, C.; Schneider, K.N.; Gosheger, G.; Dieckmann, R.; Deventer, N.; Hardes, J.; Schmidt-Braekling, T.; Andreou, D. Does the Duration of Primary and First Revision Surgery Influence the Probability of First and Subsequent Implant Failures after Extremity Sarcoma Resection and Megaprosthetic Reconstruction? *Cancers* **2021**, *13*, 2510. https://doi.org/10.3390/cancers13112510

Academic Editor: Justus P. Beier

Received: 2 April 2021
Accepted: 18 May 2021
Published: 21 May 2021

Publisher's Note: MDPI stays neutral with regard to jurisdictional claims in published maps and institutional affiliations.

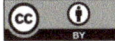

Copyright: © 2021 by the authors. Licensee MDPI, Basel, Switzerland. This article is an open access article distributed under the terms and conditions of the Creative Commons Attribution (CC BY) license (https://creativecommons.org/licenses/by/4.0/).

Simple Summary: Tumor endoprostheses are a common type of reconstruction after the resection of an extremity bone sarcoma. However, in the long-term, first and subsequent implant failures leading to revision surgery are common. One potential risk factor for implant failure is the length of surgery. This study investigates the impact of the length of surgery on prosthetic survival in 568 patients with sarcoma. Patients who had a first implant failure had a longer surgery; however, there were no differences in the infection-free survival, but only in the probability of mechanical failure. Patients with a subsequent revision surgery for infection had a shorter duration of surgery during the first revision. In conclusion, a shorter surgery appears beneficial; however, longer surgeries are not clearly associated with infection. In revision surgery, a longer operating time, indicating a more thorough debridement, may be desirable.

Abstract: Complications in megaprosthetic reconstruction following sarcoma resection are quite common. While several risk factors for failure have been explored, there is a scarcity of studies investigating the effect of the duration of surgery. We performed a retrospective study of 568 sarcoma patients that underwent megaprosthetic reconstruction between 1993 and 2015. Differences in the length of surgery and implant survival were assessed with the Kaplan–Meier method, the log-rank test and multivariate Cox regressions using an optimal cut-off value determined by receiver operating curves analysis using Youden's index. 230 patients developed a first and 112 patients a subsequent prosthetic failure. The median duration of initial surgery was 210 min. Patients who developed a first failure had a longer duration of the initial surgery (225 vs. 205 min, $p = 0.0001$). There were no differences in the probability of infection between patients with longer and shorter duration of initial surgery (12% vs. 13% at 5 years, $p = 0.492$); however, the probability of mechanical failure was higher in patients with longer initial surgery (38% vs. 23% at 5 years, $p = 0.006$). The median length of revision surgery for the first megaprosthetic failure was 101 min. Patients who underwent first revision for infection and did not develop a second failure had a longer median duration of the first revision surgery (150 min vs. 120 min, $p = 0.016$). A shorter length of the initial surgery appears beneficial, however, the notion that longer operating time increases the risk of deep infection could not be reproduced in our study. In revision surgery for infection, a longer operating time, possibly indicating a more thorough debridement, appears to be associated with a lower risk for subsequent revision.

Keywords: tumor endoprosthesis; megaprosthesis; periprosthetic joint infection; revision surgery; sarcoma

1. Introduction

The use of megaprostheses to address osteoarticular defects after limb-sparing resections of malignant bone tumors has become the reconstruction method of choice over the last few decades [1–3]. As the prognosis of extremity sarcoma patients has improved over the last few decades [1,4] more and more patients require revision surgeries for—sometimes multiple—implant failures [1,3,5]. These revisions are associated with a high disease burden [1,6] and may potentially result in the amputation of the affected limb [7,8]. As a result, there is a need to identify potential risk factors for the development of prosthetic failures that ideally would be accessible for perioperative optimization.

Previous studies on non-megaprosthetic arthroplasty have identified a longer duration of surgery as a potential risk factor for complications [9,10], possibly because the bacterial contamination of the surgical field might increase with the length of surgery [11]. Consequently, the impact of the length of surgery has also been discussed as a risk factor for megaprosthetic infection [12]. However, only very few studies have, to our knowledge, investigated this issue [13–15], with some studies finding an association between a longer surgical time and a higher probability for infections, while another did not. However, these studies were limited by the small number of implants included, while their findings were based on univariate analyses, despite the fact that several factors, such as reconstruction length may interact with the duration of a procedure. Furthermore, subsequent prosthetic failures and re-revision surgeries have become more common in oncological patients [1,3,16,17], but no study has yet investigated the impact of the length of the first revision surgery on the probability of subsequent failures.

We therefore asked whether there is an association between the length of primary or revision surgery at a tertiary bone sarcoma center and the probability of mechanical or infectious megaprosthetic complications. We hypothesized that a longer duration of a procedure might be a risk factor for further complications, especially infections.

2. Materials and Methods

2.1. Study Design

We retrospectively queried our institution's database and identified 817 patients with bone tumors who underwent resection and megaprosthetic reconstruction of the upper or lower limb using a single modular system (MUTARS™, Implantcast GmbH, Buxtehude, Germany) between 1993 and 2015. Patient demographics, tumor characteristics, surgical and oncological treatments, postoperative complications and their treatment as well as patient follow-up and oncological outcomes were retrospectively collected from the patients' medical records and entered into an electronic datasheet. All patient data were anonymized before analysis.

Patients with bone metastases, benign tumors as well as surviving patients with follow-up of less than 6 months, who were considered to be lost to follow-up, were excluded from this analysis (Figure 1). We also excluded patients undergoing revisions due to a tumor recurrence/progression, as they can potentially be associated with a multitude of factors that were not comprehensively investigated in the present study (e.g., tumor size, histology, neo-/adjuvant treatments, response etc.).

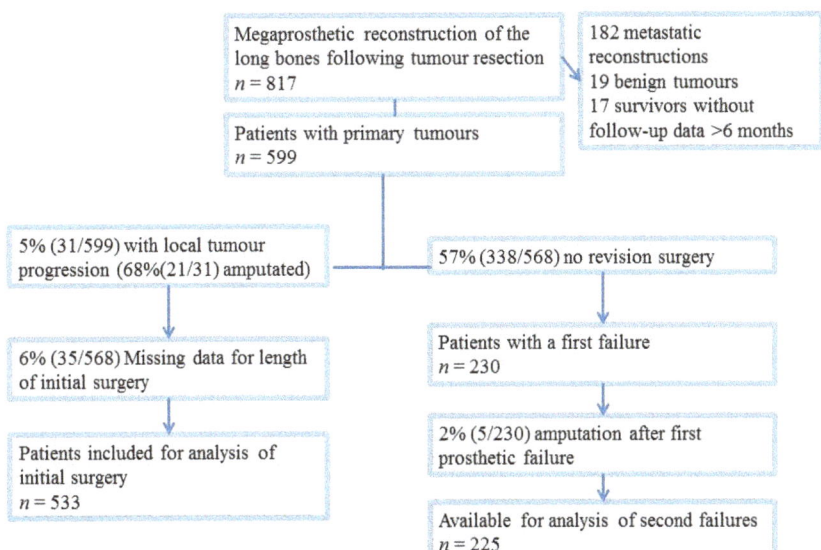

Figure 1. STROBE diagram showing inclusion of patients.

Furthermore, all patients who underwent amputation to treat a first prosthetic failure (2%, 5/230) were excluded from analysis of second failures.

The length of surgery was defined as the time from the first incision to wound closure and was retrieved from the operating theatre records. For patients with two-stage revisions the duration of the longest procedure was recorded. Patients with missing data regarding the length of the initial surgery or surgical treatment for the first complication were excluded from the respective analyses (Figure 1). As a result, 533 patients were available to evaluate whether the length of initial surgery was associated with the development of a first prosthetic failure and 225 patients were available to assess a possible association between the length of revision surgery and the development of a second failure (Figure 1). The median follow-up was 55 months (interquartile range (IQRI 25–114) for all patients and 68 months (IQR 35–127) for surviving patients. The median follow-up for patients who developed a first prosthetic failure amounted to 91 months (IQR 45–159) for all patients and 99 months (IQR 55–170) for surviving patients. Patient, tumor, and treatment characteristics of these patients are presented in Tables 1 and 2.

First and subsequent failures were classified according to the system proposed by Henderson et al. [18]. For further analysis, infections were looked at in a subgroup analysis and compared to non-infectious failures. Infections were treated using debridement, antibiotics, irrigation and implant retention (DAIR), one-stage or two-stage exchanges depending on the type of infection (early or late), soft tissue condition, stem ingrowth, culture results as well as the quality and amount of residual bone.

Table 1. Patient demographics and surgical details for all patients excluding local tumor progression as a first failure mode, patients with a first failure excluding patients who underwent amputation for the first failure and patients with a second failure.

Variable	All Patients $n = 568$	Patients with a First Failure $n = 230$
Males	63% ($n = 357$)	69% ($n = 159$)
Diabetes	2% ($n = 13$)	2% ($n = 5$)
Smoking	8% ($n = 46$)	4% ($n = 9$)
Pathological fracture	10% ($n = 55$)	4% ($n = 9$)
Previous surgery	12% ($n = 66$)	14% ($n = 31$)
Cemented stem	24% ($n = 136$)	22% ($n = 50$)
Extra-articular resection	22% ($n = 122$)	27% ($n = 61$)
Reconstruction site		
Distal femur	38% ($n = 218$)	48% ($n = 110$)
Proximal tibia	17% ($n = 96$)	26% ($n = 58$)
Proximal femur	17% ($n = 99$)	8% ($n = 19$)
Proximal humerus	16% ($n = 92$)	7% ($n = 16$)
Total femur	4% ($n = 21$)	3% ($n = 8$)
Total knee	2% ($n = 11$)	3% ($n = 8$)
Total humerus	4% ($n = 24$)	3% ($n = 6$)
Distal humerus	1% ($n = 7$)	2% ($n = 5$)

Table 2. Oncological details for all patients excluding local tumor progression as a first failure mode, patients with a first failure excluding patients who underwent amputation for the first failure and patients with a second failure.

Tumor Entity	All Patients $n = 568$	Patients with a First Failure $n = 230$
High-grade osteosarcoma	52% ($n = 295$)	61% ($n = 140$)
Ewing sarcoma	15% ($n = 87$)	12% ($n = 28$)
Chondrosarcoma	13% ($n = 74$)	8% ($n = 18$)
Pleomorphic sarcoma	11% ($n = 63$)	8% ($n = 19$)
Low-grade osteosarcoma	3% ($n = 16$)	4% ($n = 10$)
Dedifferentiated chondrosarcoma	2% ($n = 11$)	2% ($n = 5$)
Others	4% ($n = 22$)	4% ($n = 10$)
Local radiation treatment	22% ($n = 129$)	20% ($n = 46$)
Preoperative	10% ($n = 56$)	6% ($n = 14$)
Postoperative	14% ($n = 78$)	15% ($n = 34$)
Systemic chemotherapy	79% ($n = 450$)	76% ($n = 175$)
Preoperative	73% ($n = 415$)	76% ($n = 175$)
Postoperative	78% ($n = 444$)	82% ($n = 189$)
Metastasized disease	30% ($n = 170$)	19% ($n = 44$)
Primary metastases	17% ($n = 95$)	13% ($n = 29$)
Died of disease	23% ($n = 128$)	14% ($n = 31$)

2.2. First and Second Implant Failures

There was a total of 230 first implant failures after a median time of 17 months (IQR 4–60), among which structural failures were found in 15% (84/568) (Table S1), followed by infection in 10% of cases (58/568), aseptic loosening in 8% of cases (45/568) and soft tissue failures in 7% of cases (43/568). The overall revision-free implant survival probability was 74% (95% CI 70–78) after two years and 64% (95% CI 60–68) at five years. The infection-free survival probability was 91% (95% CI 88–94) after two years and 87% (95% CI 84–90) after five years, while the survivorship free from revision for a mechanical failure was 83% (95% CI 80–86) after two years and 73% (95% CI 69–77) after five years. Five of these patients underwent amputation to treat the first complication and were excluded from the analysis of second failures. Among the remaining 225 patients, 50% (112/225) had a second failure after a median time of 17 months (IQR 5–47) (20% infections (45/112), followed by 17% structural failures (38/112), 8% aseptic loosening (19/112), and 3% soft tissue failures (7/112). The implant survivorship free from revision for a second failure was 69% (95% CI 63–75%) after two years and 46% after five years (95% CI 38–53) following the first revision surgery.

2.3. Statistical Analysis

The duration of follow-up and time to implant failure were calculated from the date of the primary tumor surgery. The time to second failure was calculated from the date of final reconstruction for the previous failure. Contingency tables were analyzed using the chi-squared test. Continuous variables were checked for normality using the Shapiro–Wilk test. Medians with IQRs were calculated for non-parametric data. Non-parametric analyses were performed using the Mann–Whitney U-Test. Implant survival probabilities, with their respective 95% confidence intervals, were calculated with the Kaplan–Meier method and compared using the log-rank test. We used receiver operating characteristic (ROC) curves to analyze the association between the length of surgery and implant failure. Area under the curve (AUC) values were calculated using a non-parametric distribution assumption. The optimal cut-off value was determined using the Youden index. Hazard ratios (HR) were estimated with their respective 95% confidence intervals (CI) in multivariate Cox regression models. Multivariate analysis of risk factors was conducted including risk factors that were identified from univariate analysis and taking into consideration the findings of a previous study on subsequent failures [3].

Statistical calculations were performed with SPSS Version 25.0 (IBM Corp., Armonk, NY, USA). All p values were two-sided; a p-value < 0.05 was considered significant.

3. Results

3.1. First Implant Failures

The median length of tumor resection and megaprosthetic reconstruction was 210 min (IQR 174–255). Patients who developed an implant failure had a longer median duration of the initial surgery compared to patients with no failures (225 min (IQR 180–268) vs. 205 min (IQR 160–242), $p = 0.0001$). Contrary to our hypothesis, subgroup analysis showed that patients who developed an infection as a first failure did not have a longer primary surgery time compared to patients with no infections (210 min (IQR 173–255) vs. 200 min (IQR 170–248), $p = 0.417$). On the other hand, patients treated for a mechanical complication had a significantly longer primary surgery time compared to patients with no mechanical complications (235 min (IQR 185–278) vs. 204 (IQR 160–243), $p = 0.0001$). As there are relevant differences in median operating times for different anatomic locations, subgroup analyses were performed and presented in Table 3.

The ROC analysis showed a significant association between the length of primary surgery and first implant failure (AUC 0.592, 95% CI 0.543–0.641, $p = 0.0001$) with an optimal cut-off at 234 min. Survivorship free from revision was significantly higher in patients with a shorter surgical time (68% (95% CI 62–74) vs. 55% (95% CI 47–63) at five years, $p = 0.036$). Again, subgroup analyses showed no differences in the infection-free implant survival probability between patients with shorter and longer durations of primary surgery (88% (95% CI 83–93) vs. 87% (95% CI 83–92), $p = 0.492$). On the other hand, patients with shorter durations of primary surgery had a significantly higher implant survivorship free from revision for a mechanical failure compared to patients with longer surgical durations (77% (95% CI 72–83) vs. 62% (95% CI 54–70) at 5 years, $p = 0.006$). Multivariate analysis (Table 4) confirmed that the length of the initial surgical procedure was a significant risk factor for first implant failure taking potential further risk factors into consideration.

Table 3. Length of surgery for the different anatomic sites of reconstruction, displaying the differences between patients with or without implant failure and distinguishing between infectious and mechanical failures.

Variable	Rate of Failures	Median Length of the Initial Surgery in Minutes		
Anatomic Location and Types of Failure	% (n)	In Patients with Implant Failure	In Patients without Implant Failure	p (Mann–Whitney U-Test)
"Around the knee"	54% (176/325)	215	195	<0.0001
Mechanical	44% (142/325)	229	195	<0.0001
Infection	10% (34/325)	202	210	0.867
Distal femoral replacement	50% (110/218)	203	187	0.003
Mechanical	39% (85/218)	206	190	0.003
Infection	11% (25/218)	195	195	0.924
Proximal tibial replacement	60% (58/96)	240	220	0.127
Mechanical	53% (51/96)	235	220	0.538
Infection	7% (7/96)	270	227	0.097
Upper extremity	22% (27/123)	206	193	0.92
Mechanical	11% (13/123)	238	193	0.215
Infection	11% (14/123)	189	196	0.309
Lower extremity	45% (203/446)	225	210	0.001
Mechanical	36% (159/446)	235	209	<0.0001
Infection	10% (44/446)	203	215	0.716
Total bone or total knee	39% (22/56)	278	242	0.075
Mechanical	23% (13/56)	295	242	0.001
Infection	16% (9/56)	233	275	0.147

Table 4. Multivariate Cox regression analysis of risk factors for first prosthetic failure. * for the multivariate analysis the threshold value determined using Youden's index was used as opposed to the metric value of the duration of surgery.

Variable	Hazard Ratio	p-Value	95% CI
Extra-articular resection	1.9	<0.001	1.4–2.6
Reconstruction length in millimeters	1	0.662	1–1
Duration of initial surgery (categorized) *	1.4	0.033	1.1–1.8
Diabetes	1.1	0.839	0.4–3
Postoperative radiation	1.3	0.164	0.9–2

3.2. Second Implant Failure

The median duration of tumor resection and megaprosthetic reconstruction in patients who developed a first implant failure was 218 min (IQR 180–261). In this cohort, we found no differences in the length of the primary surgery between patients who developed a second implant failure and patients who did not (218 (IQR 180–255) vs. 220 (IQR 180–274), $p = 0.261$).

The median length of revision surgery for the first megaprosthetic failure was 101 min (IQR 64–153). Interestingly, patients who suffered a second failure had a shorter duration of revision surgery compared to patients who had no further failures (90 min (IQR 55–128) vs. 117 min (IQR 75–157), $p = 0.014$). Subgroup analyses in this cohort showed that there were no significant differences in the length of revision surgery between patients treated for a mechanical first complication (median 95 min (IQR 64–152) vs. 85 min (IQR 52–121), $p = 0.184$), whereas patients who underwent first revision for an infection and did not develop a second implant failure and had a significantly longer median duration of the first revision surgery (150 min (IQR 118–186) vs. 120 min (85–150), $p = 0.016$).

ROC analysis confirmed an association between a shorter length of revision surgery and a second implant failure (AUC 0.398, 95% CI 0.317–0.478), $p = 0.014$) with an optimal cut-off at 123 min. The implant survivorship free from revision for a second failure was significantly higher in patients with a longer duration of revision surgery (62% (95% CI 48–76) vs. 39% (95% CI 28–50) at 5 years after first revision surgery, $p = 0.004$).

In multivariate analysis (Table 5), a longer duration of the revision surgery was associated with a reduced risk for second complications.

Table 5. Multivariate Cox regression analysis of risk factors for second prosthetic failure. * for the multivariate analysis the threshold value determined using Youden's index was used as opposed to the metric value of the duration of surgery.

Variable	Hazard Ratio	p-Value	95% CI
Extra-articular resection	1.5	0.110	0.9–2.4
Reconstruction length in millimeters	1	0.425	1–1
Diabetes	5.8	0.004	1.7–19
Duration of the initial surgery (categorized) *	0.9	0.521	0.6–1.4
Duration of the revision surgery (categorized) *	0.5	0.003	0.3–0.8
Postoperative radiation	2.5	0.001	1.5–4.4

4. Discussion

Patients who undergo extremity sarcoma resection and megaprosthetic reconstruction are at a high risk for prosthetic failure and subsequent revisions [3,18,19]. Orthopaedic oncologists are therefore required to evaluate possible risk factors for failure and, ideally, identify areas of optimization potential. The length of surgery as a potential risk factor has been studied previously [20]; however, previous results have been inconclusive [13–15]. As sarcoma resection and megaprosthetic reconstructions have a longer surgical duration and are associated with a higher risk of failure compared to non-oncological arthroplasty procedures [18,21], modifying a procedure related risk factor, such as the duration of the surgery, would offer surgeons a chance to reduce the burden of megaprosthetic revision. Our study investigated the influence of the length of the initial and first revision surgery on first and subsequent megaprosthetic failures in sarcoma patients. While we found that a longer operating time in the initial surgery was generally associated with shorter revision free survival probability, it was not associated, as we expected, with a higher infection risk, but with a higher probability of non-infectious failures. On the other hand, in patients who underwent revision surgery for periprosthetic infection, a shorter duration of the revision surgery was associated with a higher risk of subsequent failures.

The results of our study should be interpreted taking its limitations into consideration. Given its retrospective design, we extracted available data from patients' records, resulting in a possible selection bias. Furthermore, the study spans a fairly long period of time, during which surgical technique, implant design and adjuvant treatments have evolved to a certain degree and which is a cause for some inhomogeneity in our cohort. On the other hand, this allowed us to achieve a long follow-up period, and we have previously demonstrated that implant survivorship in our cohort did not differ for patients treated at different points during the study period [3]. Furthermore, we attempted to partially offset the impact of such an inhomogeneity by only including patients treated at a single institution and with a single modular megaprosthetic system.

We also acknowledge that we could only include a limited number of implants in some anatomic localizations, and some of our results might not be transferable to all sites of megaprosthetic reconstruction. Nonetheless, we chose to include all localizations as they represent the typical distribution of extremity bone sarcomas as seen in everyday practice. Finally, we investigated periprosthetic infections as a failure mode, the successful management of which depends on multiple factors such as microbiological findings, antibiotic therapy as well as host and soft tissue conditions, [22–27] which could not be evaluated in detail in the present analysis. However, we believe that this is balanced out by the large number of infectious megaprosthetic failures we were able to examine.

Our results suggest that the duration of the resection of a bone sarcoma and megaprosthetic reconstruction in a tertiary center is not itself an independent risk factor for the development of megaprosthetic infections. This contradicts the findings of two previous studies by Dhanoa et al. and Peel et al., which reported a significantly longer duration of primary surgery in patients with megaprostheses who went on to develop infections in two cohorts of 105 and 121 patients, respectively [13,14]. However, these studies on the one hand included patients with benign tumors and—in the study by Dhanoa et al.—non-oncological patients, the surgical treatment of which is generally both shorter and spares much more soft tissue compared to sarcoma patients [13]. Furthermore, both studies also included patients with pelvic tumors undergoing megaprosthetic reconstructions, which are associated with both a much longer duration of surgery and a much higher probability of postoperative infection compared to patients with extremity sarcomas [28]. The latter might also explain the somewhat high infection rate particularly in the study by Peel et al. of 28% [14]. Contrary to these studies, Cho et al. [15] investigated 62 patients undergoing proximal tibial replacement for malignant and locally aggressive bone and soft tissue tumors and did not find a correlation between a duration of surgery and infections, however this study again included patients with benign tumors as well as patients with bone metastases.

Our analysis also demonstrated that mechanical complications as a first implant failure were associated with a longer length of surgery. To our knowledge, such an association has not been described previously and given the retrospective study design, we can only speculate about potential causes. A longer duration of primary tumor surgery usually occurs in more extensive tumors that may require more time for dissection and may result in a more severe soft tissue damage. The resection of a greater amount of soft tissue may lead to a reduced implant support that might render the affected limb more prone to mechanical complications.

Another interesting finding of our study regarded the influence of surgical time on the probability of subsequent failure after the surgical treatment of the first prosthetic failure. One the one hand, we found no correlation between at the duration of primary surgery and the probability of subsequent failure, suggesting that the impact of the duration of primary surgery is mostly restricted to the first complication, and on the other hand, the duration of revision surgery for first infectious complication was significantly—and relevantly—shorter in patients with subsequent infections, compared to patients without subsequent infections. To our knowledge, no study has yet examined this aspect of revision surgery as a risk factor for further complications. In recent years aggressive debridement of bradytrophic tissue around the prosthesis during revision surgery has been proposed as a means to reduce the probability of subsequent megaprosthetic infections, and has also been shown to facilitate one-stage exchange procedures in patients with infected implants [5,16,24,29,30]. The longer duration of revision surgery in the group of patients without subsequent failures might, therefore, be considered to be a surrogate for the aggressiveness of the revision surgery, although we readily acknowledge the purely hypothetical nature of this suggestion in our cohort.

5. Conclusions

In conclusion, the duration of primary tumor surgery and megaprosthetic reconstruction at an experienced tertiary bone sarcoma center appears not to be associated with the risk of first megaprosthetic infection. On the other hand, a longer duration of first revision surgery for infection was associated with a lower risk for subsequent revisions. While this finding should be confirmed in an independent cohort and possible reasons should be evaluated in future studies, we believe that aiming for a shorter surgical duration in revision surgery at the expense of the meticulousness of the procedure might not be the optimal way to avoid further prosthesis revisions.

Supplementary Materials: The following are available online at https://www.mdpi.com/article/10.3390/cancers13112510/s1, Table S1: Subtypes of structural failures for first and second prosthetic failures.

Author Contributions: Conceptualization, C.T., D.A., G.G., R.D., T.S.-B., K.N.S.; methodology, C.T., D.A., G.G.; formal analysis, C.T., D.A.; investigation, C.T., D.A., J.H.; resources, G.G., R.D., T.S.-B. data curation, C.T., D.A., J.H., G.G.; writing—original draft preparation, C.T., D.A.; writing—review and editing, C.T., D.A., G.G., J.H., K.N.S., N.D., D.A., T.S.-B., R.D. visualization, N.D., C.T., D.A.; supervision, G.G.; project administration, G.G.; funding acquisition, G.G., D.A. All authors have read and agreed to the published version of the manuscript.

Funding: The APC was funded by the Open Access Publishing Funds of the Westphalian Wilhelms University of Muenster.

Institutional Review Board Statement: The study was conducted according to the guidelines of the Declaration of Helsinki, and approved by the Ethics Committee of "Ethikkommission der Aerztekammer Westfalen-Lippe und der Westfaelischen Wilhelms Universitaet" (protocol code 2016-625-f-S and 12 December 2016).

Informed Consent Statement: Patient consent was waived due to the investigation of routine patient data.

Data Availability Statement: All relevant data is in the manuscript.

Acknowledgments: We would like to thank all the staff that was involved in the in hospital and outpatient care of the patients included in the study.

Conflicts of Interest: C.T., D.A., T.S.-B., R.D., N.D. have received travel expenses or did paid lectures during the study period but outside the submitted work from Implantcast GmbH, Buxtehude, Germany. G.G. reports a patent for silver coating of metallic endoprostheses with royalties paid by Implantcast GmbH, Buxtehude, Germany outside the submitted work. J.H. reports a research grant paid by Implantcast GmbH, Buxtehude, Germany outside the submitted work. The funders had no role in the design of the study; in the collection, analyses, or interpretation of data; in the writing of the manuscript, or in the decision to publish the results.

References

1. Grimer, R.J.; Aydin, B.K.; Wafa, H.; Carter, S.R.; Jeys, L.; Abudu, A.; Parry, M. Very long-term outcomes after endoprosthetic replacement for malignant tumours of bone. *Bone Jt. J.* **2016**, *98-B*, 857–864. [CrossRef] [PubMed]
2. Gosheger, G.; Gebert, C.; Ahrens, H.; Streitbuerger, A.; Winkelmann, W.; Hardes, J. Endoprosthetic reconstruction in 250 patients with sarcoma. *Clin. Orthop. Relat. Res.* **2006**, *450*, 164–171. [CrossRef]
3. Theil, C.; Roder, J.; Gosheger, G.; Deventer, N.; Dieckmann, R.; Schorn, D.; Hardes, J.; Andreou, D. What is the Likelihood That Tumor Endoprostheses Will Experience a Second Complication After First Revision in Patients With Primary Malignant Bone Tumors And What Are Potential Risk Factors? *Clin. Orthop. Relat. Res.* **2019**, *477*, 2705–2714. [CrossRef] [PubMed]
4. Smeland, S.; Bielack, S.S.; Whelan, J.; Bernstein, M.; Hogendoorn, P.; Krailo, M.D.; Gorlick, R.; Janeway, K.A.; Ingleby, F.C.; Anninga, J.; et al. Survival and prognosis with osteosarcoma: Outcomes in more than 2000 patients in the EURAMOS-1 (European and American Osteosarcoma Study) cohort. *Eur. J. Cancer* **2019**, *109*, 36–50. [CrossRef]
5. Wafa, H.; Grimer, R.J.; Reddy, K.; Jeys, L.; Abudu, A.; Carter, S.R.; Tillman, R.M. Retrospective evaluation of the incidence of early periprosthetic infection with silver-treated endoprostheses in high-risk patients: Case-control study. *Bone Jt. J.* **2015**, *97-B*, 252–257. [CrossRef] [PubMed]
6. Heyberger, C.; Auberger, G.; Babinet, A.; Anract, P.; Biau, D.J. Patients with Revision Modern Megaprostheses of the Distal Femur Have Improved Disease-Specific and Health-Related Outcomes Compared to Those with Primary Replacements. *J. Knee Surg.* **2018**, *31*, 822–826. [CrossRef] [PubMed]
7. Jeys, L.M.; Grimer, R.J.; Carter, S.R.; Tillman, R.M. Risk of amputation following limb salvage surgery with endoprosthetic replacement, in a consecutive series of 1261 patients. *Int. Orthop.* **2003**, *27*, 160–163. [CrossRef]
8. Suresh Nathan, S.; Tan Lay Hua, G.; Mei Yoke, C.; Mann Hong, T.; Peter Pereira, B. Outcome satisfaction in long-term survivors of oncologic limb salvage procedures. *Eur J. Cancer Care* **2021**, *30*, e13377. [CrossRef]
9. Nowak, L.L.; Schemitsch, E.H. Duration of surgery affects the risk of complications following total hip arthroplasty. *Bone Jt. J.* **2019**, *101*, 51–56. [CrossRef]

10. Orland, M.D.; Lee, R.Y.; Naami, E.E.; Patetta, M.J.; Hussain, A.K.; Gonzalez, M.H. Surgical Duration Implicated in Major Postoperative Complications in Total Hip and Total Knee Arthroplasty: A Retrospective Cohort Study. *J. Am. Acad. Orthop. Surg. Glob. Res. Rev.* **2020**, *4*, e2000043. [CrossRef]
11. Davis, N.; Curry, A.; Gambhir, A.K.; Panigrahi, H.; Walker, C.R.; Wilkins, E.G.; Worsley, M.A.; Kay, P.R. Intraoperative bacterial contamination in operations for joint replacement. *J. Bone Jt. Surg. Br.* **1999**, *81*, 886–889. [CrossRef]
12. De Gori, M.; Gasparini, G.; Capanna, R. Risk Factors for Perimegaprosthetic Infections After Tumor Resection. *Orthopedics* **2017**, *40*, e11–e16. [CrossRef]
13. Dhanoa, A.; Ajit Singh, V.; Elbahri, H. Deep Infections after Endoprosthetic Replacement Operations in Orthopedic Oncology Patients. *Surg. Infect.* **2015**, *16*, 323–332. [CrossRef] [PubMed]
14. Peel, T.; May, D.; Buising, K.; Thursky, K.; Slavin, M.; Choong, P. Infective complications following tumour endoprosthesis surgery for bone and soft tissue tumours. *Eur. J. Surg. Oncol.* **2014**, *40*, 1087–1094. [CrossRef] [PubMed]
15. Cho, W.H.; Song, W.S.; Jeon, D.G.; Kong, C.B.; Kim, J.I.; Lee, S.Y. Cause of infection in proximal tibial endoprosthetic reconstructions. *Arch. Orthop. Trauma Surg.* **2012**, *132*, 163–169. [CrossRef]
16. Sigmund, I.K.; Gamper, J.; Weber, C.; Holinka, J.; Panotopoulos, J.; Funovics, P.T.; Windhager, R. Efficacy of different revision procedures for infected megaprostheses in musculoskeletal tumour surgery of the lower limb. *PLoS ONE* **2018**, *13*, e0200304. [CrossRef]
17. Schneider, K.N.; Broking, J.N.; Gosheger, G.; Lubben, T.; Hardes, J.; Schorn, D.; Smolle, M.A.; Theil, C.; Andreou, D. What Is the Implant Survivorship and Functional Outcome After Total Humeral Replacement in Patients with Primary Bone Tumors? *Clin. Orthop. Relat. Res.* **2021**, 10–1097. [CrossRef]
18. Henderson, E.R.; Groundland, J.S.; Pala, E.; Dennis, J.A.; Wooten, R.; Cheong, D.; Windhager, R.; Kotz, R.I.; Mercuri, M.; Funovics, P.T.; et al. Failure mode classification for tumor endoprostheses: Retrospective review of five institutions and a literature review. *J. Bone Jt. Surg. Am. Vol.* **2011**, *93*, 418–429. [CrossRef]
19. Sevelda, F.; Waldstein, W.; Panotopoulos, J.; Stihsen, C.; Kaider, A.; Funovics, P.T.; Windhager, R. Survival, failure modes and function of combined distal femur and proximal tibia reconstruction following tumor resection. *Eur. J. Surg. Oncol.* **2017**, *43*, 416–422. [CrossRef]
20. Ravi, B.; Jenkinson, R.; O'Heireamhoin, S.; Austin, P.C.; Aktar, S.; Leroux, T.S.; Paterson, M.; Redelmeier, D.A. Surgical duration is associated with an increased risk of periprosthetic infection following total knee arthroplasty: A population-based retrospective cohort study. *EClinicalMedicine* **2019**, *16*, 74–80. [CrossRef]
21. Peersman, G.; Laskin, R.; Davis, J.; Peterson, M.G.; Richart, T. Prolonged operative time correlates with increased infection rate after total knee arthroplasty. *HSS J.* **2006**, *2*, 70–72. [CrossRef]
22. Fehring, K.A.; Abdel, M.P.; Ollivier, M.; Mabry, T.M.; Hanssen, A.D. Repeat Two-Stage Exchange Arthroplasty for Periprosthetic Knee Infection Is Dependent on Host Grade. *J. Bone Jt. Surg. Am.* **2017**, *99*, 19–24. [CrossRef]
23. Hardes, J.; Gebert, C.; Schwappach, A.; Ahrens, H.; Streitburger, A.; Winkelmann, W.; Gosheger, G. Characteristics and outcome of infections associated with tumor endoprostheses. *Arch. Orthop. Trauma Surg.* **2006**, *126*, 289–296. [CrossRef]
24. Jeys, L.M.; Grimer, R.J.; Carter, S.R.; Tillman, R.M. Periprosthetic infection in patients treated for an orthopaedic oncological condition. *J. Bone Jt. Surg. Am. Vol.* **2005**, *87*, 842–849. [CrossRef]
25. Akgun, D.; Muller, M.; Perka, C.; Winkler, T. A positive bacterial culture during re-implantation is associated with a poor outcome in two-stage exchange arthroplasty for deep infection. *Bone Jt. J.* **2017**, *99-B*, 1490–1495. [CrossRef]
26. Theil, C.; Freudenberg, S.C.; Gosheger, G.; Schmidt-Braekling, T.; Schwarze, J.; Moellenbeck, B. Do Positive Cultures at Second Stage Re-Implantation Increase the Risk for Reinfection in Two-Stage Exchange for Periprosthetic Joint Infection? *J. Arthroplast.* **2020**, *35*, 2996–3001. [CrossRef]
27. Theil, C.; Schneider, K.N.; Gosheger, G.; Schmidt-Braekling, T.; Ackmann, T.; Dieckmann, R.; Frommer, A.; Klingebiel, S.; Schwarze, J.; Moellenbeck, B. Revision TKA with a distal femoral replacement is at high risk of reinfection after two-stage exchange for periprosthetic knee joint infection. *Knee Surg. Sports Traumatol. Arthrosc.* **2021**, 1–8. [CrossRef]
28. Ogura, K.; Boland, P.J.; Fabbri, N.; Healey, J.H. Rate and risk factors for wound complications after internal hemipelvectomy. *Bone Jt. J.* **2020**, *102-B*, 280–284. [CrossRef]
29. Funovics, P.T.; Hipfl, C.; Hofstaetter, J.G.; Puchner, S.; Kotz, R.I.; Dominkus, M. Management of septic complications following modular endoprosthetic reconstruction of the proximal femur. *Int. Orthop.* **2011**, *35*, 1437–1444. [CrossRef]
30. Ghazavi, M.; Mortazavi, J.; Patzakis, M.; Sheehan, E.; Tan, T.L.; Yazdi, H. Hip and Knee Section, Treatment, Salvage: Proceedings of International Consensus on Orthopedic Infections. *J. Arthroplast.* **2019**, *34*, S459–S462. [CrossRef]

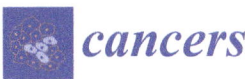

Article

Survival Analysis of 3 Different Age Groups and Prognostic Factors among 402 Patients with Skeletal High-Grade Osteosarcoma. Real World Data from a Single Tertiary Sarcoma Center

Richard E. Evenhuis [1,*], Ibtissam Acem [1,2], Anja J. Rueten-Budde [3], Diederik S. A. Karis [1], Marta Fiocco [3], Desiree M. J. Dorleijn [1], Frank M. Speetjens [4], Jakob Anninga [5], Hans Gelderblom [4] and Michiel A. J. van de Sande [1,5]

1. Department of Orthopedic Surgery, Leiden University Medical Center, 2300RC Leiden, The Netherlands; i.acem@lumc.nl (I.A.); d.s.a.karis@lumc.nl (D.S.A.K.); D.M.J.Dorleijn@lumc.nl (D.M.J.D.); M.A.J.van_de_Sande@lumc.nl (M.A.J.v.d.S.)
2. Department of Surgical Oncology and Gastrointestinal Surgery, Erasmus MC Cancer Institute, 3000CB Rotterdam, The Netherlands
3. Department of Biomedical Data Science, Section Medical Statistics and Bioinformatics, Mathematical Institute Leiden University, 2300RC Leiden, The Netherlands; a.j.ruten-budde@math.leidenuniv.nl (A.J.R.-B.); m.fiocco@math.leidenuniv.nl (M.F.)
4. Department of Medical Oncology, Leiden University Medical Center, 2300RC Leiden, The Netherlands; F.M.Speetjens@lumc.nl (F.M.S.); A.J.Gelderblom@lumc.nl (H.G.)
5. Princess Máxima Center for Pediatric Oncology, 3720AC Utrecht, The Netherlands; J.K.Anninga@prinsesmaximacentrum.nl
* Correspondence: R.e.evenhuis@lumc.nl; Tel.: +31-651672659

Citation: Evenhuis, R.E.; Acem, I.; Rueten-Budde, A.J.; Karis, D.S.A.; Fiocco, M.; Dorleijn, D.M.J.; Speetjens, F.M.; Anninga, J.; Gelderblom, H.; van de Sande, M.A.J. Survival Analysis of 3 Different Age Groups and Prognostic Factors among 402 Patients with Skeletal High-Grade Osteosarcoma. Real World Data from a Single Tertiary Sarcoma Center. *Cancers* **2021**, *13*, 486. https://doi.org/10.3390/cancers13030486

Academic Editor: Subree Subramanian
Received: 27 December 2020
Accepted: 23 January 2021
Published: 27 January 2021

Publisher's Note: MDPI stays neutral with regard to jurisdictional claims in published maps and institutional affiliations.

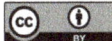

Copyright: © 2021 by the authors. Licensee MDPI, Basel, Switzerland. This article is an open access article distributed under the terms and conditions of the Creative Commons Attribution (CC BY) license (https://creativecommons.org/licenses/by/4.0/).

Simple Summary: Age is one of many prognostic factors for overall survival in patients with skeletal osteosarcoma. This retrospective study provides an overview of survival in patients with high-grade osteosarcoma in different age groups. It shows prognostic variables for survival and local control among the overall cohort. In this study, in which 402 patients with skeletal high-grade osteosarcoma were included, poor survival was associated with increasing age. Age groups, tumor size, poor histopathological response, distant metastasis at presentation, and local recurrence were independent prognostic factors associated to overall survival and event-free survival. Differences in outcome among different age groups can be partially explained by patient characteristics and treatment characteristics.

Abstract: Age is a known prognostic factor for many sarcoma subtypes, however in the literature there are limited data on the different risk profiles of different age groups for osteosarcoma survival. This study aims to provide an overview of survival in patients with high-grade osteosarcoma in different age groups and prognostic variables for survival and local control among the entire cohort. In this single center retrospective cohort study, 402 patients with skeletal high-grade osteosarcoma were diagnosed and treated with curative intent between 1978 and 2017 at the Leiden University Medical Center (LUMC). Prognostic factors for survival were analyzed using a Cox proportional hazard model. In this study poor overall survival (OS) and event-free survival (EFS) were associated with increasing age. Age groups, tumor size, poor histopathological response, distant metastasis (DM) at presentation and local recurrence (LR) were important independent prognostic factors influencing OS and EFS. Differences in outcome among different age groups can be partially explained by patient characteristics and treatment characteristics.

Keywords: osteosarcoma; survival; prognosis; age groups; chemotherapy; metastasis; local recurrence

1. Introduction

High-grade conventional osteosarcoma is a primary malignant bone tumor that has a bimodal distribution curve. The first peak is at the age of puberty and adolescence, the second curve arises after the age of 40 [1,2]. Despite being a rare disease (prevalence of 3–4 cases per million per year [3,4]), osteosarcoma is the most common primary malignant bone tumor. It continues to be a high risk malignancy and has one of the highest mortality rates of any type of cancer diagnosed around puberty [5]. Before the introduction of chemotherapy in the 1980's, survival for patients with high-grade osteosarcoma was poor with survival probabilities as low as less than 20% [3]. After the introduction of chemotherapy, the overall survival (OS) increased to an average of 60% [3,6,7].

Multiple studies conclude more favorable survival probabilities in pediatric patients compared with adolescent and young adults (AYA) or older adults [8–10]. In contrast, some studies stated that no differences in survival were found between pediatric patients and older adults [11,12]. The variation in survival probabilities among age groups might be due to differences in tumor characteristics, chemotherapy regimens, pathohistological response, or different patient characteristics [9,13–18].

The aim of this single center retrospective study is to provide an overview of survival outcome within three age groups (pediatric, AYA, adult) and for the total cohort. The second aim is to identify prognostic factors for OS and event-free survival (EFS) in patients with high-grade osteosarcoma.

2. Methods

2.1. Design, Setting, Data Source, Participants

This observational retrospective cohort study was performed at the Leiden University Medical Center (LUMC) in the Netherlands between 1978 and 2017. All consecutive patients diagnosed with histologically proven high-grade osteosarcoma treated with curative intent that met inclusion criteria were included. Patients with a skeletal high-grade primary osteosarcoma, treated with curative intent using (neo)adjuvant chemotherapy and surgery, were eligible for this study. Patients were excluded if they were diagnosed with, a low grade (parosteal) or intermediate grade osteosarcoma (peri-osteal), had a secondary osteosarcoma (i.e., radiation-induced), received a treatment with palliative intent, if data about surgery or chemotherapy were missing, or when the tumor location was facial or extra-skeletal. Patients with metastasis at presentation were eligible when curative intent was set at start of the treatment including planned metastasectomy. High-grade osteosarcoma consists of conventional osteosarcoma (osteoblastic, chondroblastic and fibroblastic), small cell and telangiectatic osteosarcoma. Apart from these subgroups, the WHO distinguishes high-grade surface osteosarcoma and secondary osteosarcoma as other types of high-grade osteosarcoma. This study was approved by the medical ethical committee of the LUMC as no patients were approached and data were handled anonymously. The approval code is G18.065/SH/gk. The used data comprised real world data.

2.2. Variables

Baseline variables were age, sex, location and size of the tumor and distant metastasis (DM) at presentation. Treatment data include LR, surgical margin, type of resection and response to chemotherapy. Patients were categorized into one of three age groups (children 0–<16, AYA 16–<40, older adults ≥ 40). Location of the primary tumor was defined as extremity (upper or lower extremity) or axial (tumors of the chest including ribs, spine or pelvis). The size of the primary tumor was divided according to the American Joint Committee on Cancer (AJCC) into small (≤8 cm) or large (>8 cm) [19]. Radical resection was defined as a wide radical resection with both macroscopic as microscopic surgical margins free of tumor and the entire dissection performed through healthy tissues. Marginal surgical margin was defined as a dissection that extended into or through the reactive zone that surrounds the tumor. Irradical or intralesional margin was defined as entering the tumor at any point during surgery [20].

The type of resection was divided into 3 subgroups; (1). reconstruction with an allo- or autograft, prosthesis or rotationplasty; (2). amputation of the affected limb or exarticulation of the joint without reconstruction; (3). resection that consisted of local resection, en-bloc resection or hemipelvectomy without reconstruction. The protocolized planned chemotherapy was either an intentional treatment with (Methotrexate, Doxorubicin, Cisplatin (MAP) or with Doxorubicin, Cisplatin (AP). Patients were treated with at least one cycle to a maximum of 6 cycles chemotherapy. Patients receiving preoperative chemotherapy were categorized in three groups (1 cycle MAP or 2 cycles AP preoperative, 2 cycles MAP or 3 cycles AP preoperative and >2 cycles MAP or >3 cycles AP preoperative). Generally, 2 cycles MAP or 3 cycles AP are used preoperatively. The other variants show patients receiving less or more cycles preoperative chemotherapy. Histopathological response on chemotherapy was obtained by a reference pathologist after histopathologic examination of the resected primary tumor. The percentage of tumor necrosis attributable to preoperative chemotherapy was defined by the Huvos grading. Huvos grading stage 1 and 2 is defined as ≤90% necrosis (bad responders). Huvos grading stage 3 and 4 defined is as >90% necrosis (good responders) [21].

Primary outcome was OS from surgery until death or until last date of follow-up. Secondary outcome was EFS; from resection to first event which consisted of LR, progression of metastasis, new metastasis, death or last date of follow-up. In patients with DM at presentation the next event was considered for EFS. LR was defined as a relapse of primary tumor situated at the same location of the primary tumor which was radically or marginally resected.

2.3. Follow-Up

Patients were followed at the outpatient clinic for local control, functional outcome and disease progression. Follow-up consisted of physical examination and radiographic control. Radiographic control comprised chest radiography and radiography of the affected bone. Follow-up visits were performed maximum 25 years after diagnosis with frequent visits in the first years after initial diagnosis and less frequent in later years according to the EURAMOS protocol [22].

2.4. Statistical Analysis

A Cox proportional hazards regression model with time fixed and time dependent covariates [23] was estimated to evaluate the association between OS, EFS and prognostic factors. Age group, location of the tumor, size of the tumor, the presence of DM at presentation, surgical margin, response to chemotherapy and local recurrence of disease were included in the Cox model. The effect of LR on survival outcomes was analyzed in two different ways, as a time-dependent covariate in the Cox model and by using the Landmark approach [24]. A landmark model only uses information available at the landmark time (t_{LM}). Only patients alive at t_{LM} are included in the analysis. In our study t_{LM} is chosen at 24 months after the date of surgery. At the landmark time patients were classified as having experienced LR before 24 months or not. Survival curves were estimated using the Kaplan–Meier (KM) methodology. Outcomes were statistically significant when the p-value was <0.05. Because of a low number of patients for some crosstabulations, the Fisher exact test was used instead of the Chi-square test when testing categorical variables. Median follow-up time was computed using the reversed KM estimator. Missing covariates were imputed using multiple imputation methods [25] for survival data with the event indicator and the Nelson–Aalen estimator of the cumulative hazard as variables in the imputation model [26]. In total 20 data sets were imputed, Rubin's rule was applied to obtain the final estimates along with their standard error. The analysis was performed by using SPSS (IBM Corp. Released 2017. IBM SPSS Statistics for Windows, Version 25.0. Armonk, NY: IBM Corp).

3. Results

3.1. Baseline Characteristics

The total LUMC-cohort contained 610 patients with osteosarcoma (Figure 1). Twenty patients were excluded due to secondary osteosarcoma, 88 patients due to low, intermediate or unknown grade osteosarcoma and 1 patient due to an inconclusive pathology report. Among 501 patients with high-grade osteosarcoma, 84 patients were not treated with curative intent, for 2 patients the date of resection was unknown, and 13 patients were excluded because the primary tumor was located facially or extra-skeletally (soft-tissue). After applying the exclusion criteria, 402 patients were included in this study. The median age at diagnosis was 19.14 years (range 3–82 years). The three age groups comprised 114 children (28.7%) aged 0 to <16 years, 218 (54.2%) adolescents and young adults (AYA) aged 16–<40 and 70 (17.4%) older adults aged ≥40 years. Among all patients 60% of them had a poor histopathological response on chemotherapy and 40% had a good histopathological response on chemotherapy.

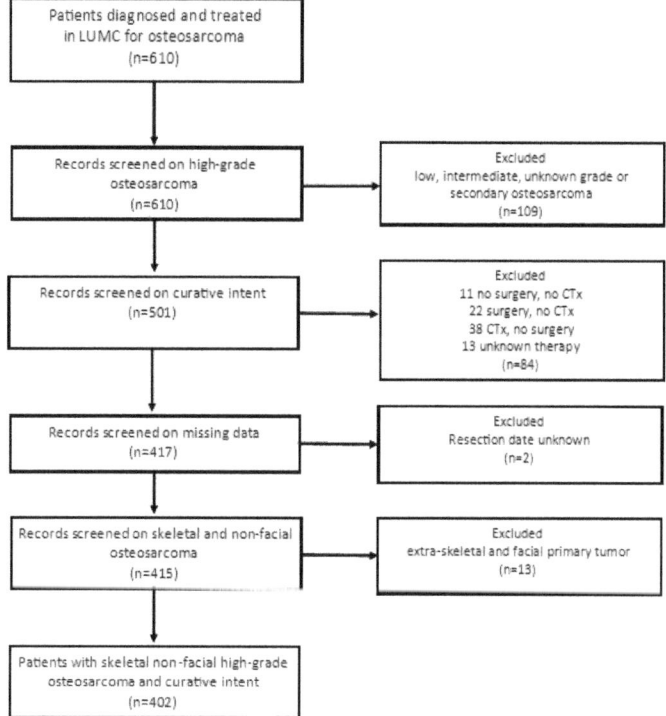

Figure 1. Flowchart patient selection. Legend; LUMC = Leiden University Medical Center, CTx = Chemotherapy.

3.2. Differences in Presentation Among Age Groups

A significant difference at presentation was found among the age groups comparing tumor location ($p < 0.001$) (Table 1). Older adults more often presented with an axial tumor compared to children and AYA. A significant difference was found among age groups and patients presenting with pathological fractures ($p = 0.007$). Of all patients, 347 (89.4%) presented without a pathological fracture of whom 102 children (90.3%), 193 AYA (92.3%) and 52 older adults (78.8%). Children were diagnosed significantly more often with DM at presentation compared to AYA and older adults ($p = 0.037$). Children, AYA and older adults, respectively, presented with at least one pulmonary metastasis in 16.5%,

12% and 5.7% of patients. Of all patients, 55 children (51.9%) underwent a radical resection compared to 99 AYA (48.3%) and 29 (42.6%) older adults. A total of 50 patients (13.2%) had an irradical resection: 7 children (6.6%), 31 AYA (15.1%) and 12 older adults (17.6%). No significant differences were found among the age groups between different types of resection ($p = 0.070$). However, the 258 patients (66.7%) receiving resection and reconstruction comprised of 77 children (71.3%), 139 AYA (66.2%), and 42 older adults (60.9%). The 56 (14.5%) patients receiving resection comprised of 7 children only (6.5%) compared to 36 AYA (17.1%) and 13 older adults (18.8%). Older adults were significantly more often treated with AP chemotherapy ($p < 0.001$), where children were more often treated with MAP ($p < 0.001$). The amount of received pre-operative chemotherapy cycles did not differ significantly among age groups. The majority of the patients (77.7%) received two MAP cycles or three AP cycles pre-operative. Finally, the response on chemotherapy differed significantly among the age groups ($p = 0.005$). Children had a good histopathological response significantly more often on pre-operative chemotherapy compared with AYA and older adults.

Table 1. Characteristics of the overall cohort diagnosed with skeletal high-grade osteosarcoma.

Characteristic	N (%)	Children (0–<16 yrs)	AYA (16–<40 yrs)	Older Adults (≥40 yrs)	p-Value
Gender	402	114 (28.7)	218 (54.2)	70 (17.4)	0.092
Male	228 (56.7)	64 (56.1)	132 (57.9)	32 (45.7)	
Female	174 (43.3)	50 (43.9)	86 (39.4)	38 (54.3)	
Location tumor	402	114 (28.4)	218 (54.2)	70 (17.4)	<0.001
Extremities	372 (92.5)	112 (98.2)	203 (93.1)	57 (81.4)	
Axial (pelvis, chest, spine)	30 (7.5)	2 (1.8)	15 (6.9)	13 (18.6)	
Tumor size	375	107 (28.5)	200 (53.3)	68 (18.1)	0.377
Small (≤8 cm)	154 (41.1)	43 (40.2)	78 (39)	33 (48.5)	
Large (≥8 cm)	221 (58.9)	64 (59.8)	122 (61)	35 (51.5)	
Pathologic fracture	388	113 (29.1)	209 (53.9)	66 (17)	0.007
No	347 (89.4)	102 (90.3)	193 (92.3)	52 (78.8)	
Yes	41 (10.6)	11 (9.7)	16 (7.7)	14 (21.2)	
Distant metastasis at presentation	391	111 (28.4)	210 (53.7)	70 (17.9)	0.037
No	325 (83.1)	87 (78.4)	173 (82.4)	65 (92.9)	
Yes	66 (16.9)	24 (21.6)	37 (17.6)	5 (7.1)	
*No. of lungmets at presentation	388	109 (28.1)	209 (53.9)	70 (18)	0.389
None	341 (87.9)	91 (83.5)	184 (88)	66 (94.3)	
1	9 (2.3)	3 (2.8)	6 (2.9)	0 (0)	
2–5	30 (7.7)	11 (10.1)	16 (7.7)	3 (4.3)	
>5	8 (2.1)	4 (3.7)	3 (1.4)	1 (1.4)	
Surgical margin	379	106 (28)	205 (54.1)	68 (17.9)	0.178
Radical	183 (48.3)	55 (51.9)	99 (48.3)	29 (42.6)	
Marginal	146 (38.5)	44 (41.5)	75 (36.6)	27 (39.7)	
Irradical	50 (13.2)	7 (6.6)	31 (15.1)	12 (17.6)	
Type of resection	387	108 (27.9)	210 (54.3)	69 (17.8)	0.070
Resection/reconstruction	258 (66.7)	77 (71.3)	139 (66.2)	42 (60.9)	
Amputation/exarticulation	73 (18.9)	24 (22.2)	35 (16.7)	14 (20.3)	
Resection only	56 (14.5)	7 (6.5)	36 (17.1)	13 (18.8)	
Chemotherapy treatment	359	98 (27.3)	198 (55.6)	63 (17.5)	<0.001
Intention AP	225 (62.7)	43 (43.9)	125 (55.6)	57 (90.5)	
Intention MAP	134 (37.3)	55 (56.1)	73 (36.9)	6 (9.5)	
*Pre-op CTx cycles	309	89 (28.8)	176 (57)	44 (14.2)	0.256
1 MAP or 2 AP	41 (13.3)	12 (13.5)	22 (12.5)	7 (15.9)	
2 MAP or 3 AP	240 (77.7)	74 (83.1)	134 (76.1)	32 (72.7)	
>2 MAP or >3 AP	28 (9.1)	3 (3.4)	20 (11.4)	5 (11.4)	
*Response on chemotherapy	337	105 (31.2)	184 (54.6)	48 (14.2)	0.005
Poor (Huvos 1,2)	202 (59.9)	51 (48.6)	115 (62.5)	36 (75)	
Good (Huvos 3,4)	135 (40.1)	54 (51.4)	69 (37.5)	12 (25)	
*/** Local recurrence	391	106 (27.1)	215 (55)	70 (17.9)	
No	346 (88.5)	102 (96.2)	190 (88.4)	54 (77.1)	
Yes	45 (11.5)	4 (3.8)	25 (11.6)	16 (22.9)	

Legend: AYA = Adolescent and Young Adult, Lungmets = lung metastasis, AP = Adriamycine-CisPlatin, MAP = Methotrexate-Adriamycine-CisPlatin, CTx = Chemotherapy, pre-op = pre-operative, * Fisher exact test because number of patients <5, ** No p-value because of time dependent variable.

3.3. Overall Survival in Total Cohort

Median follow-up time for the overall cohort containing 402 patients, was 136 months (95%CI 116.4–155.6). Among these patients, 5-year OS was 59.1% (95%CI 54.2–64.0). The 5-year OS for 114 children, 218 AYA and 70 older adults was, respectively, 67.2% (95%CI 58.18–76.22), 56.5% (49.84–63.16), 54.3% (42.34–66.26) as can be seen in Figure 2 and Table 3. The 5-year OS for 325 patients (83.1%) without DM at presentation was 66.1% (95%CI 60.81–71.40). OS for 66 patients (16.9%) with DM at presentation was significantly lower ($p < 0.001$) with a 5-year OS of 30% (95%CI 18.63–41.37) (Table 2, Figure 3). Among patients presenting without DM, OS differed significantly between the three age groups ($p = 0.006$). Children, AYA and older adults had, respectively, a 5-year OS of 78.5% (95%CI 87.32–69.68), 63.8% (95%CI 56.35–71.25) and 55.4% (95%CI 43.05–67.75).

Table 2. Overall survival (OS) among different age groups with or without distant metastasis (DM) at presentation.

Factors	N (%)	5-yr OS among M0 (%)	p-Value	N (%)	5-yr OS among M1 (%)	p-Value
Overall group	325 (83.1)	66.1		66 (16.9)	30	
			0.006			0.971
Child (0–<16)	87 (26.8)	78.5		24 (36.4)	21.7	
AYA (16–<40)	173 (53.2)	63.8		37 (56.1)	32.4	
Older adults ≥40	65 (20)	55.4		5 (7.6)	40	

Legend: M0 = patients without metastasis at presentation, M1 = patients with metastasis at presentation.

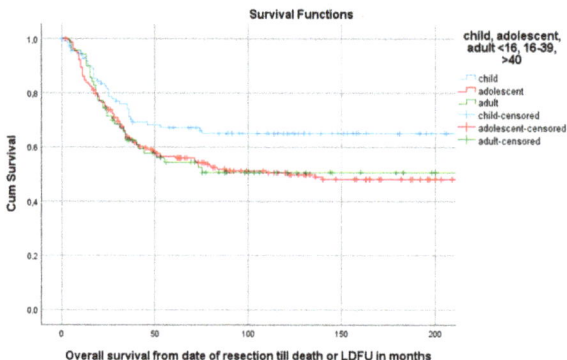

Figure 2. Kaplan–Meier (KM) estimation of OS in the total cohort divided by age group. Legend: OS = overall survival, cum survival = cumulative survival, LDFU = last date of follow-up.

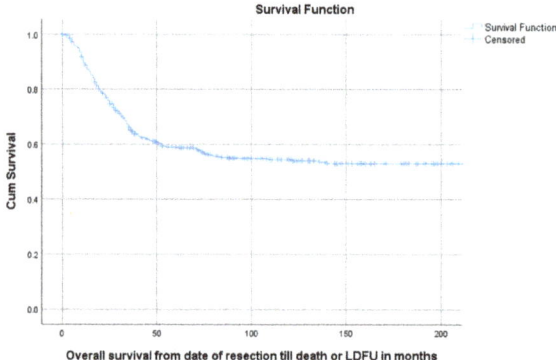

Figure 3. Cont.

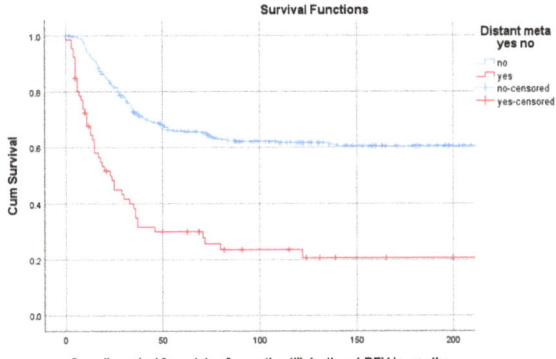

Figure 3. KM estimation of OS in the total cohort (upper panel) and of patients with and without distant metastasis (lower panel). Legend: OS = overall survival, DM = distant metastasis at presentation, cum survival = cumulative survival, LDFU = last date of follow-up.

3.4. Event Free Survival

Of all 402 patients, 55.5% (223/402) experienced an event defined as LR, progression of metastasis, diagnosis of new metastasis or death. The 5-year EFS for 114 children, 218 AYA and 70 older adults was, respectively, 58.5% (95%CI 49.29–67.71), 40.6% (95%CI 33.94–47.26), 38.9% (95%CI 27.34–50.46) as can be seen in Table 3 and Figure 4. A total of 1, 3 and 5 years after surgery the event-free survival was, respectively, 71.6% (95%CI 67.1–76.1), 49.2% (95%CI 44.3–54.1) and 45.3% (95%CI 40.4–50.2) (Figure 5).

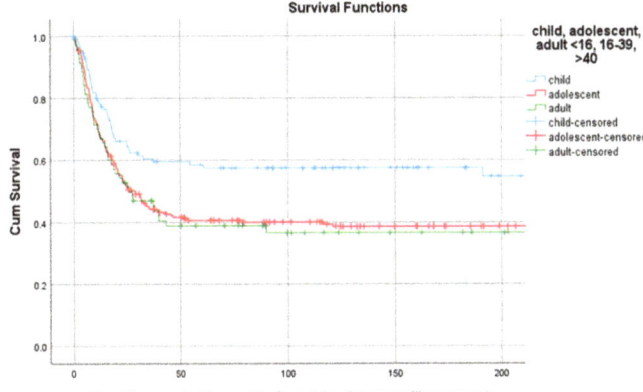

Figure 4. KM estimation of EFS in total cohort divided by age group. Legend: EFS = event-free survival, cum survival = cumulative survival.

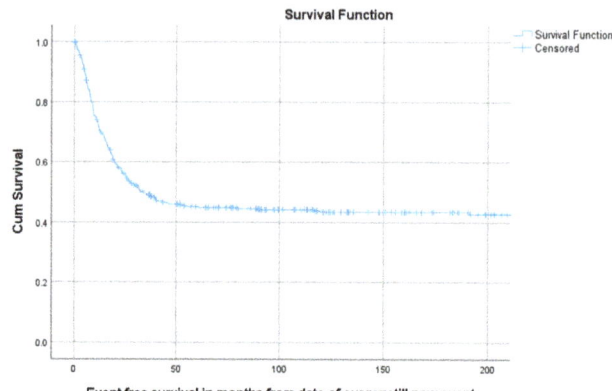

Figure 5. KM estimation of EFS of total cohort. Legend: EFS = Event-free survival, cum survival = cumulative survival.

Table 3. OS and EFS at 5 years along with 95% confidence interval (CI).

Factors	N (%)	5-Year OS (%) with 95%CI	p-Value	N (%)	5-Year EFS (%) with 95%CI	p-Value
Sex	402		0.126	402		0.033
Male	228 (56.7)	55.5 (48.8–62.16)		228 (56.7)	40.7 (34.23–47.17)	
Female	174 (43.3)	63.6 (56.35–70.85)		174 (43.3)	51.3 (43.85–58.75)	
Age group	402		0.044	402		0.007
Child (0–<16)	114 (28.4)	67.2 (58.18–76.22)		114 (28.4)	58.5 (49.29–67.71)	
AYA (16–<40)	218 (54.2)	56.5 (49.84–63.16)		218 (54.2)	40.6 (33.94–47.26)	
Older adults ≥40	70 (17.4)	54.3 (42.34–66.26)		70 (17.4)	38.9 (27.34–50.46)	
Location	402		0.960	402		0.361
Extremities	372 (92.5)	59.1 (54.0–64.2)		372 (92.5)	45.8 (40.70–50.90)	
Axial (chest, spine, pelvis)	30 (7.5)	60 (42.56–77.44)		30 (7.5)	40 (22.56–57.44)	
Tumor size	375		<0.001	375		<0.001
Small ≤8 cm	154 (41.1)	72.4 (65.15–79.65)		154 (41.1)	70.1 (52.26–67.94)	
Large ≥8 cm	221 (58.9)	50.2 (43.34–57.06)		221 (58.9)	34.5 (28.03–40.97)	
Surgical margin	379		0.037	379		0.030
Radical	183 (48.3)	60.7 (53.45–67.95)		183 (48.3)	48.2 (40.75–55.65)	
Marginal	146 (38.5)	62.3 (54.26–70.34)		146 (38.5)	47.5 (39.27–55.73)	
Irradical	50 (13.2)	45.4 (31.48–59.32)		50 (13.2)	29.9 (17.16–42.64)	
Type of resection	387		0.002	387		0.004
Resection/reconstruction	258 (66.7)	60.6 (54.52–66.68)		258 (66.7)	47.1 (40.83–53.37)	
Amputation/exarticulation	73 (18.9)	45.7 (34.14–57.26)		73 (18.9)	33.6 (22.62–44.58)	
Resection only	56 (14.5)	72.2 (60.24–84.16)		56 (14.5)	56.7 (43.57–69.83)	
Response on chemotherapy	337		<0.001	337		<0.001
Poor (Huvos 1,2)	202 (59.9)	46.6 (39.54–53.66)		202 (59.9)	31.2 (24.73–37.67)	
Good (Huvos 3,4)	135 (40.1)	74.5 (67.05–81.95)		135 (40.1)	66.9 (58.86–74.94)	
Distant metastasis at presentation	391		<0.001	391		<0.001
No	325 (83.1)	66.1 (60.81–71.39)		325 (83.1)	50.9 (45.41–56.39)	
Yes	66 (16.9)	30 (18.63–41.37)		66 (16.9)	20.9 (10.71–31.09)	

Legend: CTx = Chemotherapy.

3.5. Landmark Analysis

Survival from landmark time at 24 months post-surgery was estimated for patients with and without LR at t_{LM}. In this analysis 304 patients were included; 20 patients (6.6%) had an LR within 24 months post-surgery. Patients with LR at t_{LM} had a poor survival compared to patients without ($p < 0.001$) (Figure 6).

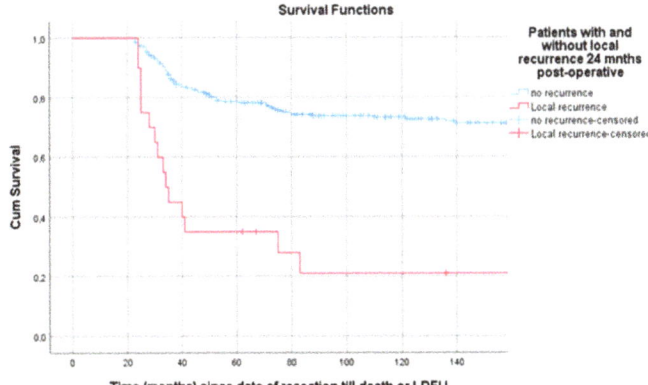

Figure 6. Landmark analysis of patients with and without LR 24 months post-surgery. Legend: LR = local recurrence, cum survival = cumulative survival, LDFU = last date of follow-up.

3.6. Prognostic Factors

Size of the tumor (HR 1.711, 95%CI 1.193–2.455), the response to chemotherapy (HR 0.422, 95%CI 0.276–0.646), the presence of distant metastasis at presentation (HR 3.578, 95%CI 2.492–5.138) and local recurrence of disease (HR 4.456, 95%CI 2.911–6.682) were significantly associated with OS (Table 4). Age group (AYA vs. children, HR 1.499, 95%CI 1.067–2.108), (older adults vs. children, HR 1.708, 95%CI 1.094–2.666), size of the tumor (HR 1.836 95%CI 1.335–2.527), response on chemotherapy (HR 0.407, 95%CI 0.288–0.574) and distant metastasis at presentation (HR 2.575, 95%CI 1.859–3.565) were associated with EFS. Age group was found to be an independent prognostic factor of EFS but not for OS. An HR of 1.313 on OS was found comparing AYA and children (95%CI 0.891–1.935). An HR of 1.326 on OS was found comparing older adults and children (95%CI 0.802–2.193).

Table 4. Hazard ratio for prognostic factors on OS and EFS along with the 95% confidence interval estimated with the Cox proportional hazards regression model.

Factors	HR$_{OS}$	95% CI	*p*-Value	HR$_{EFS}$	95% CI	*p*-Value
Sex			0.490			0.097
Male						
Female	0.891	0.642–1.237		0.786	0.592–1.044	
Age group						
Child (0–<16)		*Reference group*			*Reference group*	
AYA (16–<40)	1.313	0.891–1.935	0.168	1.499	1.067–2.108	0.020
Older adults ≥40	1.326	0.802–2.193	0.272	1.708	1.094–2.666	0.018
Location			0.678			0.346
Extremities						
Axial (chest, spine, pelvis)	0.868	0.446–1.692		1.277	0.768–2.123	
Tumor size			0.004			<0.001
Small ≤8 cm						
Large ≥8 cm	1.711	1.193–2.455		1.836	1.335–2.527	
Surgical margin						
Radical		*Reference group*			*Reference group*	
Marginal	0.839	0.586–1.203	0.340	0.941	0.689–1.285	0.702
Irradical	1.248	0.783–1.988	0.351	1.141	0.769–1.693	0.513
Response on chemotherapy			<0.001			<0.001
Poor (Huvos 1,2)						
Good (Huvos 3,4)	0.422	0.276–0.646		0.407	0.288–0.574	
Distant metastasis at presentation			<0.001			<0.001
No						
Yes	3.578	2.492–5.138		2.575	1.859–3.565	
** Local recurrence			<0.001			
No						
Yes	4.456	2.911–6.682				

Legend: CTx = Chemotherapy, ** = *time dependent variable*, HR = Hazard Ratio.

4. Discussion

This study shows significant differences in tumor characteristics, treatment characteristics and outcome survival outcomes as OS and EFS among children, AYA and older adult population in patients with high-grade osteosarcoma. Children and AYA had better OS and EFS compared to the older adults. These results are in line with previous studies [8,11,14,15,17,18]. Older adults present more often with an axial located tumor, pathological fracture and the protocolized treatment consists more often of AP instead of MAP. Furthermore, a good histopathological response on chemotherapy is less often seen in older adults.

In line with previous studies [3,17] age group was found to be an independent prognostic factor for EFS, resulting in poor EFS among older patients. When comparing AYA vs. children and older adults vs. children, respectively, an HR of 1.499 (95%CI 1.067–2.108) and 1.708 (95%CI 1.094–2.666) was found. A possible explanation for a poor EFS in older patients is that older patients suffer more often of axial located tumors that are technically more difficult to operate on and could lead to a higher risk of incomplete surgical resection [3,4,14,15,17].

A higher frequency of AP chemotherapy among an older group was possibly due to the fact that the older adults tolerate a less intensive chemotherapy protocol. Dose limitations due to comorbidities, age-related organ dysfunction or chemotherapy related toxicity might be associated to poorer response to chemotherapy compared with younger patients [8,17]. Finally, osteosarcoma in older adults seems to have another biological behavior and tends to be more resistant to chemotherapy than that in younger patients [3,8,9]. All these factors can (partly) lead to a decreased EFS in older patients.

DM at presentation is another important prognostic factor resulting in poor survival [11,27]. In this study children present more often with DM at presentation compared to AYA and older adults. Our findings are in contrast with the studies of Hagleitner et al. and Tsuda et al. [8,9], both stating that metastasis presented less frequently in younger patients. However, Hagleitner et al. and Tsuda et al. both used a different distribution of age groups (respectively, patients aged 0–14 yrs, 15–19 yrs, 20–40 yrs and patients aged <40 yrs, 41–64 yrs, >65 yrs). It is of methodological importance in which categorial variable age has been converted and therefore outcomes can vary fairly [10,17]. Another explanation could be the inclusion criteria of this study possibly resulting in a low number of older adults who are more likely to develop DM. As a result of the inclusion criteria, the number of excluded older adults with DM at presentation might be higher. Comorbidities in older adults could lead to restrictions in chemotherapy regimens and therefore have a higher risk of palliative therapy [15,28]. In the study of Tsuda et al. patients with palliative therapy were taken into account as well. In the study of Hagleitner et al. it is not clearly described if patients received palliative therapy. This led to the fact that care should be taken while comparing this study with the studies of Hagleitner et al. and Tsuda et al.

The factors associated with OS were tumor size, histopathological response to chemotherapy, DM at presentation and LR. The factors associated with an effect on EFS were age group, tumor size, histopathological response to chemotherapy and DM at presentation. These results are in line with previous studies [3,9,17,18,29,30]. Age groups were found to be an independent prognostic factor for EFS but not for OS. These results are not in line with the studies of Hagleitner et al. and Mankin et al. [8,31]. This could be explained by the fact that Hagleitner et al. performed a study with only 102 patients. Therefore, adjustment for all important variables in the multivariate analysis could not be done. Furthermore, both studies used different inclusion criteria, therefore a proper comparison could not be made. Finally, care should be taken when interpreting the effect of histopathological response on OS and EFS. In the multivariate analysis, both AP as MAP chemotherapy were taken into account while analyzing the effect on histopathological response. The histopathological response in patients receiving AP chemotherapy is evaluated earlier (after 6 weeks) in comparison to patients receiving MAP (after 10 weeks). In addition,

MAP is a more intensive chemotherapy regimen compared to AP and therefore possibly influencing the effect on the primary outcome.

After 40 years of (neo)adjuvant chemotherapy for osteosarcoma, whose benefits in terms of survival are well established but have not improved, this paper clearly shows that it is time to change the approach and consider additional therapeutic options. In recent years there have been no major results in phase 3 trials in the (neo)adjuvant treatment of patients with resectable osteosarcoma. Phase-2 trials so far have shown no effective trials for poor prognosis osteosarcoma [32–34]. The international community of physicians involved in this disease awaits results of the investigation of the complete genomic landscape of osteosarcoma [35]. Insights from pan-genomic studies could gain a better insight into the development and clonal evolution of this malignancy, that hopefully will lead to the development of more specific drugs for osteosarcoma [36]. These results should guide the development of new (neo)adjuvant trials.

Strengths and Limitations

Our study is one of the largest single center studies investigating prognostic factors on survival. This cohort offers a long median follow-up time of 136 months. In addition, it is one of the few studies describing patient and treatment characteristics in three different age groups and therefore it could be directive to future studies. Other studies describe small study populations or present data from prospective or randomized controlled trials with different pre-empted endpoints and inclusion criteria [8,9,14–18].

Due to the retrospective nature of this study, several limitations were present. In this study we were unable to assess histopathological response per type of chemotherapy regimen. Although histopathological response is an important prognostic factor influencing OS and EFS, care should be taken be taken while interpreting these data. Furthermore, we were unable to assess the association of chemotherapy treatment with survival in the multivariate analysis. Finally, not all known pathological and biochemical features of osteosarcoma patients were taken into account in this paper. The retrospective nature of this study explains for the lack of some possibly important prognostic factors that could not be retrieved for most of the patients.

5. Conclusions

In this single center study, we found poor OS and EFS in older adults with high-grade osteosarcoma compared to AYA and children. Large tumor size, a poor histopathological response, DM at presentation and LR are important independent prognostic factors influencing OS negatively. Age group (older adults), large tumor size, a poor histopathological response and DM at presentation were found to be important independent prognostic factors influencing EFS negatively. DM and LR can make a significant difference in prognosis and is therefore key in the approach of patients suffering high-grade skeletal osteosarcoma. Differences in outcome among different age groups can be partially explained by patient and treatment characteristics.

Author Contributions: Conceptualization, R.E.E. and M.A.J.v.d.S.; methodology, R.E.E., A.J.R.-B., M.F. and M.A.J.v.d.S.; software, R.E.E.; validation, R.E.E., M.F., D.M.J.D., F.M.S., J.A., H.G. and M.A.J.v.d.S.; formal analysis, R.E.E., A.J.R.-B. and M.F.; investigation, R.E.E., D.S.A.K.; resources, not applicable; data curation, R.E.E. and D.S.A.K.; writing—original draft preparation, R.E.E.; writing—review and editing, R.E.E., I.A., A.J.R.-B., D.S.A.K., M.F., D.M.J.D., F.M.S., J.A., H.G. and M.A.J.v.d.S.; visualization, R.E.E. and I.A.; supervision, M.A.J.v.d.S.; project administration, R.E.E. All authors have read and agreed to the published version of the manuscript.

Funding: This research received no external funding.

Institutional Review Board Statement: The study was conducted according to the guide-lines of the Declaration of Helsinki, and approved by the Institutional Ethics Committee of the Leiden University Medical Center. The date of approval is September 6th 2018, and the approv-al code is G18.065/SH/gk.

Informed Consent Statement: Patient consent was waived due to the fact that this retro-spective cohort study was not obligatory for the Wet medisch-wetenschappelijk onderzoek met mensen (WMO; Medical Research Involving Human Subjects Act).

Data Availability Statement: The data presented in this study are available on request from the corresponding author. The data are not publicly available since the database consists of single center data and other studies are currently being conducted with this data.

Acknowledgments: This research did not receive any specific grant from funding agencies in the public, commercial, or not-for-profit sectors.

Conflicts of Interest: The authors declare no conflict of interest.

References

1. The ESMO/European Sarcoma Network Working Group. Bone sarcomas: ESMO Clinical Practice Guidelines for diagnosis, treatment and follow-up. *Ann. Oncol.* **2014**, *25*, iii113–iii123. [CrossRef] [PubMed]
2. Ferrari, S.; Bertoni, F.; Mercuri, M.; Picci, P.; Giacomini, S.; Longhi, A.; Bacci, G. Predictive factors of disease-free survival for non-metastatic osteosarcoma of the extremity: An analysis of 300 patients treated at the Rizzoli Institute. *Ann. Oncol.* **2001**, *12*, 1145–1150. [CrossRef]
3. Smeland, S.; Bielack, S.S.; Whelan, J.; Bernstein, M.; Hogendoorn, P.; Krailo, M.D.; Gorlick, R.; Janeway, K.A.; Ingleby, F.C.; Anninga, J.; et al. Survival and prognosis with osteosarcoma: Outcomes in more than 2000 patients in the EURAMOS-1 (European and American Osteosarcoma Study) cohort. *Eur. J. Cancer* **2019**, *109*, 36–50. [CrossRef] [PubMed]
4. Bielack, S.S.; Kempf-Bielack, B.; Delling, G.; Exner, G.U.; Flege, S.; Helmke, K.; Kotz, R.; Salzer-Kuntschik, M.; Werner, M.; Winkelmann, W.; et al. Prognostic Factors in High-Grade Osteosarcoma of the Extremities or Trunk: An Analysis of 1,702 Patients Treated on Neoadjuvant Cooperative Osteosarcoma Study Group Protocols. *J. Clin. Oncol.* **2002**, *20*, 776–790. [CrossRef] [PubMed]
5. Zhang, C.; Guo, X.; Xu, Y.; Han, X.; Cai, J.; Wang, X.; Wang, G. Lung metastases at the initial diagnosis of high-grade osteo-sarcoma: Prevalence, risk factors and prognostic factors. A large population-based cohort study. *Sao Paulo Med. J.* **2019**, *137*, 423–429. [CrossRef] [PubMed]
6. Mirabello, L.; Troisi, R.J.; Savage, S.A. Osteosarcoma incidence and survival rates from 1973 to 2004. *Cancer* **2009**, *115*, 1531–1543. [CrossRef] [PubMed]
7. Berner, K.; Johannesen, T.B.; Berner, A.; Haugland, H.K.; Bjerkehagen, B.; Bøhler, P.J.; Bruland, Ø.S. Time-trends on incidence and survival in a nationwide and unselected cohort of patients with skeletal osteosarcoma. *Acta Oncol.* **2014**, *54*, 25–33. [CrossRef]
8. Hagleitner, M.M.; Hoogerbrugge, P.M.; Van Der Graaf, W.T.; Flucke, U.; Schreuder, H.B.; Loo, D.M.M.W.T. Age as prognostic factor in patients with osteosarcoma. *Bone* **2011**, *49*, 1173–1177. [CrossRef]
9. Tsuda, Y.; Ogura, K.; Shinoda, Y.; Kobayashi, H.; Tanaka, S.; Kawai, A. The outcomes and prognostic factors in patients with osteosarcoma according to age: A Japanese nationwide study with focusing on the age differences. *BMC Cancer* **2018**, *18*, 614. [CrossRef]
10. Harting, M.T.; Lally, K.P.; Andrassy, R.J.; Vaporciyan, A.A.; Cox, C.S., Jr.; Hayes-Jordan, A.; Blakely, M.L. Age as a prognostic factor for patients with osteosarcoma: An analysis of 438 patients. *J. Cancer Res. Clin. Oncol.* **2009**, *136*, 561–570. [CrossRef]
11. Aljubran, A.; Griffin, A.; Pintilie, M.; Blackstein, M. Osteosarcoma in adolescents and adults: Survival analysis with and without lung metastases. *Ann. Oncol.* **2009**, *20*, 1136–1141. [CrossRef] [PubMed]
12. Glasser, D.B.; Lane, J.M.; Huvos, A.G.; Marcove, R.C.; Rosen, G. Survival, prognosis, and therapeutic response in osteogenic sarcoma. The memorial hospital experience. *Cancer* **1992**, *69*, 698–708. [CrossRef]
13. Hanafy, E.; Al Jabri, A.; GadElkarim, G.; Dasaq, A.; Nazim, F.; Al Pakrah, M. Tumor histopathological response to neoadjuvant chemotherapy in childhood solid malignancies: Is it still impressive? *J. Investig. Med.* **2017**, *66*, 289–297. [CrossRef] [PubMed]
14. Imura, Y.; Takenaka, S.; Kakunaga, S.; Nakai, T.; Wakamatsu, T.; Outani, H.; Tanaka, H.; Tamiya, H.; Oshima, K.; Hamada, K.; et al. Survival analysis of elderly patients with osteosarcoma. *Int. Orthop.* **2019**, *43*, 1741–1747. [CrossRef] [PubMed]
15. Ferrari, S.; Bielack, S.S.; Smeland, S.S.; Longhi, A.; Egerer, G.; Hall, K.S.; Donati, D.; Kevric, M.; Brosjö, O.; Comandone, A.; et al. EURO-B.O.S.S.: A European study on chemotherapy in bone-sarcoma patients aged over 40: Outcome in primary high-grade osteosarcoma. *Tumori J.* **2018**, *104*, 30–36. [CrossRef]
16. Ali, B.A.; Salman, M.; Ghanem, K.M.; Boulos, F.; Haidar, R.; Saghieh, S.; Akel, S.; Muwakkit, S.A.; El-Solh, H.; Saab, R.; et al. Clinical Prognostic Factors and Outcome in Pediatric Osteosarcoma: Effect of Delay in Local Control and Degree of Necrosis in a Multidisciplinary Setting in Lebanon. *J. Glob. Oncol.* **2019**, *5*, 1–8. [CrossRef]
17. Janeway, K.A.; Barkauskas, D.A.; Krailo, M.D.; Meyers, P.A.; Schwartz, C.L.; Ebb, D.H.; Seibel, N.L.; Grier, H.E.; Gorlick, R.; Marina, N. Outcome for adolescent and young adult patients with osteosarcoma. *Cancer* **2012**, *118*, 4597–4605. [CrossRef]
18. Nagano, A.; Ishimaru, D.; Nishimoto, Y.; Akiyama, H.; Kawai, A. Primary bone sarcomas in patients over 40 years of age: A retrospective study using data from the Bone Tumor Registry of Japan. *J. Orthop. Sci.* **2017**, *22*, 749–754. [CrossRef]
19. Amin, M.B.; Greene, F.L.; Edge, S.B.; Compton, C.C.; Gershenwald, J.E.; Brookland, R.K.; Meyer, L.; Gress, D.M.; Byrd, D.R.; Winchester, D.P. *AJCC Cancer Staging Manual*, 8th ed.; American Joint Commission on Cancer: Chicago, IL, USA, 2017.

20. Enneking, W.F.; Spanier, S.S.; Goodman, M.A. A system for the surgical staging of musculoskeletal sarcoma. *Clin. Orthop. Relat. Res.* **1980**, *153*, 106–120. [CrossRef]
21. Rosen, G.; Caparros, B.; Huvos, A.G.; Kosloff, C.; Nirenberg, A.; Cacavio, A.; Marcove, R.C.; Lane, J.M.; Mehta, B.; Urban, C. Preoperative chemotherapy for osteogenic sarcoma: Selection of postoperative adjuvant chemotherapy based on the re-sponse of the primary tumor to preoperative chemotherapy. *Cancer* **1982**, *49*, 1221–1230. [CrossRef]
22. Whelan, J.S.; Bielack, S.S.; Marina, N.; Smeland, S.; Jovic, G.; Hook, J.M.; Krailo, M.; Anninga, J.K.; Butterfass-Bahloul, T.; Böhling, T.; et al. EURAMOS-1, an international randomised study for osteosarcoma: Results from pre-randomisation treatment. *Ann. Oncol.* **2015**, *26*, 407–414. [CrossRef] [PubMed]
23. Barr, L.C.; Stotter, A.T.; A'Hern, R.P. Influence of local recurrence on survival: A controversy reviewed from the perspective of soft tissue sarcoma. *BJS* **1991**, *78*, 648–650. [CrossRef]
24. Van Houwelingen, H.C. Dynamic Prediction by Landmarking in Event History Analysis. *Scand. J. Stat.* **2007**, *34*, 70–85. [CrossRef]
25. Rubin, D.B. Multiple Imputation After 18+ Years. *J. Am. Stat. Assoc.* **1996**, *91*, 473. [CrossRef]
26. Li, P.; Stuart, E.A.; Allison, D.B. Multiple Imputation. *JAMA* **2015**, *314*, 1966–1967. [CrossRef] [PubMed]
27. Petrilli, A.S.; De Camargo, B.; Filho, V.O.; Bruniera, P.; Brunetto, A.L.; Jesus-Garcia, R.; Camargo, O.P.; Pena, W.; Péricles, P.; Davi, A.; et al. Results of the Brazilian Osteosarcoma Treatment Group Studies III and IV: Prognostic Factors and Impact on Survival. *J. Clin. Oncol.* **2006**, *24*, 1161–1168. [CrossRef]
28. Aggerholm-Pedersen, N.; Maretty-Nielsen, K.; Keller, J.; Baerentzen, S.; Safwat, A. Comorbidity in Adult Bone Sarcoma Patients: A Population-Based Cohort Study. *Sarcoma* **2014**, *2014*, 1–9. [CrossRef] [PubMed]
29. Weeden, S.; Grimer, R.; Cannon, S.; Taminiau, A.; Uscinska, B. The effect of local recurrence on survival in resected osteosarcoma. *Eur. J. Cancer* **2001**, *37*, 39–46. [CrossRef]
30. Hauben, E.; Weeden, S.; Pringle, J.; Van Marck, E.; Hogendoorn, P.C. Does the histological subtype of high-grade central osteosarcoma influence the response to treatment with chemotherapy and does it affect overall survival? A study on 570 patients of two consecutive trials of the European Osteosarcoma Intergroup. *Eur. J. Cancer* **2002**, *38*, 1218–1225. [CrossRef]
31. Mankin, H.J.; Hornicek, F.J.; Rosenberg, A.E.; Harmon, D.C.; Gebhardt, M.C. Survival Data for 648 Patients with Osteosarcoma Treated at One Institution. *Clin. Orthop. Relat. Res.* **2004**, *429*, 286–291. [CrossRef]
32. Van Maldegem, A.M.; Bhosale, A.; Gelderblom, H.; Hogendoorn, P.C.; Hassan, A.B. Comprehensive analysis of published phase I/II clinical trials between 1990-2010 in osteosarcoma and Ewing sarcoma confirms limited outcomes and need for translational investment. *Clin. Sarcoma Res.* **2012**, *2*, 5. [CrossRef] [PubMed]
33. Lagmay, J.P.; Krailo, M.D.; Dang, H.; Kim, A.; Hawkins, D.S.; Beaty, O.; Widemann, B.C.; Zwerdling, T.; Bomgaars, L.; Langevin, A.-M.; et al. Outcome of Patients With Recurrent Osteosarcoma Enrolled in Seven Phase II Trials Through Children's Cancer Group, Pediatric Oncology Group, and Children's Oncology Group: Learning From the Past to Move Forward. *J. Clin. Oncol.* **2016**, *34*, 3031–3038. [CrossRef] [PubMed]
34. Omer, N.; Le Deley, M.-C.; Piperno-Neumann, S.; Marec-Berard, P.; Italiano, A.; Corradini, N.; Bellera, C.; Brugières, L.; Gaspar, N. Phase-II trials in osteosarcoma recurrences: A systematic review of past experience. *Eur. J. Cancer* **2017**, *75*, 98–108. [CrossRef] [PubMed]
35. Roberts, R.D.; Lizardo, M.M.; Reed, D.R.; Hingorani, P.; Glover, J.; Allen-Rhoades, W.; Fan, T.; Khanna, C.; Sweet-Cordero, E.A.; Cash, T.; et al. Provocative questions in osteosarcoma basic and translational biology: A report from the Children's Oncology Group. *Cancer* **2019**, *125*, 3514–3525. [CrossRef]
36. Tirtei, E.; Cereda, M.; De Luna, E.; Quarello, P.; Asaftei, S.D.; Fagioli, F. Omic approaches to pediatric bone sarcomas. *Pediatr. Blood Cancer* **2019**, *67*, e28072. [CrossRef]

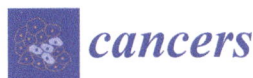

Article

Treatment of Angiosarcoma with Pazopanib and Paclitaxel: Results of the EVA (Evaluation of Votrient® in Angiosarcoma) Phase II Trial of the German Interdisciplinary Sarcoma Group (GISG-06)

Daniel Pink [1,2,*,†], Dimosthenis Andreou [3,†], Sebastian Bauer [4], Thomas Brodowicz [5], Bernd Kasper [6], Peter Reichardt [7], Stephan Richter [8], Lars H. Lindner [9], Joanna Szkandera [10], Viktor Grünwald [4,11], Maxim Kebenko [12], Marietta Kirchner [13] and Peter Hohenberger [14]

1. Department of Hematology, Oncology and Palliative Medicine, Helios Hospital Bad Saarow, Sarcoma Center Berlin-Brandenburg, 15526 Bad Saarow, Germany
2. Department of Internal Medicine C, University Hospital Greifswald, 17475 Greifswald, Germany
3. Division of Orthopedic Oncology and Sarcoma Surgery, Helios Hospital Bad Saarow, Sarcoma Center Berlin-Brandenburg, 15526 Bad Saarow, Germany; dimosthenis.andreou@helios-gesundheit.de
4. Department of Medical Oncology, University Hospital Essen, Sarcoma Center, University of Duisburg-Essen, 45147 Essen, Germany; sebastian.bauer@uk-essen.de (S.B.); viktor.gruenwald@uk-essen.de (V.G.)
5. Department of Interal Medicine 1/Oncology, Medical University Vienna-General Hospital, 1090 Vienna, Austria; thomas.brodowicz@meduniwien.ac.at
6. Interdisciplinary Tumor Center, Sarcoma Unit, University Medical Center Mannheim, University of Heidelberg, 68167 Mannheim, Germany; bernd.kasper@medma.uni-heidelberg.de
7. Department of Oncology and Palliative Medicine, Helios Hospital Berlin-Buch, Sarcoma Center Berlin-Brandenburg, 13125 Berlin, Germany; peter.reichardt@helios-gesundheit.de
8. Department of Internal Medicine I, University Hospital Carl Gustav Carus, Technical University Dresden, 01307 Dresden, Germany; stephan.richter@uniklinikum-dresden.de
9. Department of Medicine III, University Hospital Munich, Ludwig Maximilians University, 81377 Munich, Germany; lars.lindner@med.uni-muenchen.de
10. Clinical Division of Oncology, Department of Medicine, Medical University of Graz, 8036 Graz, Austria; joanna.szkandera@medunigraz.at
11. Department of Hematology, Hemostasis and Oncology, Hannover Medical School, 30625 Hannover, Germany
12. Department of Hematology and Oncology, University Hospital Schleswig-Holstein, 23538 Lübeck, Germany; maxim.kebenko@uksh.de
13. Institute of Medical Biometry and Informatics, University of Heidelberg, 69120 Heidelberg, Germany; kirchner@imbi.uni-heidelberg.de
14. Division of Surgical Oncology and Thoracic Surgery, University Medical Center Mannheim, University of Heidelberg, 68167 Mannheim, Germany; peter.hohenberger@umm.de
* Correspondence: daniel.pink@helios-gesundheit.de; Tel.: +49-33631-3527
† These authors share the first authorship.

Citation: Pink, D.; Andreou, D.; Bauer, S.; Brodowicz, T.; Kasper, B.; Reichardt, P.; Richter, S.; Lindner, L.H.; Szkandera, J.; Grünwald, V.; et al. Treatment of Angiosarcoma with Pazopanib and Paclitaxel: Results of the EVA (Evaluation of Votrient® in Angiosarcoma) Phase II Trial of the German Interdisciplinary Sarcoma Group (GISG-06). *Cancers* **2021**, *13*, 1223. https://doi.org/10.3390/cancers13061223

Academic Editors: Maurizio D'Incalci and Mohammed M. Milhem

Received: 14 February 2021
Accepted: 8 March 2021
Published: 11 March 2021

Publisher's Note: MDPI stays neutral with regard to jurisdictional claims in published maps and institutional affiliations.

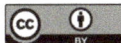

Copyright: © 2021 by the authors. Licensee MDPI, Basel, Switzerland. This article is an open access article distributed under the terms and conditions of the Creative Commons Attribution (CC BY) license (https:// creativecommons.org/licenses/by/ 4.0/).

Simple Summary: There are very few systemic treatment options for patients with advanced angiosarcomas. We therefore examined whether combined treatment with paclitaxel and pazopanib was active and well tolerated. However, we did not meet a preplanned interim target of 6/14 patients without progression of the disease at 6 months, after which finding we stopped recruitment, having enrolled a total of 26 patients. Of the patients enrolled, 46% were progression-free at 6 months. Two patients showed a complete and seven patients a partial tumor response to treatment. The progression-free survival of patients with superficial tumors was significantly longer compared to the patients with visceral tumors. A total of 10 drug-related serious adverse effects were reported in 5 patients, including a fatal hepatic failure. The results in patients with superficial tumors appear promising. Future studies should evaluate the safety and efficacy of vascular endothelial growth factor receptor (VEGFR) and immune checkpoint inhibitors with or without paclitaxel in a randomized, multiarm setting.

Abstract: We aimed to evaluate the efficacy and toxicity of paclitaxel combined with pazopanib in advanced angiosarcoma (AS). The primary end point was progression-free survival (PFS) rate at six months (PFSR6). Planned accrual was 44 patients in order to detect a PFSR6 of >55%, with an interim futility analysis of the first 14 patients. The study did not meet its predetermined interim target of 6/14 patients progression-free at 6 months. At the time of this finding, 26 patients had been enrolled between July 2014 and April 2016, resulting in an overrunning of 12 patients. After a median follow-up of 9.5 (IQR 7.7–15.4) months, PFSR6 amounted to 46%. Two patients had a complete and seven patients a partial response. Patients with superficial AS had a significantly higher PFSR6 (61% vs. 13%, $p = 0.0247$) and PFS (11.3 vs. 2.7 months, $p < 0.0001$) compared to patients with visceral AS. The median overall survival in the entire cohort was 21.6 months. A total of 10 drug-related serious adverse effects were reported in 5 patients, including a fatal hepatic failure. Although our study did not meet its primary endpoint, the median PFS of 11.6 months in patients with superficial AS appears to be promising. Taking recent reports into consideration, future studies should evaluate the safety and efficacy of VEGFR and immune checkpoint inhibitors with or without paclitaxel in a randomized, multiarm setting.

Keywords: angiosarcoma; paclitaxel; pazopanib; efficacy; toxicity; progression-free survival

1. Introduction

Angiosarcomas (AS) are very rare malignant mesenchymal tumors with morphological and functional features resembling endothelial cells [1]. They account for ca. 2% of all soft tissue sarcomas, with an estimated incidence of 3/1,000,000/year [2,3]. Approximately two-thirds of AS affect the skin, most commonly of the head and neck region, but they can develop anywhere in the body [4,5]. While most tumors arise spontaneously, some AS are associated with endogenous and exogenous risk factors, mainly previous radiotherapy and chronic lymphedema [4]. Their prognosis is worse compared to most soft tissue sarcomas, with reported 5-year overall survival (OS) probabilities of 35–40% for patients with localized tumors treated with curative intent and a median survival of 8–12 months for patients with metastases [4]. The course of the disease appears to be influenced by the site of origin, with visceral AS in particular showing a poorer outcome, although it remains unclear whether this is a result of differences in tumor biology or clinical presentation [4,5].

There are very few established systemic treatment options for patients with advanced AS [6]. The weekly administration of paclitaxel, a mitotic inhibitor with additional antiangiogenic activity, was evaluated in a prospective phase II trial and achieved a 6-month progression-free survival (PFS) rate of 24% and a median OS of 8.3 months [2]. Furthermore, a potential role of inhibitors of vascular endothelial growth factor receptor (VEGFR) in the treatment of advanced AS has been suggested based on the results of in vitro studies demonstrating that AS show a distinct up-regulation of vascular-specific receptor tyrosine kinases [4,7]. However, treatment with sorafenib alone, a VEGFR and RAS tyrosine kinase inhibitor (TKI), was associated with only limited antitumor activity in pretreated AS patients and a short duration of tumor control in a phase II study from the French Sarcoma Group [8]. Pazopanib, on the other hand, has demonstrated promising results in pretreated metastatic soft tissue sarcoma [9].

We decided to evaluate the efficacy and toxicity of paclitaxel combined with pazopanib and therefore conducted a multicenter open-label phase II trial in patients with advanced AS.

2. Materials and Methods

2.1. Study Population

Patients were eligible if they were 18 years of age or older and had a histologically confirmed, unresectable, locally advanced or metastatic primary or secondary AS with a documented progression in the last 6 months prior to screening. They were required to have adequate bone marrow, cardiac, gastrointestinal, liver and renal functions, an Eastern Cooperative Oncology Group (ECOG) performance status score of ≤2 and an estimated life expectancy of >3 months. At least one measurable skin lesion or one target lesion measurable with computed tomography (CT) scans or magnetic resonance imaging (MRI) was required as per the Response Evaluation Criteria in Solid Tumors (RECIST) 1.1 [10]. Women of childbearing potential and sexually active men were required to agree to the use of adequate contraception throughout the study and for 30 days after the last dose of study drug.

Exclusion criteria included: active treatment for malignant disease other than AS; prior treatment with taxanes in the last 12 months prior to study entry; any chemotherapy or radiotherapy within 14 days before start of study medication; major surgery or trauma within 28 days prior to first dose and/or presence of any nonhealing wound, fracture, ulcer or uncontrolled infection; history or clinical evidence of central nervous system metastases or leptomeningeal sarcomatosis; evidence of active bleeding or bleeding diathesis, as well as known endobronchial lesions and/or lesions infiltrating major pulmonary vessels; pregnant or breastfeeding women.

2.2. Study Design, Treatment and Outcomes

This phase II trial (EudraCT number:2012-005846-39, ClinicalTrials.gov Identifier: NCT02212015) was a multicenter, open-label, prospective, single-arm study conducted at 9 sites in 2 countries. Paclitaxel was administered at a dose of 70 mg/m^2 as a 2-h intravenous infusion on days 1, 8 and 15 of a 28-day treatment cycle, after intravenous premedication with dexamethasone, diphenhydramine and cimetidine. Standard antiemetics (mainly granisetron and ondansetron) were also recommended prior to paclitaxel administration. Pazopanib was concurrently administered at a daily dose of 800 mg to be taken orally without food at least one hour before or two hours after a meal. Patients received a total of 6 cycles of paclitaxel, unless disease progression or limiting toxicity—especially peripheral neuropathy grade 2 or higher—occurred. Pazopanib was continued beyond the 6 cycles of paclitaxel treatment, until disease progression or limiting toxicities occurred. In case of side effects under combination treatment attributable to pazopanib, paclitaxel was continued as monotherapy until the end of the 6th cycle, unless patients developed disease progression or limiting toxicities under monotherapy. The protocol specified criteria for dose reductions and delays in case of limiting toxicities.

The objective of this trial was to evaluate efficacy and safety of the experimental treatment given by a combination of pazopanib with paclitaxel for patients with advanced or metastatic angiosarcoma (AS). The primary study endpoint was PFS rate at 6 months after start of study treatment, evaluated on a predefined set of target and nontarget lesions based on the RECIST.1.1 criteria. Radiographical assessments were recommended every 8 weeks or sooner, when clinically indicated, by CT or MRI scans of the chest, abdomen, and all other tumor localizations. The diameter of skin lesions was measured clinically and documented with photographs in the patient files. The evaluation of the PFS rate at 6 months had to take place at 182 days ± 32 days after the beginning of treatment. Patients who had no available evaluation at this time and no documented CR, PR, or SD at a later point, were classified per-protocol as having PD for the purposes of the primary endpoint—a definition which led to a divergence between PFS rate at 6 months and median PFS.

Secondary endpoints were OS defined as start of therapy until death, best overall response (BOR), and toxicity according to the National Cancer Institute Common Terminology Criteria for Adverse Events (CTCAE) version 4.0. The endpoint PFS rate at 3 months was added to the statistical analysis plan prior to the final study report, in order to improve the comparability of the trial's results to previous studies. PFS was defined as start of therapy until first PD or death, whatever came first. Two subgroup analyses were planned in the protocol for primary and secondary endpoints: superficial vs. visceral and primary vs. secondary AS.

2.3. Sample Size

The primary statistical analysis addressed the question whether the 6-month PFS rate was higher than 35%. The sample size was calculated to detect a 6-month PFS rate of >55%, defined as a clinically relevant success, at a one-sided significance level of $\alpha = 0.05$

with a power of ≥80%. The study used Simon's two-stage optimal design with a planned interim futility analysis after enrolment of the first 14 patients and a maximal sample size of 44 patients in case of proceeding to the second stage. The second stage would have been completed, if at least 6 of the first 14 patients were progression-free and alive (defined as success) at 6 months. According to the study protocol, recruitment was not stopped, however it was specified that additional patients would not be included in the interim analysis. At the time of the interim analysis, a total of 26 patients had already been enrolled, resulting in an overrunning of 12 patients. The study was closed on 31 December 2019 without any further enrolment of patients for futility reasons.

2.4. Statistical Analysis

Baseline demographics were summarized by median with interquartile range (IQR) or frequencies in the full analysis set (FAS) of all 26 patients. The analysis of the primary endpoint was conducted at the interim analysis for the first 14 patients, as specified by the study protocol (PP set) and for all 26 patients enrolled as FAS. To guarantee the defined significance level of $\alpha = 0.05$ in the FAS, the method to handle overrunning by Engler and Kieser was applied [11], leading to the following amendment: if $\leq 17/26$ successes were observed, the trial would be stopped with the conclusion that the study treatment should not be further investigated. If $\geq 18/26$ successes were observed, the trial would be stopped with the conclusion that the study treatment should be further investigated in this histology. The point estimate for PFS rate at 6 month with 90% exact Clopper-Person confidence intervals (CI), in line with a one-sided $\alpha = 0.05$, were provided for the PP set and the FAS.

All secondary endpoints were analyzed in the FAS with all $n = 26$ patients included after the end of study. The point estimate for PFS rate at 3 months with 95% exact Clopper-Person CI was provided. Differences in proportions between subgroups were assessed by Barnard's exact test due to the small sample size. Analyses of OS and PFS were performed with the Kaplan–Meier method and survival distributions between subgroups were compared with the log-rank test. Descriptive statistics were used for the analysis of toxicities and BOR, while differences in proportions was assessed by exact Pearson's chi-square test. Reported p-values for the secondary endpoints are interpreted descriptively and a p-value < 0.05 is considered statistically significant. All analyses were performed in SAS® System 9.4 (SAS Inc., Cary, NC, USA).

3. Results

3.1. Baseline Demographics

Between July 2014 and April 2016, 26 AS patients were enrolled in this study. Baseline demographics are presented in Table 1. The median age at enrollment amounted to 60.5 (IQR, 48–70) years. The median time between AS diagnosis and start of treatment in this trial was 6 (IQR, 1–43) months. The majority of the patients were female ($n = 23$), had an ECOG performance status score of 0 ($n = 20$) and a superficial AS primary ($n = 18$). The rate of primary versus secondary AS was exactly balanced. Of the secondary AS, eight tumors arose in irradiated fields of previous malignancies. 69% of patients had a cutaneous angiosarcoma manifestation, 31% of patients had a visceral manifestation. Distant metastases were observed in 21 patients, the majority of which were localized in the liver ($n = 9$), the bones ($n = 7$) and the lungs ($n = 6$). Only 3 patients (12%) had received systemic chemotherapy for AS prior to study enrollment.

Table 1. Baseline demographics and disease characteristics.

Variable	n	%
Study cohort	26	100%
Sex		
Female	23	88%
Male	3	12%
ECOG performance status score		
0	20	77%
1	5	19%
Not available	1	4%
Tumor site		
Superficial AS	18	69%
Visceral AS	8	31%
Tumor origin		
Primary AS	13	50%
Secondary AS	13	50%
Disease status at presentation		
Locally advanced	5	19%
Metastatic	21	81%
Liver	9	35%
Bone	7	27%
Lung	6	23%
Lymph nodes	3	12%
Other	9	35%
Prior treatments		
Surgery	14	54%
Radiotherapy	3	12%
Chemotherapy	3	12%
No prior treatments	11	42%

ECOG, Eastern Cooperative Oncology Group; AS, angiosarcoma.

3.2. Safety and Toxicity

A total of 127 cycles of paclitaxel concurrent to pazopanib were administered. The median number of cycles amounted to 6 (IQR, 4–6 cycles), with a median of 17 (IQR, 10–18) infusions. Twenty-four patients (92%) received at least 2 cycles. Paclitaxel was discontinued due to toxicity in 3 patients (12%; 1× liver toxicity, 1× allergic reaction, 1× polyneuropathy). In 23 patients with full data available, pazopanib was administered for a median of 22 (IQR, 9–35) weeks, and was discontinued due to toxicity or withdrawal of consent in 7 patients (35%; 3× liver toxicity, 2× withdrawal of consent, 1× pneumothorax, 1× poor tolerance).

Table 2 lists all related and unrelated adverse events with a toxicity grade ≥ 3. A total of 10 drug-related serious adverse effects were reported in 5 patients (19%). These events were increased hepatic enzymes ($n = 3$), hepatic failure, pneumothorax, dehydration, reduced general condition, gastrointestinal bleeding, fever of unknown origin and severe neutropenia. The hepatic failure occurred in a patient with a visceral secondary AS of the liver, a medical history of myelodysplastic syndrome, and previous whole body irradiation and allogenic stem cell transplantation 2 days after of start of treatment with pazopanib and 1 application of paclitaxel. It was fatal and related to the study treatment.

3.3. Efficacy

The primary endpoint of PFS rate at 6 months amounted to 29% (90% CI, 10–54%) in the PP set with 14 patients and to 46% (90% CI, 29–64%) in the FAS with 26 patients. The following results are reported for the FAS.

The median follow-up was 9.5 (IQR 7.7–15.4) months. The 3-month PFS rate was 62% (95%CI, 41–80%). Patients with superficial AS had a significantly higher PFS rate at 6 months of 61% (95% CI, 35.8–82.7%), compared to 13% (95% CI, 3.2–52.7%) for patients with visceral AS ($p = 0.0247$).

There was no difference in the 6-months PFS between primary and secondary AS with 46% each. The median PFS amounted to 8 (95% CI, 4.6–11.3) months. Patients with superficial AS had a significantly higher median PFS of 11.3 (95% CI, 5.5–21.1) months, compared to patients with visceral AS (2.7 (95% CI 1.2–5.5) months; $p < 0.0001$, Figure 1). There were no statistically significant differences in median PFS between patients with primary AS of 5.5 months (95% CI 3.9–12.5) and secondary AS of 9.5 months (95% CI 4.6–21.1; $p = 0.32$).

Table 2. All adverse events (AE) grade ≥3.

Toxicity	Grade III/IV		Grade V	
	AE	Affected Patients (%)	AE	Affected Patients (%)
Increased alanine aminotransferase	11	3 (12%)	0	0 (0%)
Increased aspartate aminotransferase	3	1 (4%)	0	0 (0%)
Allergic reaction	1	1 (4%)	0	0 (0%)
Reduced general condition	2	2 (8%)	0	0 (0%)
Anemia	1	1 (4%)	0	0 (0%)
Arterial hypertension	7	2 (8%)	0	0 (0%)
Dehydration	2	1 (4%)	0	0 (0%)
Increased gamma-glutamyl transferase	6	1 (4%)	0	0 (0%)
Hepatic failure	0	0	1	1 (4%)
Anorexia	1	1 (4%)	0	0 (0%)
Catheter-related infection	1	1 (4%)	0	0 (0%)
Leukopenia	20	3 (12%)	0	0 (0%)
Fatigue	5	2 (8%)	0	0 (0%)
Neutropenia	16	3 (12%)	0	0 (0%)
Pneumothorax	1	1 (4%)	0	0 (0%)
Pleuritic pain	1	1 (4%)	0	0 (0%)
Back pain	5	2 (8%)	0	0 (0%)

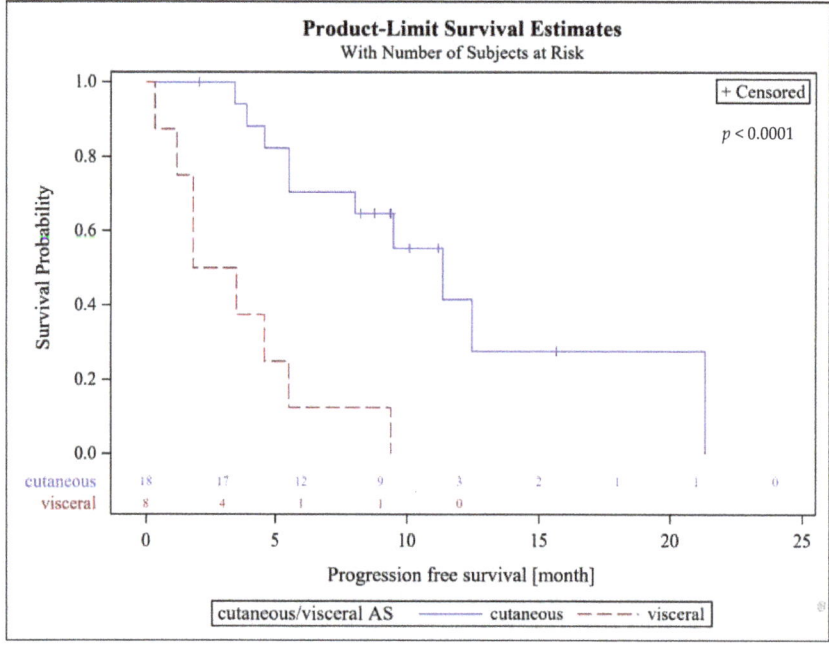

Figure 1. Progression free survival probability of patients with superficial (cutaneous) and visceral AS.

The BOR could be evaluated in all but one patient, who developed a fatal hepatic failure prior to first assessment of response. Two patients (8%) presented with CR after 4 and 5 months, seven patients (27%) had a PR after 5 to 7 months, 6 patients (23%) presented with SD and 10 patients (38%) developed progressive disease (PD). The BOR for the subgroups superficial vs. visceral and primary vs. secondary AS are presented at Table 3.

Table 3. Best overall response in absolute and relative (%) frequencies for subgroup analyses.

Best Overall Response (BOR)	Superficial AS, $n = 18$	Visceral AS, $n = 8$
CR	2 (11%)	0 (0%)
PR	6 (34%)	1 (12.5%)
SD	4 (22%)	2 (25%)
PD	6 (33%)	4 (50%)
n.e.	0 (0%)	1 (12.5%)
Best Overall Response (BOR)	Primary AS, $n = 13$	Secondary AS, $n = 13$
CR	0 (0%)	2 (15%)
PR	5 (38.5%)	2 (15%)
SD	3 (23%)	3 (23%)
PD	5 (38.5%)	5 (39%)
n.e.	0 (0%)	1 (8%)

CR, complete response; PR, partial response; SD, stable disease; PD, progressive disease; n.e., not evaluated.

Eight deaths were observed during the follow-up period. The median OS in the entire cohort was 21.6 (95% CI, 20.5—not estimable) months. There were no statistically significant differences in median OS between patients with superficial (21.6 (95% CI, 10–21.6) months) and visceral AS (20.5 (95% CI, 2.8–not estimable) months; $p = 0.752$), or between patients with primary (20.5 (95% CI, 10–not estimable) months) and secondary AS (21.6 (95% CI not estimable) months; $p = 0.621$).

4. Discussion

The prognosis of patients with advanced AS is poor and only a few active systemic treatment options are available [6]. Our prospective phase II trial evaluating the efficacy and toxicity of paclitaxel combined with pazopanib did not meet its predetermined interim target of 6/14 patients progression-free at 6 months. However, at the time of this finding 26 patients had already been enrolled in the study, as a recruitment stop after completion of Simon's stage I was not stipulated in the study protocol. The resulting overrunning necessitated an amendment of the statistical analysis plan. After a long evaluation of the feasibility of possible amendments, the study committee had to decide to terminate the trial for futility reasons at the end of 2019, as it could not be expected to meet its primary endpoint even with a modest increase of the recruitment target.

A post hoc in-depth review of the study protocol and the collected data revealed limitations of the trial design. The target group of the study was superficial AS of the extremities and scalp and secondary AS. The interim analysis had been introduced primarily under safety and toxicity aspects and the study committee expected that these patients would easily clear the threshold of 6/14 successes after 6 months. This was the reason why a recruitment stop after the first stage of the study was not included in the protocol. However, the protocol inclusion criteria did not restrict recruitment to patients with superficial AS only and several of the first 14 patients had a visceral AS, a subgroup known to have a considerably worse prognosis [4,5]. Furthermore, while previous AS studies had defined a PFS rate at 6 months of 30% [2] or 40% [12] as clinically relevant, our protocol set the bar at 55%—again based on the data on superficial AS. Thus, the early recruitment of a nonintended group of patients carrying a worse prognosis compromised the trial and led to early discontinuation for futility reasons despite the fact that the PFS rate at 6 months for the whole cohort was 46%.

It is therefore difficult to draw definitive conclusions on the role of combined paclitaxel and pazopanib treatment in AS patients. However, our results with a 6-months PFS rate in the superficial AS group of 61.1% and a median PFS of 11.6 months (Figure 1) compare favorably with the data of the EORTC STBSG group reporting a 9.5 months PFS for taxane-based therapy in superficial AS and 7 months for the overall group.

A previous phase-II trial (ANGIOTAX [2]) assessed the efficacy and toxicity of weekly paclitaxel in patients with advanced AS including visceral sites in 26% of the patients and demonstrated a median PFS of 4 months. The nonprogression rate was 74% at 2 months and 24% at 6 months. The authors concluded that the treatment regimen constitutes a good comparator for further clinical trials [2]. The follow-up study (ANGIOTAX-PLUS) was designed as a randomized, phase-II trial aiming to assess the efficacy and safety of adding bevacizumab (BWP) to weekly paclitaxel (WP) in advanced AS [12]. The median PFS amounted to 6.6 months for both arms, and there were no differences in median OS either, so that the authors concluded that both treatment arms were active but that the study results did not support additional clinical investigation of the BWP regime in patients with advanced AS [12].

Taking the results of these studies into consideration, the median PFS of 8 months observed in our trial suggests that the combination of paclitaxel with pazopanib is an active treatment of advanced AS, but it remains unclear whether the combined treatment offers advantages compared to single-agent treatment with paclitaxel. Conflicting results regarding the possible advantages of the paclitaxel/pazopanib combination compared to paclitaxel alone have previously been reported for ovarian cancer as well, with one small randomized phase-II trial demonstrating a better outcome for patients treatment with the combined regimen [13], while another small randomized phase-II trial later reported no benefit for the combined regimen [14].

An interesting finding of our analysis was that patients with superficial AS had a significantly higher median PFS of 11.3 months vs. 2.7 months for patients with visceral AS. These results confirm the findings of the ANGIOTAX-PLUS study, demonstrating a median PFS of 8 months in patients with superficial AS vs. 3.6 months in patients with visceral AS for both arms combined [12]. This did not, however, translate into significant differences in median OS between patients with superficial and visceral AS, which might be attributed to effective further treatments after progression, which were not documented in our trial. Taking these findings into consideration, we believe that future clinical trials on AS should stratify patients according to the localization of their primary tumor and perform separate analyses of the results of patients with superficial and visceral AS.

Interestingly, while the ANGIOTAX-PLUS study did not perform subgroup analyses for median OS, it did report a median OS of 19.5 months for the WP regimen, which was considerably longer compared to a median OS of 8 months for the WP regimen in the ANGIOTAX study [2,12]. This finding underlines the critical role of randomization using a concurrent internal control arm in rare diseases [12], and illustrates why it is not prudent to compare the PFS and OS rates achieved in our trial with those reported for previous studies.

In terms of toxicity of the combined paclitaxel and pazopanib regimen, only 19% of the patients in our trial developed serious adverse effects, compared to 32% of the patients treated with BWP in the ANGIOTAX-PLUS study developing drug-related serious adverse effects and no patients treated with WP [12]. Furthermore, we were able to administer slightly more paclitaxel infusions (median, 17), compared to the WP arm (median, 16) and the BWP arm (median, 14) of the ANGIOTAX-PLUS study [12]. The duration of treatment with pazopanib in our study was also slightly longer compared to the duration of bevacizumab treatment in the ANGIOTAX-PLUS study (22 vs. 18 weeks) [12]. Treatment delays and treatment discontinuation due to toxicity are important aspects of phase-II trials, as PFS and OS often depend on the dose intensity and cumulative dose achieved.

5. Conclusions

In conclusion, our analysis does not allow any definitive conclusions on the efficacy of combined treatment of paclitaxel and pazopanib in patients with advanced AS, although the median PFS of 11.6 months in patients with superficial AS in our study appears to be promising. On the other hand, recent case series have suggested that immune checkpoint inhibitors may be active in the treatment of advanced AS [15], while the combination of VEGFR and checkpoint inhibitors, already established in the treatment of several solid tumors, also appears to be a promising treatment option in soft tissue sarcoma patients in general [16]. We therefore believe that future studies should evaluate the safety and efficacy of VEGFR and immune checkpoint inhibitors with or without paclitaxel in a randomized, multiarm setting, as is the case in the currently recruiting NCT04339738 trial [17].

Author Contributions: Conceptualization: D.P., P.R. and P.H.; methodology: D.P., P.R., M.K. (Marietta Kirchner), and P.H.; software: M.K. (Marietta Kirchner); validation: D.P., D.A., M.K. (Marietta Kirchner), and P.H.; formal analysis: D.P., D.A., M.K. (Marietta Kirchner), and P.H.; investigation: D.P., S.B., T.B., B.K., P.R., S.R., L.H.L., J.S., V.G., M.K. (Maxim Kebenko), and P.H.; resources: D.P., S.B., T.B., B.K., P.R., S.R., L.H.L., J.S., V.G., M.K. (Maxim Kebenko), and P.H.; data curation: D.P., D.A., M.K. (Marietta Kirchner), and P.H.; writing—original draft preparation: D.P., D.A., M.K. (Marietta Kirchner), P.H.; writing—review and editing: D.P., D.A., S.B., T.B., B.K., P.R., S.R., L.H.L., J.S., V.G., M.K. (Maxim Kebenko), M.K. (Marietta Kirchner), and P.H.; visualization: D.P., D.A., M.K. (Marietta Kirchner), and P.H.; supervision: D.P. and P.H.; project administration: D.P. and P.H.; funding acquisition: D.P., P.H. All authors have read and agreed to the published version of the manuscript.

Funding: This research was funded by the German Interdisciplinary Sarcoma Group (GISG) through a grant by GSK (later Novartis). The funding source had no role in the design and conduct of the study; the collection, management, analysis, and interpretation of the data; the preparation, review, or approval of the manuscript; and decision to submit the manuscript for publication.

Institutional Review Board Statement: The study was conducted according to the guidelines of the Declaration of Helsinki and approved by the Ethics Committee II of the Medical Faculty Mannheim, University of Heidelberg (Reference #2012-005846-39; approval date: 22 July 2014).

Informed Consent Statement: Informed consent was obtained from all subjects involved in the study.

Data Availability Statement: The data presented in this study are available on request from the corresponding author. The data are not publicly available, in accordance with the study protocol.

Acknowledgments: We thank the patients and their families who participated in the EVA trial and the physicians, nurses, data managers, and support staff of the collaborating centers. We further thank Monika Sommer and Marion Bergmann, of the Medical Faculty Mannheim of the University Heidelberg for data management and study coordination assistance.

Conflicts of Interest: D.P. reports institutional fees from Roche (advisory role), Lilly (advisory role), PharmaMar (advisory role, lecture fee), Blueprint Medicines (lecture fee) and research grants from Lilly, PharmaMar, Novartis, Clinigen, BMS, EUSA Pharma, Roche. S.B. reports personal fees from Deciphera, grants from Incyte, grants and personal fees from Blueprint Medicines, personal fees from Lilly, grants and personal fees from Novartis, personal fees from Daichii-Sankyo, personal fees from Plexxikon, personal fees from Exelixis, personal fees from Bayer, and others from Pfizer, during the course of the study; personal fees from PharmaMar, personal fees from Lilly, personal fees from Roche, personal fees from GSK, outside the submitted work. T.B. reports personal fees from Roche (lecture fee), personal fees from Amgen (lecture fee, advisory board), personal fees from Bayer (lecture fee, advisory board), personal fees from Novartis (lecture fee, advisory board), personal fees from PharmaMar (lecture fee, advisory board), personal fees from Eisai (lecture fee, advisory board), personal fees from Eli Lilly (lecture fee, advisory board), outside the submitted work. V.G.: reports grants, personal fees and nonfinancial support from Astra Zeneca, grants, personal fees and nonfinancial support from Bristol-Myers Squibb, personal fees from MSD Sharp & Dohme, grants, personal fees and nonfinancial support from Ipsen, personal fees from Merck Serono, grants, personal fees and nonfinancial support from Pfizer, personal fees from EUSAPharm, personal fees from Novartis, personal fees from Eisai; grants and nonfinancial support from Astra Zeneca, grants, personal fees and nonfinancial support from Bristol-Myers Squibb, personal fees and nonfinancial support from Bayer, grants and personal fees from MSD Sharp & Dohme, personal fees from Roche, personal fees from Janssen-Cilag, personal fees from Asklepios Clinic, personal fees from Diakonie Clinic, personal fees from Lilly, personal fees from PharmaMar, personal fees from Dortmund Hospital, personal fees from Clinic of Oldenburg, personal fees from Onkowissen, grants from Novartis, personal fees from Janssen-Cilag, grants and personal fees from MSD Sharp & Dohme.

P.R. received honoraria from Bayer, Clinigen, BMS, Roche, MSD, and Deciphera for a position on advisory boards and received honoraria for speaking at symposia from Novartis, Pfizer, PharmaMar, Lilly, and Amgen. The remaining authors (D.A., B.K., S.R., L.H.L., J.S., M.K. (Maxim Kebenko), M.K. (Marietta Kirchner), P.H.) have no conflicts of interest to declare.

References

1. Fletcher, C.; Bridge, J.; Hogendoorn, P.; Mertens, F. *WHO Classification of Tumours of Soft Tissue and Bone*; International Agency for Research on Cancer: Lyon, France, 2013; p. 468.
2. Penel, N.; Bui, B.N.; Bay, J.-O.; Cupissol, D.; Ray-Coquard, I.; Piperno-Neumann, S.; Kerbrat, P.; Fournier, C.; Taieb, S.; Jimenez, M.; et al. Phase II Trial of Weekly Paclitaxel for Unresectable Angiosarcoma: The ANGIOTAX Study. *J. Clin. Oncol.* **2008**, *26*, 5269–5274. [CrossRef] [PubMed]
3. Ressing, M.; Wardelmann, E.; Hohenberger, P.; Jakob, J.; Kasper, B.; Emrich, K.; Eberle, A.; Blettner, M.; Zeissig, S.R. Strengthening health data on a rare and heterogeneous disease: Sarcoma incidence and histological subtypes in Germany. *BMC Public Health* **2018**, *18*, 1–11. [CrossRef]
4. Penel, N.; Marréaud, S.; Robin, Y.-M.; Hohenberger, P. Angiosarcoma: State of the art and perspectives. *Crit. Rev. Oncol.* **2011**, *80*, 257–263. [CrossRef] [PubMed]
5. Young, R.J.; Brown, N.J.; Reed, M.W.; Hughes, D.; Woll, P.J. Angiosarcoma. *Lancet Oncol.* **2010**, *11*, 983–991. [CrossRef]
6. Schlemmer, M.; Reichardt, P.; Verweij, J.; Hartmann, J.; Judson, I.; Thyss, A.; Hogendoorn, P.; Marreaud, S.; Van Glabbeke, M.; Blay, J. Paclitaxel in patients with advanced angiosarcomas of soft tissue: A retrospective study of the EORTC soft tissue and bone sarcoma group. *Eur. J. Cancer* **2008**, *44*, 2433–2436. [CrossRef] [PubMed]
7. Antonescu, C.R.; Yoshida, A.; Guo, T.; Chang, N.-E.; Zhang, L.; Agaram, N.P.; Qin, L.-X.; Brennan, M.F.; Singer, S.; Maki, R.G. KDR Activating Mutations in Human Angiosarcomas Are Sensitive to Specific Kinase Inhibitors. *Cancer Res.* **2009**, *69*, 7175–7179. [CrossRef] [PubMed]
8. Ray-Coquard, I.; Italiano, A.; Bompas, E.; Le Cesne, A.; Robin, Y.; Chevreau, C.; Bay, J.; Bousquet, G.; Piperno-Neumann, S.; Isambert, N.; et al. Sorafenib for Patients with Advanced Angiosarcoma: A Phase II Trial from the French Sarcoma Group (GSF/GETO). *Oncologist* **2012**, *17*, 260–266. [CrossRef] [PubMed]
9. van der Graaf, W.T.; Blay, J.-Y.; Chawla, S.P.; Kim, D.-W.; Bui-Nguyen, B.; Casali, P.G.; Schöffski, P.; Aglietta, M.; Staddon, A.P.; Beppu, Y.; et al. Pazopanib for metastatic soft-tissue sarcoma (PALETTE): A randomised, double-blind, placebo-controlled phase 3 trial. *Lancet* **2012**, *379*, 1879–1886. [CrossRef]
10. Eisenhauer, E.A.; Therasse, P.; Bogaerts, J.; Schwartz, L.H.; Sargent, D.; Ford, R.; Dancey, J.; Arbuck, S.; Gwyther, S.; Mooney, M.; et al. New response evaluation criteria in solid tumours: Revised RECIST guideline (version 1.1). *Eur. J. Cancer* **2009**, *45*, 228–247. [CrossRef] [PubMed]
11. Englert, S.; Kieser, M. Methods for proper handling of overrunning and underrunning in phase II designs for oncology trials. *Stat. Med.* **2015**, *34*, 2128–2137. [CrossRef] [PubMed]
12. Ray-Coquard, I.L.; Domont, J.; Tresch-Bruneel, E.; Bompas, E.; Cassier, P.A.; Mir, O.; Piperno-Neumann, S.; Italiano, A.; Chevreau, C.; Cupissol, D.; et al. Paclitaxel Given Once Per Week With or Without Bevacizumab in Patients With Advanced Angiosarcoma: A Randomized Phase II Trial. *J. Clin. Oncol.* **2015**, *33*, 2797–2802. [CrossRef] [PubMed]
13. Pignata, S.; Lorusso, D.; Scambia, G.; Sambataro, D.; Tamberi, S.; Cinieri, S.; Mosconi, A.M.; Orditura, M.; A Brandes, A.; Arcangeli, V.; et al. Pazopanib plus weekly paclitaxel versus weekly paclitaxel alone for platinum-resistant or platinum-refractory advanced ovarian cancer (MITO 11): A randomised, open-label, phase 2 trial. *Lancet Oncol.* **2015**, *16*, 561–568. [CrossRef]
14. Richardson, D.L.; Sill, M.W.; Coleman, R.L.; Sood, A.K.; Pearl, M.L.; Kehoe, S.M.; Carney, M.E.; Hanjani, P.; Van Le, L.; Zhou, X.C.; et al. Paclitaxel With and Without Pazopanib for Persistent or Recurrent Ovarian Cancer: A Randomized Clinical Trial. *JAMA Oncol.* **2018**, *4*, 196–202. [CrossRef] [PubMed]
15. Florou, V.; Rosenberg, A.E.; Wieder, E.; Komanduri, K.V.; Kolonias, D.; Uduman, M.; Castle, J.C.; Buell, J.S.; Trent, J.C.; Wilky, B.A. Angiosarcoma patients treated with immune checkpoint inhibitors: A case series of seven patients from a single institution. *J. Immunother. Cancer* **2019**, *7*, 213. [CrossRef] [PubMed]
16. A Wilky, B.; Trucco, M.M.; Subhawong, T.K.; Florou, V.; Park, W.; Kwon, D.; Wieder, E.D.; Kolonias, D.; E Rosenberg, A.; A Kerr, D.; et al. Axitinib plus pembrolizumab in patients with advanced sarcomas including alveolar soft-part sarcoma: A single-centre, single-arm, phase 2 trial. *Lancet Oncol.* **2019**, *20*, 837–848. [CrossRef]
17. Chen, T.W.-W.; Burns, J.; Jones, R.L.; Huang, P.H. Optimal Clinical Management and the Molecular Biology of Angiosarcomas. *Cancers* **2020**, *12*, 3321. [CrossRef] [PubMed]

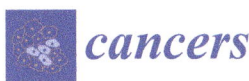

Article

Genomic Landscape of Angiosarcoma: A Targeted and Immunotherapy Biomarker Analysis

Andrea P. Espejo-Freire [1], Andrew Elliott [2], Andrew Rosenberg [3], Philippos Apolinario Costa [1], Priscila Barreto-Coelho [1], Emily Jonczak [1], Gina D'Amato [1], Ty Subhawong [4], Junaid Arshad [5], Julio A. Diaz-Perez [3], Wolfgang M. Korn [6], Matthew J. Oberley [7], Daniel Magee [8], Don Dizon [9], Margaret von Mehren [10], Moh'd M. Khushman [11], Atif Mahmoud Hussein [12], Kirsten Leu [13] and Jonathan C. Trent [1,*]

1. Department of Medicine, Hematology & Oncology, Sylvester Comprehensive Cancer Center, Jackson Memorial Hospital, Miller School of Medicine, University of Miami, Miami, FL 33136, USA; andrea.espejofreire@jhsmiami.org (A.P.E.-F.); philippos.costa@jhsmiami.org (P.A.C.); priscila.barretocoe@jhsmiami.org (P.B.-C.); eej18@med.miami.edu (E.J.); gina.damato@med.miami.edu (G.D.)
2. Department of Clinical and Translational Research, Caris Life Sciences, Phoenix, AZ 85040, USA; aelliott@carisls.com
3. Department of Pathology, Sylvester Comprehensive Cancer Center, Jackson Memorial Hospital, Miller School of Medicine, University of Miami, Miami, FL 33136, USA; arosenberg@med.miami.edu (A.R.); julio.diazperez@jhsmiami.org (J.A.D.-P.)
4. Department of Radiology, Sylvester Comprehensive Cancer Center, Jackson Memorial Hospital, Miller School of Medicine, University of Miami, Miami, FL 33136, USA; tsubhawong@med.miami.edu
5. Department of Medicine, Medical Oncology, The University of Arizona College of Medicine, University of Arizona Cancer Center, Tucson, AZ 85724, USA; junaidarshad@email.arizona.edu
6. Department of Medical Affairs, Caris Life Sciences, Phoenix, AZ 85040, USA; wmkorn@carisls.com
7. Department of Pathology and Genetics, Caris Life Sciences, Phoenix, AZ 85040, USA; moberley@carisls.com
8. Department of Cognitive Computing, Caris Life Sciences, Phoenix, AZ 85040, USA; dmagee@carisls.com
9. Department of Medical Oncology and Gynecologic Medical Oncology, Lifespan Cancer Institute, Rode Island Hospital, Providence, RI 02903, USA; don.dizon@lifespan.org
10. Department of Hematology & Oncology, Fox Chase Cancer Center, Temple Health, Philadelphia, PA 19111, USA; margaret.vonmehren@fccc.edu
11. O'Neal Comprehensive Cancer Center, Department of Medicine, Hematology & Oncology, The University of Alabama at Birmingham, Birmingham, AL 35233, USA; mkhushman@uabmc.edu
12. Department of Hematology & Oncology, Memorial Health Care System, Memorial Cancer Institute, Hollywood, FL 33021, USA; ahussein@mhs.net
13. Medical Oncology, Nebraska Cancer Specialists, Omaha, NE 68114, USA; kleu@nebraskacancer.com
* Correspondence: jtrent@med.miami.edu

Simple Summary: Angiosarcomas (AS) are rare, highly aggressive sarcomas with limited therapeutic options. Genomic sequencing techniques have identified recurrent genetic abnormalities. Nevertheless, the association of these findings with etiology, site of origin, prognosis, and therapeutic implications is not well understood. We analyzed Next Generation Sequencing (NGS) and Whole Transcriptome Sequencing (WTS) data in a cohort of 143 AS cases. We identified distinct genomic biology according to the AS primary site. Head and neck AS cases primarily have Immunotherapy (IO) response markers and mutations in *TP53* and *POT1*. On the other hand, breast AS is enriched for cell cycle alterations, predominately *MYC* amplification. Additionally, a microenvironment with abundant immune cells is present in a minority of cases but distributed evenly among primary sites. Our findings can facilitate the design and optimization of therapeutic strategies for AS according to its biology at different primary sites.

Abstract: We performed a retrospective analysis of angiosarcoma (AS) genomic biomarkers and their associations with the site of origin in a cohort of 143 cases. Primary sites were head and neck (31%), breast (22%), extremity (11%), viscera (20%), skin at other locations (8%), and unknown (9%). All cases had Next Generation Sequencing (NGS) data with a 592 gene panel, and 53 cases had Whole Exome Sequencing (WES) data, which we used to study the microenvironment phenotype. The immunotherapy (IO) response biomarkers Tumor Mutation Burden (TMB), Microsatellite Instability

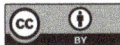

(MSI), and PD-L1 status were the most frequently encountered alteration, present in 36.4% of the cohort and 65% of head and neck AS (H/N-AS) ($p < 0.0001$). In H/N-AS, TMB-High was seen in 63.4% of cases ($p < 0.0001$) and PDL-1 positivity in 33% of cases. The most common genetic alterations were *TP53* (29%), *MYC* amplification (23%), *ARID1A* (17%), *POT1* (16%), and *ATRX* (13%). H/N-AS cases had predominantly mutations in *TP53* (50.0%, $p = 0.0004$), *POT1* (40.5%, $p < 0.0001$), and *ARID1A* (33.3%, $p = 0.5875$). In breast AS, leading alterations were *MYC* amplification (63.3%, $p < 0.0001$), *HRAS* (16.1%, $p = 0.0377$), and *PIK3CA* (16.1%, $p = 0.2352$). At other sites, conclusions are difficult to generate due to the small number of cases. A microenvironment with a high immune signature, previously associated with IO response, was evenly distributed in 13% of the cases at different primary sites. Our findings can facilitate the design and optimization of therapeutic strategies for AS.

Keywords: Angiosarcoma; biomarkers; tumor microenvironment; immunotherapy; next-generation sequencing; whole transcriptome sequencing

1. Introduction

Angiosarcomas (AS) are highly aggressive sarcomas that account for only 2% of all soft-tissue-sarcomas (STS) [1]. Unfortunately, even when patients present with localized disease, over 50% will relapse after initial treatment, resulting in a five-year OS of only 60%. Furthermore, once patients have locally advanced or metastatic disease, the median OS is only 9–15 month [2–4]. Cytotoxic chemotherapy frequently shows activity, but tumor responses are short-lived, and most patients ultimately die from metastatic disease [3,4]. Moreover, despite evidence of upregulation of vascular-specific receptor tyrosine kinases, VEGF blockade provides at most a 2–4-month survival benefit [5–9]. Lately, growing evidence of immunotherapy (IO) activity in AS has emerged [10,11]. However, not all AS primary sites show uniform responses, and ultimately IO's role in the treatment of AS is not clearly defined.

At the different sites of origin, cases of AS show different clinical features and prognosis. The most common AS location is head and neck AS (H/N-AS), followed by breast AS (B-AS), visceral, other cutaneous sites, and the extremities. The majority of cases of AS occur sporadically (primary) or are related to radiation therapy or chronic lymphedema (secondary) [12]. A French retrospective multicenter study of 161 patients reported that visceral (heart, liver, and spleen) and primary bone sites were associated with worse prognosis [13]. In a study of 200 AS cases from China that also showed biological differences, the worst prognosis was seen in H/N-AS (5-year OS of 28%), followed by visceral (37%), and B-AS (87%) [14]. Evidence shows that patients with secondary B-AS have a more aggressive tumor phenotype and worse survival outcome than patients with primary B-AS [14,15]. A study of over 470 patients extracted from the SEER database described that secondary B-AS appears in older patients and presents with more locally advanced stage (57% vs. 18%) and high grade (58% vs. 32%). In this cohort, the median OS was 93 months for primary B-AS and 32 months for secondary B-AS [15].

Along with the differences in clinical behavior, some small cohorts in the literature show genomic differences within AS. The first identified genetic alteration was *KDR* (AKA *VEGFR2*), which harbors point mutations in 10% of primary or secondary B-AS [16]. Other recurrent alterations are *TP53*, *PIK3CA*, *POT1*, *RAS*, *BRAF*, *PTPRB*, *PLCG1*, and *APC* [2,11,17]. Some mutations appear to be distinct to cases of primary and secondary AS. *MYC* amplification was reported in 50 to 100% of radiation-associated AS cases but not in primary AS [18–20]. Most recently, Whole Exome Sequencing (WES) results of 47 samples from 36 patients self-registered to the Angiosarcoma Project were published. In this cohort, the authors reported that *TP53* and *KDR* mutations are mutually exclusive, with 89% of *KDR* mutations in primary B-AS compared to 82% of TP53 in non-primary B-AS ($p = 0.02$). Nine out of ten *PIK3CA* alterations were also seen in primary B-AS ($p = 0.0003$) [11]. Despite sequencing techniques allowing the identification of recurrent somatic genetic abnormalities, the rarity of AS challenges our efforts to establish strong associations with the site of origin, etiology, and therapeutic implications.

There is growing evidence that IO is highly active for some patients with AS and that IO activity is likely dependent on the site of origin. First, a phase II study on the use of immunotherapy for advanced STS (Alliance A091401) showed that one AS patient had an objective response [21]. Subsequently, a retrospective analysis of seven AS cases treated with immunotherapy revealed a response rate of 71% (5/7) at 12 weeks, including one case of complete response [10]. Here H/N-AS cases were four out of five responders. Finally, in The Angiosarcoma Project, 3 out of 10 patients with H/N-AS received immunotherapy (IO), and two achieved exceptional responses. In contrast, none of the three patients with AS other than H/N treated with immunotherapy responded to the therapy [11].

As responses to IO are not homogeneous for specific histology, efforts to determine potential IO response markers are in progress. The Angiosarcoma Project identified that the median tumor mutation burden (TMB) was significantly higher in patients with H/N-AS ($p = 1.10 \times 10^{-5}$). In this cohort, both cases benefiting from IO had very high TMB, with 78 and 138 mutations/MB [11]. However, experience in IO for STS trials has taught us that classic IO response markers, TMB and PDL-1, are not the sole determinants of response. Transcriptomic analysis is now available to estimate the relative abundance of immune and stromal cells within tumor samples. Using this technique, Petiprez et al. described a classification of STS based on their tumor microenvironment. In the SARC028 trial for the use of PDL-1 blockage for STS, they identified that an immune-rich microenvironment, particularly a B cell abundance, correlated with better response rate and improved PFS [22]. Interestingly, the overall TMB appeared similar across all classes of microenvironment phenotypes. In other histologies, microenvironment analysis also shows predictive capabilities for IO and other targeted therapies. For example, in renal cell carcinoma, gene expression signatures of angiogenesis, T-effector, and myeloid cells are predictive of PFS for IO alone or combined with anti-VEGF blockage [23]. Whether these methods can be applied similarly to patients with AS needs further investigation.

Here, we analyzed genomic data of Next Generation Sequencing (NGS) and Whole Transcriptome Sequencing (WTS) from 143 cases. To our knowledge, this is the largest cohort of AS cases with genomic data. In addition, we described a particular AS biology according to the primary site and showed potential biomarkers, including a description of the microenvironment to guide future therapeutic studies.

2. Materials and Methods

We retrospectively analyzed the data of 143 AS tumors profiled by Caris Life Sciences from 2015–2019. We included the annotations of "Angiosarcoma", "Angiomyosarcoma", or "Lymphangiosarcoma". Clinical characteristics including age, sex, site of origin, site of biopsy, and the status of metastatic vs. primary were tabulated. No data on prior exposure to radiation therapy were available. NGS enriched for 592 cancer-related whole-gene targets was performed on each tumor. We included pathogenic mutations and copy number amplification in the analysis.

WTS was performed on 53 tumors and used for microenvironment cell population (MCP)-counter analysis, as described by Becht et al. [24]. First, we estimated a cell population of interest using transcriptomic markers (TMs). TMs are gene expression features expressed in one and only one cell population. The method generates an abundance score for CD3+ T cells, CD8+ T cells, cytotoxic lymphocytes, NK cells, B lymphocytes, monocyte lineage cells, endothelial cells, and fibroblasts [24]. Next, we identified subgroups based on tumor microenvironment profiles by hierarchical clustering of MCP-counter Z-scores [22].

Biomarkers classically associated with response to IO (TMB-High ($\geq$10/Mb), MSI-High, and PD-L1 (IHC $\geq$2+ and 5%) were included. A sarcoma pathologist at Sylvester Comprehensive Cancer Center reviewed the hematoxylin and eosin (H&E) slides to confirm the diagnosis. Additionally, we annotated data of cell morphology, anatomical biopsy site, grade, necrosis, lumen formation, and intra and peritumoral inflammatory infiltrate.

The inflammatory infiltrates were graded as follows: 0—no inflammatory cells observed, 1—corresponding to <5% of the cellularity, 2—corresponding to 5–30% of the cellularity, and 3—corresponding to >30% of the cellularity.

Cytologic, molecular, and genomic results were evaluated according to the primary tumor site. Statistical analyses were performed using Chi-square or Fisher's exact tests, where appropriate. The Wilcoxon Method was used to compare groups, and p-values were adjusted for multiple hypothesis testing using the Benjamini and Hochberg procedure.

3. Results

The cohort's median age was 67 (range 22–89); 61% were female and 29% were metastatic/recurrent. The number of cases by location were head and neck ($n = 44$, 31%), breast ($n = 31$, 22%), extremity ($n = 16$, 11%), viscera ($n = 28$, 20%), skin at other locations ($n = 11$, 8%), and unknown ($n = 13$, 9%). Table 1 shows the H&E histologic characteristics of the cases. Figure 1 shows the spectrum of the density of inflammation within cases of AS.

Table 1. Primary site distribution and histologic characteristics of cases.

Angiosarcoma Subgroup	All	Head and Neck	Breast	Visceral	Extremity	Cutaneous	Unknown	p-Value
Sample size, N (%)	143 (100%)	44 (30.8%)	31 (21.7%)	28 (19.6%)	16 (11.2%)	11 (7.7%)	13 (9.1%)	
Morphology								
Epithelioid	46 (32.9%)	19 (43.2%)	8 (26.7%)	9 (32.1%)	3 (18.8%)	3 (30.0%)	4 (36.4%)	
Spindle	9 (6.4%)	0 (0.0%)	3 (10.0%)	4 (14.3%)	0 (0.0%)	1 (10.0%)	1 (9.1%)	0.16
Mixed	85 (60.7%)	25 (56.8%)	19 (63.3%)	15 (53.6%)	13 (81.3%)	6 (60.0%)	6 (54.5%)	
Grade								
1	2 (1.4%)	0 (0.0%)	1 (3.3%)	1 (3.6%)	0 (0.0%)	0 (0.0%)	0 (0.0%)	
2	78 (55.7%)	21 (47.7%)	21 (70.0%)	15 (53.6%)	8 (50.0%)	5 (50.0%)	8 (72.7%)	0.52
3	60 (42.9%)	23 (52.3%)	8 (26.7%)	12 (42.9%)	8 (50.0%)	5 (50.0%)	3 (27.3%)	
Vessel formation								
Yes	117 (83.6%)	35 (79.5%)	28 (93.3%)	23 (82.1%)	12 (75.0%)	9 (90.0%)	9 (81.8%)	0.43
No	23 (16.4%)	9 (20.5%)	2 (6.7%)	5 (17.9%)	4 (25.0%)	1 (10.0%)	2 (18.2%)	
Inflammatory infiltrate								
0	8 (5.7%)	1 (2.3%)	2 (6.7%)	3 (10.7%)	2 (12.5%)	0 (0.0%)	0 (0.0%)	
1	105 (75.0%)	31 (70.5%)	28 (93.3%)	19 (67.9%)	11 (68.8%)	8 (80.0%)	7 (63.6%)	0.11
2	25 (17.9%)	10 (22.7%)	0 (0.0%)	6 (21.4%)	3 (18.8%)	2 (20.0%)	4 (36.4%)	
3	2 (1.4%)	2 (4.5%)	0 (0.0%)	0 (0.0%)	0 (0.0%)	0 (0.0%)	0 (0.0%)	
Location of infiltrate								
Periphery	8 (6.1%)	2 (4.7%)	1 (3.6%)	3 (12.0%)	1 (7.1%)	0 (0.0%)	1 (9.1%)	
Intratumoral	31 (23.5%)	11 (25.6%)	4 (14.3%)	6 (24.0%)	4 (28.6%)	3 (30.0%)	3 (27.3%)	0.73
Both	92 (69.7%)	30 (69.8%)	23 (82.1%)	16 (64.0%)	9 (64.3%)	7 (70.0%)	7 (63.6%)	
Neutrophils present								
Yes	30 (22.7%)	11 (25.6%)	3 (10.7%)	8 (32.0%)	5 (35.7%)	1 (10.0%)	2 (18.2%)	0.29
No	102 (77.3%)	32 (74.4%)	25 (89.3%)	17 (68.0%)	9 (64.3%)	9 (90.0%)	9 (81.8%)	

Note: Four samples (one breast, one cutaneous, and two unknown) did not have hematoxylin and eosin (H&E) slides available for review.

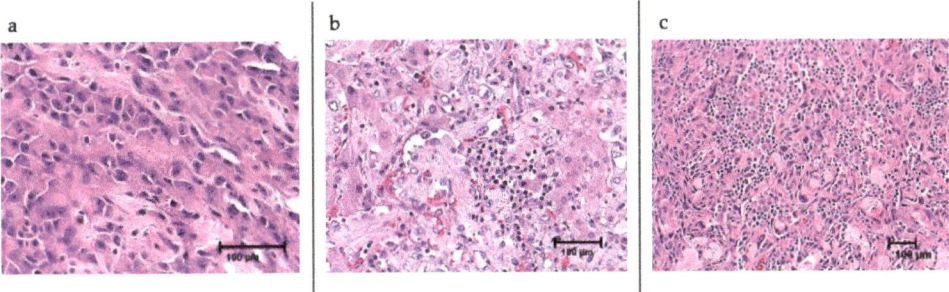

Figure 1. B cell abundance and PDL-1 positivity are present in cases with grade 2 and 3 inflammatory infiltrate by hematoxylin and eosin (H&E). Here, we illustrate the spectrum of the density of inflammation within angiosarcomas. (**a**) Grade 1—<5% of cells are inflammatory cells. (**b**) Grade 2—<30% of cells are inflammatory cells. (**c**) Grade 3—>30% of cells are inflammatory cells.

3.1. Markers of Immunotherapy Response

Predictive IO-response biomarkers were the most common marker in the entire cohort, present in 36.4% of cases (TMB-High in 26%, PD-L1+ 21.8%, MSI-High 0.7%). Predictive IO-response biomarkers were the highest in the H/N-AS subgroup, with TMB-High observed in 63.4% of H/N-AS cases ($n = 26/41$; $p < 0.0001$), a significant increase compared to other sites. Fourteen cases of H/N-AS (33%) were positive for PD-L1 by IHC, 11 of which were concurrently TMB-High. Only one case of H/N-AS had dMMR/MSI-high status. TMB-High was present in a few cases at other locations: four visceral AS cases and one case in breast, extremity, and other cutaneous site. Similarly, PDL-1 positivity is present in six cases of visceral AS, three cases of B-AS, two cases of extremity AS, and one case of other cutaneous AS. Of note, B-AS had the lowest frequency of IO-response biomarkers. Figure 2 shows IO-response biomarkers.

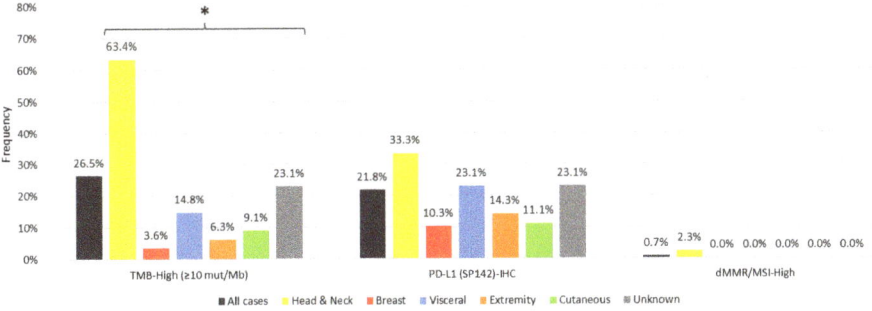

Figure 2. Immunotherapy response biomarkers vary according to the primary site. * Head and neck angiosarcoma cases have a higher predominance of TMB-High (>10 muts/MB), with $p < 0.0001$. In addition, PDL-1 positivity is present at the different sites. AS cases rarely are dMMR/MSI-High.

3.2. Genetic Alterations

The most common genetic alterations were *TP53* (29%), *MYC* amplification (23%), *ARID1A* (17%), *POT1* (16%), and *ATRX* (13%). Genetic alterations were distinct according to the primary site. In H/N-AS, *TP53* mutations were present in 48.8% ($n = 21/43$; $p = 0.0002$), *POT1* in 41.9% ($n = 18/43$; $p < 0.0001$), and *ARID1A* in 31.3% ($n = 5/16$; $p = 0.7331$). On the other hand, in B-AS, cell cycle pathway aberrations were common, with *MYC* amplification present in 63.3% ($n = 19/30$; $p < 0.0001$). Mutations in *HRAS* were present in 16.1% ($n = 5/31$; $p = 0.0155$) and *PIK3CA* in 16.1% ($n = 5/31$; $p = 0.1489$) of B-AS cases. Interestingly, *MYC* amplification was also seen in 45.5% (5/11) of cutaneous cases at other locations than H/N or breast, and 37.5% (6/16) of extremity AS cases, but not seen in H/N or visceral AS cases. *MYC* amplification has been described in radiation-associated AS of the breast [17–19]; future studies are needed to investigate further whether *MYC* amplification is an etiologic factor at other sites of secondary AS. Unfortunately, our cohort did not include annotation of whether the patient had a prior history of radiation exposure. Finally, some distinct alterations appeared more commonly at other cutaneous, visceral, and extremity locations; however, conclusions are difficult to obtain due to the small number of cases at these sites. Figure 3 shows the genetic alterations in AS.

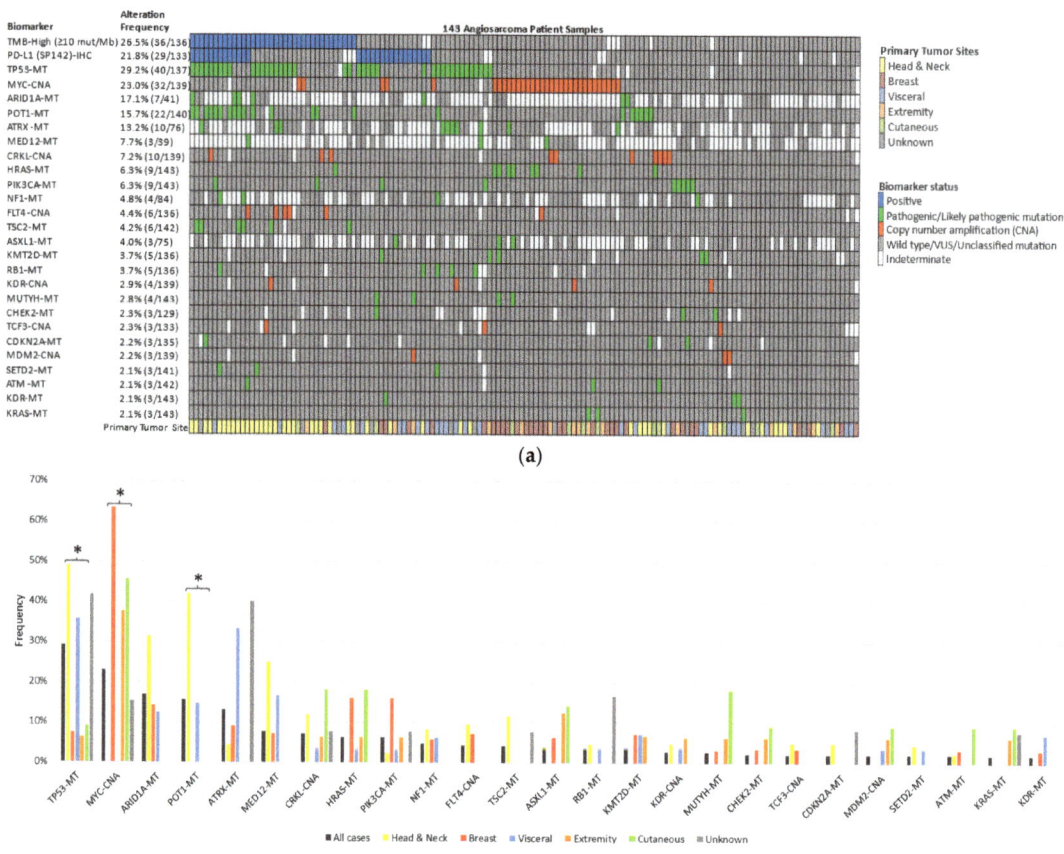

Figure 3. The genomic landscape of angiosarcoma shows a distinct pattern according to the primary site. (**a**) Oncoprint for the entire cohort of 143 cases showing the most common alterations: *TP53* (29%), *MYC* amplification (23%), *ARID1A* (17%), *POT1* (16%), and *ATRX* (13%). (**b**) Genetic alterations vary by primary site. *TP53* and *POT1* are significantly higher in H/N-AS; *MYC* amplification is primarily seen in B-AS. * $p < 0.0001$.

3.3. Microenvironment Phenotype

Using the MCP-counter method, we defined four distinct immune classes based on microenvironment cell population abundance. Hierarchical clustering identified subgroups with distinct microenvironment profiles consistent with those described by Petitprez et al. [22]. Fifty-three cases with available WTS data were distributed as follows: Immune-High—B lineage high (13.2%), Vascularized—Endothelial cells high (24.5%),

Immune-Desert (41.5%), and Heterogeneous—Moderate abundance (20.8%). Immune class signatures were evenly distributed among different primary sites. Interestingly, the Immune-High group had the lowest median TMB: 6 muts/MB (range 3–17). See Figure 4.

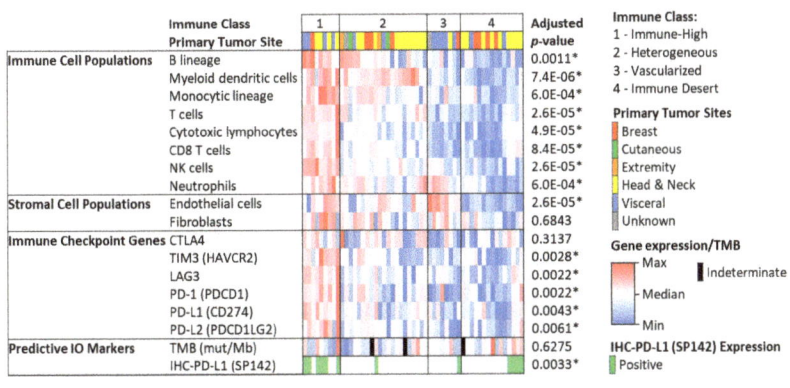

(a)

(b)

Figure 4. (a) Microenvironment phenotype in angiosarcoma. Immune-High phenotype is present in 13% of cases and seen among different primary sites, and this phenotype follows the expression of immune checkpoint genes. (b) Comparison of tumor microenvironment between angiosarcoma and melanoma showing a similar abundance of immune cells. * p value < 0.05.

Next, we compared the microenvironment of the AS cohort with a cohort of melanoma ($n = 1255$). Of all tumors in humans, melanomas have one of the highest burdens of somatic genetic alterations [25]. Moreover, particularly in cutaneous melanoma, an extensive CD8+ T-cell infiltration has been described and associated with better prognosis and response to IO [26]. Interestingly, the microenvironment of angiosarcoma has a similar immune profile to melanoma but with enrichment of endothelial and myeloid dendritic cells (Figure 4b). While the median abundance of CD8+ T cell and B cell populations was lower in AS than melanoma, the difference was not statistically significant. Neutrophils, NK cells, and monocytic lineage cells had a comparable abundance.

Finally, when analyzing the microenvironment according to the tabulated histologic characteristics observed by H&E, we observed that the cases with an inflammatory infiltrate of grade 2 or 3 had a higher number of T cells, CD8+ cells, cytotoxic T cells, NK, and B cells using the MCP counter method. Importantly, B-cell abundance in cases with grade 2 or 3 infiltrate was significantly higher than in cases of grade 0 or 1 ($p = 0.034$). In addition, expression of immune-related markers TIM3, LAG3, PD-1 (PDCD1), PD-L1 (CD274), and PD-L2 (PDCD1LG2) was also more abundant in the cases with grade 2 or 3 inflammatory infiltrate. For PDL-1, this was statistically significant ($p = 0.038$). See Figure 5.

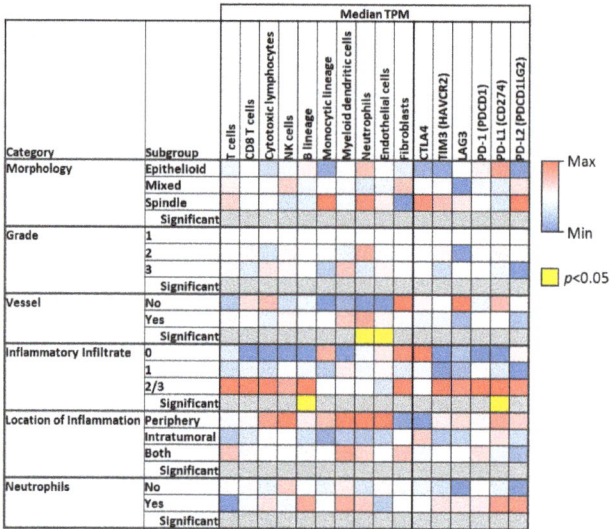

Figure 5. The presence of a grade 2 or 3 inflammatory infiltrate observed on H&E microscopy correlates significantly with higher B cell abundance and PDL-1 expression. In addition, the expression of other immune checkpoint-related genes (CTLA4, TIM3, LAG3, PD1, PD-L1, PD-L2) follows that of the immune cells.

4. Discussion

To our knowledge, this is the largest cohort of AS genomic biology described to date.

Our findings confirm previous studies that show that AS has distinct biology depending on its primary site and etiology. Here, we confirm that classical IO-response markers are common in AS, present in about one-third of the cases. We found that over 60% of cases of H/N-AS had markers of IO-response. Our findings corroborate the previously described cohorts where high TMB was clustered in 50–60% of cases of H/N-AS [11,27,28]. In these prior reports, UV light mutational signatures were described in cases of H/N-AS through whole genome and whole exome sequencing analysis. Unfortunately, our data comes from a specific 592 gene panel that involves sequencing a significantly smaller part of the genome. As such, we have limited power to present the results of mutational signatures. However, the consistency of other findings suggests that a UV mutational signature is likely to be found in cases of H/N-AS associated with high TMB. These factors may explain why H/N-AS cases benefit more from IO. The retrospective series by Florou et al. showed that most responders were cases of H/N-AS (four out of five cases) [10]. Similarly, the two cases of outstanding responses noted in the Angiosarcoma Project had TMB High H/N-AS [11].

In our cohort, TMB-High was also present in a few cases at other locations (in four cases of visceral AS and in one case of B-AS, extremity, cutaneous). PDL-1 positivity was present in 14 cases of H/N-AS, six cases of visceral AS, three cases of B-AS, two cases of extremity AS, and one case of cutaneous AS. Interestingly, in the cohort described by Florou et al., the case that achieved a long-lasting complete response had low TMB with only 0.9 muts/MB, and a patient with RT-associated B-AS also had a PR. These findings should indicate that IO-response markers are not the sole determinant of IO response. The opportunity for responses is not only seen at the H-N location.

A microenvironment with a high immune signature and abundance of B-cells was present in about 13% of the cases and evenly distributed among different primary sites. A signature of B-cell lineage abundance, regardless of high or low CD8+ T cell infiltration, appears to predict response to PD1 blockade and PFS in STS [22]. Interestingly, in this immune-high group, overall, the cases had a low TMB. The contribution of each of these factors and the dynamic microenvironment changes to IO response are still unknown. In other solid tumors, distinct microenvironment characteristics show predictor capabilities of IO and other targeted therapies [23,29]. However, not a single phenotype across solid tumors has yielded similar prognostic and predictive capabilities. Further studies are warranted to determine if a phenotype with an abundance of B cells in AS results in similar predictive capabilities to what has been seen for other STS. Additionally, the dynamics of the microenvironment upon treatment could potentially have better predictive capabilities. In melanoma, a highly immunogenic tumor where IO is active, INF-gamma driven infiltration of CD8+ lymphocytes upon treatment predicts responses [26,29]. In our cohort, we described a similar microenvironment to that of melanoma. Future studies should further examine the predictive capabilities of microenvironment analysis in AS to move forward to incorporating this method into clinical practice. WTS is commonly performed when profiling solid tumors; however, immune cell abundance and microenvironment cell counter results are not routinely reported to treating physicians. As more evidence of the predictive capabilities of this method emerges, we may be able to incorporate this information into clinical decision making as we move forward in tailoring effective therapies for rare tumors. Importantly, we reviewed the H&E slides of 138 of the patients (four cases had no available H&E slide) and described the tumor inflammatory infiltrate. We saw that B-cell abundance by WTS and PDL-1 expression was associated with the presence of an inflammatory infiltrate of grade 2 or 3, as assessed by light microscopy. Thus, we could optimize this strategy by incorporating immunohistochemistry to compare the predictive phenotypes determined by the MCP-counter method.

Certain genetic alterations of AS are more common at specific primary sites. Consequently, further studies to overcome IO resistance and increase the effectiveness of targeted therapies accounting for specific alterations are warranted. Therapeutic strategies that target *TP53*, *POT1*, and *ARID1A* could be of value in H/N-AS. *TP53* tumor suppressor activity triggers cell cycle arrest, death by apoptosis, and senescence by regulation of multiple pathways. Even though *TP53* is widely mutated in cancer, targeting it has been challenging. Recently, the study of small molecules to reestablish the activity of mutant p53 has shown promising results. In particular, APR-246 (eprenetapopt), which refolds mutant p53 to induce p53 target genes, demonstrated clinical activity in myeloid malignancies [30,31]. This promising strategy is currently under investigation in combination with IO, chemotherapy, and other targeted agents. In cases with a *TP53* mutation, we found that 67% had concomitant markers of IO response. Therefore, it may be essential to investigate if the use of this molecule could overcome IO resistance in H/N-AS. *ARID1A* is one of the most common alterations encountered in our cohort and is also seen predominately in H/N-AS. Being part of the chromatin remodeling complex SWI/SNF, its deficiency results in EZH2 overactivity. In epithelioid sarcoma, we observed success using EZH2 inhibitor tazemetostat [32–34]. This strategy has shown efficacy in *ARID1A* mutated ovarian and endometrioid cell carcinomas [35]. Therefore, prospective evaluation of tazemetostat in ARID1A mutated AS should be considered [36]. Lastly, *POT1* is involved in telomere maintenance, and its regular activity results in cell aging and apoptosis. Three percent of malignancies have *POT1* mutations; however, its prevalence is higher in AS (23%) and is described among the top predisposition genes for familial melanoma and cardiac AS [37]. In our cohort, it was predominately present in cases of H/N-AS. Unfortunately, the therapeutic role of *POT1* inhibition in cancer is currently unknown.

The molecular alterations in B-AS give additional opportunities for other therapeutic strategies. Over 60% of cases of B-AS show *MYC* amplification. In our cohort, we do not have data about the association of the cases with prior radiation therapy. However, strong evidence shows that *MYC* amplification is almost exclusively seen in radiation-associated AS [18,20]. MYC proteins coordinate transcription, DNA replication, and cell cycle progression. Strategies to target cell cycle by CDK inhibition have shown promising results in *MYC* amplified tumors. In neuroblastoma cell lines, CDK/CDK1 inhibitors show an ability to downregulate *MYC* [38]. Recently, fadraciclib, a potent inhibitor of CDK9 showed an ability to repress *MYC* and is currently in early-phase clinical trials for solid tumors and hematologic malignancies [39,40]. Additionally, bromodomain inhibitors (BET) have proven efficacy in *MYC* amplified lymphoma. Their use in combination with CDK2 inhibitor is being studied in *MYC*-driven medulloblastoma [41–43]. Finally, in ovarian cancer, *MYC* amplification predicted synergistic benefit from a combination of PARP inhibition with olaparib and CDK-4 inhibition with palbociclib [44]. These strategies deserve further study for *MYC* amplified AS. Other common mutations found in B-AS are *PIK3CA* and *HRAS*. Prior reports indicate that *PIK3CA* mutations are primarily found in cases of primary B-AS. PI3K inhibition is efficacious in *PIK3CA* mutated breast cancer. These mutations found in primary breast AS suggest that site of origin may predispose to overactive *PIK3CA*-driven AS. Here, evaluation of the use of alpelisib or other PI3K inhibitors is necessary for cases of primary breast AS [45]. These differences should be accounted for when devising differential strategies to treat RT-associated B-AS and primary B-AS. On the other hand, mutations in *RAS* usually result in downstream activation of MAPK and PI3K. Several compounds targeting downstream effects of RAS, such as MEK, AKT, and PI3K are available and should be considered in these cases [46]. This agent's synergistic effects in combination with IO are also being studied [46,47].

Finally, we acknowledge that an important constraint of our study is the limited clinical data obtained from the requisition forms submitted by the ordering physician. Because preclinical models of AS are limited, this type of genomic analysis should be performed in retrospective and prospective cohorts, with available clinical data of responses to the different therapeutic strategies to understand the therapeutic implications further. Importantly, a recent study showed similarities of the AS genomic landscape to that of canine hemangiosarcoma. In canine hemangiosarcoma, the recurrent oncogenic mutations were *TP53* (66%), *PIK3CA* (46%), *NRAS* (24%), *PTEN* (6%), and *PLCG1* (4%) [48]. Both species share some recurrent genetic alterations, which creates an opportunity to develop effective treatment strategies.

5. Conclusions

Herein, we provide robust data showing that the genomic landscape of AS varies according to the site of origin. The particularities likely represent a different etiologic phenomenon and biologic behavior. For this reason, we need further studies of retrospective cohorts to confirm and expand on the therapeutic implications. Additionally, these findings should be accounted for when designing prospective trials for AS. Finally, incorporating similar genomic testing in the correlative studies of prospective trials can help us build practical predictive tools to combat this deadly aggressive disease.

Author Contributions: Conceptualization, A.P.E.-F. and J.C.T.; Data curation, A.E., A.R. and W.M.K.; Formal analysis, A.E., W.M.K., M.J.O. and D.M.; Investigation, A.P.E.-F., A.E. and A.R.; Project administration, A.P.E.-F. and J.C.T.; Supervision, J.C.T.; Writing—original draft, A.P.E.-F.; Writing—review and editing, A.E., A.R., P.A.C., P.B.-C., E.J., G.D., T.S., J.A., J.A.D.-P., W.M.K., M.J.O., D.M., D.D., M.v.M., M.M.K., A.M.H., K.L. and J.C.T. All authors have read and agreed to the published version of the manuscript.

Funding: This research received no external funding.

Institutional Review Board Statement: This study was conducted in accordance with guidelines of the Declaration of Helsinki, Belmont report, and U.S. Common rule. In keeping with 45 CFR 46.101(b)(4), this study was performed utilizing retrospective, de-identified clinical data. Therefore, this study is considered IRB exempt.

Informed Consent Statement: Patient consent was waived due to the retrospective nature of this study and use of de-identified data.

Data Availability Statement: Data is contained within the article.

Conflicts of Interest: A.E.—Caris employee; W.M.K.—Caris employee, consultant for Merck; M.O.—Caris employee with equity; D.M.—Caris employee with stock. The remaining authors declare no conflict of interest with the data presented herein.

References

1. Ducimetière, F.; Lurkin, A.; Ranchère-Vince, D.; Decouvelaere, A.-V.; Peoc'H, M.; Istier, L.; Chalabreysse, P.; Muller, C.; Alberti, L.; Bringuier, P.-P.; et al. Incidence of Sarcoma Histotypes and Molecular Subtypes in a Prospective Epidemiological Study with Central Pathology Review and Molecular Testing. *PLoS ONE* **2011**, *6*, e20294. [CrossRef]
2. Florou, V.; Wilky, B.A. Current and Future Directions for Angiosarcoma Therapy. *Curr. Treat. Options Oncol.* **2018**, *19*, 14. [CrossRef]
3. Mito, J.K.; Mitra, D.; Barysauskas, C.M.; Mariño-Enriquez, A.; Morgan, E.A.; Fletcher, C.D.; Raut, C.P.; Baldini, E.H.; Doyle, L.A. A Comparison of Outcomes and Prognostic Features for Radiation-Associated Angiosarcoma of the Breast and Other Radiation-Associated Sarcomas. *Int. J. Radiat. Oncol.* **2019**, *104*, 425–435. [CrossRef] [PubMed]
4. Fury, M.G.; Antonescu, C.R.; Van Zee, K.; Brennan, M.; Maki, R.G. A 14-Year Retrospective Review of Angiosarcoma. *Cancer J.* **2005**, *11*, 241–247. [CrossRef] [PubMed]
5. Agulnik, M.; Yarber, J.; Okuno, S.; von Mehren, M.; Jovanovic, B.; Brockstein, B.; Evens, A.; Benjamin, R. An open-label, multicenter, phase II study of bevacizumab for the treatment of angiosarcoma and epithelioid hemangioendotheliomas. *Ann. Oncol.* **2013**, *24*, 257–263. [CrossRef] [PubMed]
6. Kollár, A.; Jones, R.L.; Stacchiotti, S.; Gelderblom, H.; Guida, M.; Grignani, G.; Steeghs, N.; Safwat, A.; Katz, D.; Duffaud, F.; et al. Pazopanib in advanced vascular sarcomas: An EORTC Soft Tissue and Bone Sarcoma Group (STBSG) retrospective analysis. *Acta Oncol.* **2016**, *56*, 88–92. [CrossRef] [PubMed]
7. Maki, R.G.; D'Adamo, D.R.; Keohan, M.L.; Saulle, M.; Schuetze, S.M.; Undevia, S.D.; Livingston, M.B.; Cooney, M.M.; Hensley, M.L.; Mita, M.M.; et al. Phase II Study of Sorafenib in Patients With Metastatic or Recurrent Sarcomas. *J. Clin. Oncol.* **2009**, *27*, 3133–3140. [CrossRef] [PubMed]
8. Ray-Coquard, I.L.; Domont, J.; Tresch-Bruneel, E.; Bompas, E.; Cassier, P.A.; Mir, O.; Piperno-Neumann, S.; Italiano, A.; Chevreau, C.; Cupissol, D.; et al. Paclitaxel Given Once Per Week With or Without Bevacizumab in Patients With Advanced Angiosarcoma: A Randomized Phase II Trial. *J. Clin. Oncol.* **2015**, *33*, 2797–2802. [CrossRef]
9. Agulnik, M.; Schulte, B.; Robinson, S.; Hirbe, A.C.; Kozak, K.; Chawla, S.P.; Attia, S.; Rademaker, A.; Zhang, H.; Abnbinati, S.; et al. An open-label single-arm phase II study of regorafenib for the treatment of angiosarcoma. *Eur. J. Cancer* **2021**, *154*, 201–208. [CrossRef] [PubMed]
10. Florou, V.; Rosenberg, A.E.; Wieder, E.; Komanduri, K.V.; Kolonias, D.; Uduman, M.; Castle, J.C.; Buell, J.S.; Trent, J.C.; Wilky, B.A. Angiosarcoma patients treated with immune checkpoint inhibitors: A case series of seven patients from a single institution. *J. Immunother. Cancer* **2019**, *7*, 213. [CrossRef] [PubMed]
11. Painter, C.A.; Jain, E.; Tomson, B.N.; Dunphy, M.; Stoddard, R.E.; Thomas, B.S.; Damon, A.L.; Shah, S.; Kim, D.; Zañudo, J.G.T.; et al. The Angiosarcoma Project: Enabling genomic and clinical discoveries in a rare cancer through patient-partnered research. *Nat. Med.* **2020**, *26*, 181–187. [CrossRef]
12. Young, R.J.; Brown, N.; Reed, M.W.; Hughes, D.J.; Woll, P. Angiosarcoma. *Lancet Oncol.* **2010**, *11*, 983–991. [CrossRef]
13. Fayette, J.; Martin, E.; Piperno-Neumann, S.; Le Cesne, A.; Robert, C.; Bonvalot, S.; Ranchère, D.; Pouillart, P.; Coindre, J.M.; Blay, J.Y. Angiosarcomas, a heterogeneous group of sarcomas with specific behavior depending on primary site: A retrospective study of 161 cases. *Ann. Oncol.* **2007**, *18*, 2030–2036. [CrossRef]
14. Wang, L.; Lao, I.W.; Yu, L.; Wang, J. Clinicopathological features and prognostic factors in angiosarcoma: A retrospective analysis of 200 patients from a single Chinese medical institute. *Oncol. Lett.* **2017**, *14*, 5370–5378. [CrossRef]
15. Yin, M.; Wang, W.; Drabick, J.J.; Harold, H.A. Prognosis and treatment of non-metastatic primary and secondary breast angiosarcoma: A comparative study. *BMC Cancer* **2017**, *17*, 295. [CrossRef] [PubMed]
16. Antonescu, C.R.; Yoshida, A.; Guo, T.; Chang, N.-E.; Zhang, L.; Agaram, N.P.; Qin, L.-X.; Brennan, M.; Singer, S.; Maki, R.G. KDR Activating Mutations in Human Angiosarcomas Are Sensitive to Specific Kinase Inhibitors. *Cancer Res.* **2009**, *69*, 7175–7179. [CrossRef]
17. Behjati, S.; Tarpey, P.S.; Sheldon, H.; Martincorena, I.; Van Loo, P.; Gundem, G.; Wedge, D.; Ramakrishna, M.; Cooke, S.L.; Pillay, N.; et al. Recurrent PTPRB and PLCG1 mutations in angiosarcoma. *Nat. Genet.* **2014**, *46*, 376–379. [CrossRef]

18. Guo, T.; Zhang, L.; Chang, N.-E.; Maki, S.S.R.G.; Antonescu, C.R. Consistent MYC and FLT4 Gene Amplification in Radiation-Induced Angiosarcoma But Not in Other Radiation-Associated Atypical Vascular Lesions Tianhua. *Cancer* 2011, *396*, 389–396.
19. Motaparthi, K.; Lauer, S.R.; Patel, R.M.; Vidal, C.I.; Linos, K. MYC gene amplification by fluorescence in situ hybridization and MYC protein expression by immunohistochemistry in the diagnosis of cutaneous angiosarcoma: Systematic review and appropriate use criteria. *J. Cutan. Pathol.* 2020, *48*, 578–586. [CrossRef]
20. Manner, J.; Radlwimmer, B.; Hohenberger, P.; Mössinger, K.; Küffer, S.; Sauer, C.; Belharazem, D.; Zettl, A.; Coindre, J.-M.; Hallermann, C.; et al. MYC High Level Gene Amplification Is a Distinctive Feature of Angiosarcomas after Irradiation or Chronic Lymphedema. *Am. J. Pathol.* 2010, *176*, 34–39. [CrossRef] [PubMed]
21. D'Angelo, S.P.; Mahoney, M.R.; A Van Tine, B.; Atkins, J.; Milhem, M.; Jahagirdar, B.N.; Antonescu, C.R.; Horvath, E.; Tap, W.D.; Schwartz, G.K.; et al. Nivolumab with or without ipilimumab treatment for metastatic sarcoma (Alliance A091401): Two open-label, non-comparative, randomised, phase 2 trials. *Lancet Oncol.* 2018, *19*, 416–426. [CrossRef]
22. Petitprez, F.; De Reyniès, A.; Keung, E.Z.; Chen, T.W.-W.; Sun, C.-M.; Calderaro, J.; Jeng, Y.-M.; Hsiao, L.-P.; Lacroix, L.; Bougoüin, A.; et al. B cells are associated with survival and immunotherapy response in sarcoma. *Nature* 2020, *577*, 556–560. [CrossRef]
23. McDermott, D.F.; Huseni, M.A.; Atkins, M.B.; Motzer, R.J.; Rini, B.I.; Escudier, B.; Fong, L.; Joseph, R.W.; Pal, S.K.; Reeves, J.A.; et al. Clinical activity and molecular correlates of response to atezolizumab alone or in combination with bevacizumab versus sunitinib in renal cell carcinoma. *Nat. Med.* 2018, *24*, 749–757. [CrossRef] [PubMed]
24. Becht, E.; Giraldo, N.; Lacroix, L.; Buttard, B.; Elarouci, N.; Petitprez, F.; Selves, J.; Laurent-Puig, P.; Sautes-Fridman, C.; Fridman, W.H.; et al. Estimating the population abundance of tissue-infiltrating immune and stromal cell populations using gene expression. *Genome Biol.* 2016, *17*, 1–20. [CrossRef]
25. Alexandrov, L.; Initiative, A.P.C.G.; Nik-Zainal, S.; Wedge, D.; Aparicio, S.A.J.R.; Behjati, S.; Biankin, A.; Bignell, G.R.; Bolli, N.; Borg, A.; et al. Signatures of mutational processes in human cancer. *Nature* 2013, *500*, 415–421. [CrossRef] [PubMed]
26. Luke, J.J.; Flaherty, K.T.; Ribas, A.; Long, G. Targeted agents and immunotherapies: Optimizing outcomes in melanoma. *Nat. Rev. Clin. Oncol.* 2017, *14*, 463–482. [CrossRef]
27. Boichard, A.; Wagner, M.J.; Kurzrock, R. Angiosarcoma heterogeneity and potential therapeutic vulnerability to immune checkpoint blockade: Insights from genomic sequencing. *Genome Med.* 2020, *12*, 1–6. [CrossRef]
28. Chan, J.Y.; Lim, J.Q.; Yeong, J.; Ravi, V.; Guan, P.; Boot, A.; Tay, T.K.Y.; Selvarajan, S.; Nasir, N.D.M.; Loh, J.H.; et al. Multiomic analysis and immunoprofiling reveal distinct subtypes of human angiosarcoma. *J. Clin. Investig.* 2020, *130*, 5833–5846. [CrossRef]
29. Riaz, N.; Havel, J.; Makarov, V.; Desrichard, A.; Urba, W.J.; Sims, J.S.; Hodi, F.S.; Martín-Algarra, S.; Mandal, R.; Sharfman, W.H.; et al. Tumor and Microenvironment Evolution during Immunotherapy with Nivolumab. *Cell* 2017, *171*, 934–949.e16. [CrossRef]
30. Bykov, V.J.N.; Eriksson, S.E.; Bianchi, J.; Wiman, K. Targeting mutant p53 for efficient cancer therapy. *Nat. Rev. Cancer* 2017, *18*, 89–102. [CrossRef]
31. Cluzeau, T.; Sebert, M.; Rahmé, R.; Cuzzubbo, S.; Walter-Petrich, A.; Che, J.L.; Peterlin, P.; Beve, B.; Attalah, H.; Chermat, F.; et al. APR-246 Combined with Azacitidine (AZA) in TP53 Mutated Myelodysplastic Syndrome (MDS) and Acute Myeloid Leukemia (AML). a Phase 2 Study By the Groupe Francophone Des Myélodysplasies (GFM). *Blood* 2019, *134*, 677. [CrossRef]
32. Makita, S.; Tobinai, K. Targeting EZH2 with tazemetostat. *Lancet Oncol.* 2018, *19*, 586–587. [CrossRef]
33. Stacchiotti, S.; Schoffski, P.; Jones, R.; Agulnik, M.; Villalobos, V.M.; Jahan, T.M.; Chen, T.W.-W.; Italiano, A.; Demetri, G.D.; Cote, G.M.; et al. Safety and efficacy of tazemetostat, a first-in-class EZH2 inhibitor, in patients (pts) with epithelioid sarcoma (ES) (NCT02601950). *J. Clin. Oncol.* 2019, *37*, 11003. [CrossRef]
34. Blay, J.-Y.; Toulmonde, M.; Penel, N.; Mir, O.; Chevreau, C.; Anract, P.; Bompas, E.; Rios, M.; Firmin, N.; Italiano, A.; et al. Natural history of sarcomas and impact of reference centers in the nationwide NETSARC study on 35,784 patients (pts) from 2010 to 2017. *Ann. Oncol.* 2018, *29*, viii576. [CrossRef]
35. Alldredge, J.K.; Eskander, R.N. EZH2 inhibition in ARID1A mutated clear cell and endometrioid ovarian and endometrioid endometrial cancers. *Gynecol. Oncol. Res. Pract.* 2017, *4*, 1–9. [CrossRef]
36. Caumanns, J.J.; Wisman, G.B.A.; Berns, K.; van der Zee, A.G.; de Jong, S. ARID1A mutant ovarian clear cell carcinoma: A clear target for synthetic lethal strategies. *Biochim. et Biophys. Acta (BBA) - Bioenerg.* 2018, *1870*, 176–184. [CrossRef]
37. Wu, Y.; Poulos, R.C.; Reddel, R.R. Role of POT1 in Human Cancer. *Cancers* 2020, *12*, 2739. [CrossRef]
38. Delehouze, C.; Godl, K.; Loaec, N.; Bruyere, C.; Desban, N.; Oumata, N.; Galons, H.; Roumeliotis, T.I.; Giannopoulou, E.G.; Grenet, J.; et al. CDK/CK1 inhibitors roscovitine and CR8 downregulate amplified MYCN in neuroblastoma cells. *Oncogene* 2013, *33*, 5675–5687. [CrossRef]
39. Frame, S.; Saladino, C.; Mackay, C.; Atrash, B.; Sheldrake, P.; McDonald, E.; Clarke, P.A.; Workman, P.; Blake, D.; Zheleva, D. Fadraciclib (CYC065), a novel CDK inhibitor, targets key pro-survival and oncogenic pathways in cancer. *PLoS ONE* 2020, *15*, e0234103. [CrossRef]
40. Horiuchi, D.; Kusdra, L.; Huskey, N.E.; Chandriani, S.; Lenburg, M.; Gonzalez-Angulo, A.M.; Creasman, K.J.; Bazarov, A.V.; Smyth, J.; Davis, S.E.; et al. MYC pathway activation in triple-negative breast cancer is synthetic lethal with CDK inhibition. *J. Exp. Med.* 2012, *209*, 679–696. [CrossRef]
41. Bolin, S.; Borgenvik, A.; Persson, C.; Sundström, A.; Qi, J.; Bradner, J.E.; Weiss, W.; Cho, Y.-J.; Weishaupt, H.; Swartling, F.J. Combined BET bromodomain and CDK2 inhibition in MYC-driven medulloblastoma. *Oncogene* 2018, *37*, 2850–2862. [CrossRef] [PubMed]

42. Li, W.; Gupta, S.K.; Han, W.; Kundson, R.A.; Nelson, S.; Knutson, D.; Greipp, P.T.; Elsawa, S.F.; Sotomayor, E.M.; Gupta, M. Targeting MYC activity in double-hit lymphoma with MYC and BCL2 and/or BCL6 rearrangements with epigenetic bromodomain inhibitors. *J. Hematol. Oncol.* **2019**, *12*, 1–13. [CrossRef] [PubMed]
43. Delmore, J.E.; Issa, G.C.; Lemieux, M.; Rahl, P.B.; Shi, J.; Jacobs, H.M.; Kastritis, E.; Gilpatrick, T.; Paranal, R.M.; Qi, J.; et al. BET Bromodomain Inhibition as a Therapeutic Strategy to Target c-Myc. *Cell* **2011**, *146*, 904–917. [CrossRef] [PubMed]
44. Yi, J.; Liu, C.; Tao, Z.; Wang, M.; Jia, Y.; Sang, X.; Shen, L.; Xue, Y.; Jiang, K.; Luo, F.; et al. MYC status as a determinant of synergistic response to Olaparib and Palbociclib in ovarian cancer. *EBioMedicine* **2019**, *43*, 225–237. [CrossRef]
45. Andre, F.; Ciruelos, E.; Rubovszky, G.; Campone, M.; Loibl, S.; Rugo, H.S.; Iwata, H.; Conte, P.; Mayer, I.A.; Kaufman, B.; et al. Alpelisib for PIK3CA-Mutated, Hormone Receptor–Positive Advanced Breast Cancer. *N. Engl. J. Med.* **2019**, *380*, 1929–1940. [CrossRef]
46. Moore, A.R.; Rosenberg, S.C.; McCormick, F.; Malek, S. RAS-targeted therapies: Is the undruggable drugged? *Nat. Rev. Drug Discov.* **2020**, *19*, 533–552. [CrossRef]
47. Hong, D.S.; Fakih, M.G.; Strickler, J.H.; Desai, J.; Durm, G.A.; Shapiro, G.I.; Falchook, G.S.; Price, T.J.; Sacher, A.; Denlinger, C.S.; et al. KRASG12C Inhibition with Sotorasib in Advanced Solid Tumors. *N. Engl. J. Med.* **2020**, *383*, 1207–1217. [CrossRef]
48. Megquier, K.; Turner-Maier, J.; Swofford, R.; Kim, J.-H.; Sarver, A.L.; Wang, C.; Sakthikumar, S.; Johnson, J.; Koltookian, M.; Lewellen, M.; et al. Comparative Genomics Reveals Shared Mutational Landscape in Canine Hemangiosarcoma and Human Angiosarcoma. *Mol. Cancer Res.* **2019**, *17*, 2410–2421. [CrossRef]

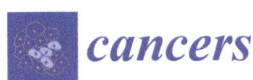

Review

Tumor and Peripheral Immune Status in Soft Tissue Sarcoma: Implications for Immunotherapy

Luana Madalena Sousa [1,2], Jani Sofia Almeida [3,4,5,6,7], Tânia Fortes-Andrade [1], Manuel Santos-Rosa [3,4,5,6,7], Paulo Freitas-Tavares [7,8], José Manuel Casanova [4,5,6,7,8] and Paulo Rodrigues-Santos [1,3,4,5,6,7,*]

1. Laboratory of Immunology and Oncology, Center for Neuroscience and Cell Biology (CNC), University of Coimbra, 3004-504 Coimbra, Portugal; luana.sousa@student.uc.pt (L.M.S.); tania.andrade@student.fmed.uc.pt (T.F.-A.)
2. Life Sciences Department, Faculty of Sciences and Technology (FCTUC), University of Coimbra, 3000-456 Coimbra, Portugal
3. Institute of Immunology, Faculty of Medicine (FMUC), University of Coimbra, 3004-504 Coimbra, Portugal; jani.almeida@student.uc.pt (J.S.A.); msrosa@fmed.uc.pt (M.S.-R.)
4. Center of Investigation in Environment, Genetics and Oncobiology (CIMAGO), Faculty of Medicine, University of Coimbra, 3000-548 Coimbra, Portugal; jmcasanova@fmed.uc.pt
5. Coimbra Institute for Clinical and Biomedical Research (iCBR), Faculty of Medicine, University of Coimbra, 3000-548 Coimbra, Portugal
6. Center for Innovation in Biomedicine and Biotechnology (CIBB), University of Coimbra, 3000-548 Coimbra, Portugal
7. Clinical Academic Centre of Coimbra (CACC), 3000-075 Coimbra, Portugal; pftavares@chuc.min-saude.pt
8. Coimbra Hospital and University Center (CHUC), Tumor Unit of the Locomotor Apparatus (UTAL), University Clinic of Orthopedics, Orthopedics Service, 3000-075 Coimbra, Portugal
* Correspondence: paulo.santos@fmed.uc.pt; Tel.: +351-239-857-777 (ext. 242844)

Simple Summary: Soft Tissue Sarcomas are a rare and heterogeneous group of tumors, which have a characteristic complexity, leading to a difficult diagnosis and a lack of response to treatment. The aim of this review is to summarize the role of immune cells, soluble plasmatic factors, immune checkpoints; and the expression of immune-related genes predicting survival, response to therapy, and potential immunotherapeutic agents or targets in Soft Tissue Sarcomas.

Abstract: Soft Tissue Sarcomas (STS) are a heterogeneous and rare group of tumors. Immune cells, soluble factors, and immune checkpoints are key elements of the complex tumor microenvironment. Monitoring these elements could be used to predict the outcome of the disease, the response to therapy, and lead to the development of new immunotherapeutic approaches. Tumor-infiltrating B cells, Natural Killer (NK) cells, tumor-associated neutrophils (TANs), and dendritic cells (DCs) were associated with a better outcome. On the contrary, tumor-associated macrophages (TAMs) were correlated with a poor outcome. The evaluation of peripheral blood immunological status in STS could also be important and is still underexplored. The increased lymphocyte-to-monocyte ratio (LMR) and neutrophil-to-lymphocyte ratio (NLR), higher levels of monocytic myeloid-derived suppressor cells (M-MDSCs), and Tim-3 positive CD8 T cells appear to be negative prognostic markers. Meanwhile, NKG2D-positive CD8 T cells were correlated with a better outcome. Some soluble factors, such as cytokines, chemokines, growth factors, and immune checkpoints were associated with the prognosis. Similarly, the expression of immune-related genes in STS was also reviewed. Despite these efforts, only very little is known, and much research is still needed to clarify the role of the immune system in STS.

Keywords: soft tissue sarcoma; immune monitoring; immunophenotyping; cytokines; immune checkpoints; gene expression

1. Soft Tissue Sarcoma

Soft Tissue Sarcomas (STS) are a heterogeneous group of diseases of mesenchymal origin. STS represent approximately 1% of solid tumors [1]. This group comprises over 50 different histologic subtypes that affect patients of all ages [2]. Although they can occur anywhere in the body, the most common anatomic sites are the extremities (60–70%) and the abdomen and retroperitoneum (20%) [3]. In addition to being highly heterogeneous in anatomical localization and histology, they are also heterogeneous in terms of molecular characteristics and prognosis [4].

STS diagnosis is mainly based on histological interpretations, including immunohistochemistry, cytogenetic, and molecular analysis [5]. However, due to their rarity and heterogeneity, the diagnosis is challenging and requires expert analysis [6]. Therefore, a consensus and reproducible diagnostic criteria are crucial. The WHO classification provides an organization by tumor type, considering morphologic, immunohistochemical, and genetic features [7,8]. This classification also stratifies STS according to clinical behavior into benign, intermediate locally aggressive, intermediate rarely metastasizing, and malignant [7,8].

The increased availability of genomic technologies has provided a better understanding of sarcoma biology. STS can be divided into two groups based on genetic profiles: STS associated with specific genetic alterations and STS with nonspecific and nonrecurrent genetic alterations [5]. The first group includes chromosomal translocations that produce chimeric fusion genes, often encoding aberrant transcription factors, oncogenic mutations, or recurrent gene amplifications. These alterations may be tumor-specific or shared by several histological tumors with different histomorphologies and behaviors. In contrast to the STS associated with specific genetic alterations, the second group tends to have complex karyotypes, such as changes in chromosome number, unbalanced translocations, genetic deletions, and amplifications [5]. Concerning etiology, even though the majority is unknown, there are some genetic predisposal syndromes, such as Li-Fraumeni syndrome, Von Recklinghausen disease, or RB1 tumor-suppressor gene mutations that can lead to STS. Environmental factors, such as ionization, radiation, and chemical exhibitors, may also promote these sarcomas [6].

For localized STS, surgical resection with or without radiotherapy is the standard treatment. Unfortunately, STS recurs frequently as a locally inoperable or metastatic disease. For a locally advanced or metastatic disease, the usual treatment is chemotherapy [9]. Single-agent anthracycline is the first-line therapy and, for the second-line treatment, trabectedin and eribulin have demonstrated efficacy for some subtypes of STS [4].

Despite the remarkable improvement in cancer diagnosis and treatment, many patients do not respond to therapy. This limited effectiveness of current strategies is often attributed to the complexity of the disease. That is, at least partly, supported by the complex microenvironment where the tumor is growing and defeating the immune system

There is a growing interest in studying the immunological status of STS patients. The tumor microenvironment (TME) includes different populations of non-tumor cells, such as endothelial, stromal, cancer-associated fibroblasts and adipocytes, and immune cells [9]. The study of tumor-infiltrating and peripheral immune cells and mediators of the immune response may help to reveal the mechanisms related to tumor immunity. Moreover, such a study could identify potential biomarkers that favor an accurate prognosis, effective therapy response monitoring, and a refined approach to treatment. Recently, a transcriptomic analysis of >10,000 patients identified four distinct TME subtypes conserved across 20 different cancers: immune-enriched, fibrotic (IE/F); immune-enriched, non-fibrotic (IE); fibrotic (F); and immune-depleted (D). This TME subtyping strongly correlated with survival in most of the cancer types analyzed. The IE/F and IE TME were correlated with a better prognosis, while the F TME was linked to a worse prognosis. Furthermore, this study has also showed that patients with immune-favorable TME subtypes could benefit the most from immunotherapeutic approaches [10].

Concerning sarcomas, critical elements of peripheral blood and TME also play an essential role in predicting the response to therapy and are potential therapeutic agents or targets. Furthermore, a study from The Cancer Genome Atlas (TCGA) consortium proposed an association of the TME with prognosis in different STS histotypes [11]. Regarding the TME, the immune cells play an important role in controlling the progression of multiple tumor types. Nevertheless, in human STS, their characterization remains poorly defined. In a later study, Petitprez et al. developed a new classification and stratification of STS based on the composition of the immune microenvironment [12]. This classification was made up of five sarcoma immune classes with clearly different profiles and significantly different TME compositions. Each histological subtype was identified in each class, making it clear that the immune profile varies even between tumors with the same histology. This work also confirmed that the simplistic characterization of STS as "non-immunogenic" tumors does not apply to all, given that two sarcoma immune classes showed an elevated expression of genes specific to immune populations and the expression of immune-checkpoint-related genes. Furthermore, they also demonstrated that the immune microenvironment could be used to evaluate the prognosis and predict the response to immunotherapy.

The aim of this review was to summarize the prognostic and therapy response prediction value of immune cells, soluble plasmatic factors, immune checkpoints, and the expression of immune-related genes in STS patients, as well as their role in immunotherapeutic approaches.

2. The Role of Immune Cells in STS

2.1. Tumor-Associated Macrophages

Macrophages are vital innate immune cells present in tissues, and it has been suggested that they play a role in tumor development and progression [13]. They are differentiated by the local microenvironment into M1 or M2 macrophages, developing a pro- or anti-inflammatory response, respectively. Macrophages that are differentiated by the TME are called tumor-associated macrophages (TAMs). Due to several factors, for example, IL-4 and IL-13, an M2-like differentiation occurs in the TME, which facilitates tumor immune escape and metastasis [14,15]. M2-like TAMs block CD8 T cell-mediated anti-tumor immune response either directly, through their expression of inhibitor ligands, such as the programmed death-ligand 1 (PD-L1), or indirectly, via the C-C motif chemokine ligand 22 (CCL-22)-mediated recruitment of regulatory T cells (Tregs). A recent study detected, through immunohistochemistry, M2-like TAMs in all STS samples, while M1-like TAMs were only found in a few tumors and in a low density [16]. The presence of TAMs polarized toward a pro-tumoral phenotype in all the STS samples analyzed supports the possibility of targeting TAMs for STS treatment. TAMs could also be used to predict the clinical outcome. In several tumor types, this prognostic significance has already been shown [17,18]. However, concerning sarcomas, little is currently known. Still, the high density of M2-like macrophages, expressing CD163, and M1-like macrophages, identified by CD68 staining, were both significantly correlated with a poor outcome in non-gynecologic leiomyosarcomas [19]. Later, Kostine et al. also evaluated M2 and M1-like macrophages, and only the M2 phenotype was associated with worse survival rates for leiomyosarcoma [20]. Similarly, in myxoid liposarcoma (MLS), high levels of TAMs were also associated with poor survival [21]. More recently, a study performed with different types of STS identified TAMs as a poor prognostic for local recurrence, confirming the negative prognostic value of TAMs [22].

2.2. Tumor-Associated Neutrophils

Neutrophils make up a substantial proportion of the immune infiltrate in cancer, and their role has long been a matter of controversy. Similar to TAMs, in mouse models, it has been demonstrated that tumor-associated neutrophils (TANs) can retain some functional plasticity and can acquire different phenotypes based on specific features of the TME. In a

TGF-β-rich environment, neutrophils usually acquire an N2 phenotype associated with a pro-tumor activity. On the contrary, in the presence of IFN-β or inhibition of TGF-β, neutrophils switch to an N1 profile, which is usually associated with anti-tumor activity. Although the tumor-promoting effects of N2 TANs have been demonstrated, human TANs remain underexplored [23]. Ponzetta et al. have shown that mice with profound neutropenia presented an earlier tumor development compared with wild-type mice [24]. Moreover, the adoptive cell transfer of neutrophils into sarcoma-bearing mice restores tumor growth to the level of the control group. These results prove that TANs are essential to restrain sarcomagenesis. The same study also showed a correlation between the high density of TANs and a better outcome in undifferentiated pleomorphic sarcomas (UPS). However, this correlation was not observed in other STS subtypes, such as dedifferentiated liposarcoma, leiomyosarcoma, and myxofibrosarcoma.

2.3. Tumor-Infiltrating Lymphocytes

Tumor-infiltrating lymphocytes (TILs) are strong indicators of tumor immunogenicity. TILs have been described in various malignant tumors, including STS, and some studies support the influence of TILs on the progression of some tumors [25]. It was observed that most STS patients had low TIL infiltration. However, in STS, TILs have been only reported considering a few STS subtypes in limited sample size studies. For these reasons, although the presence of TILs and their impact on positive outcomes have been demonstrated in several sarcoma subtypes, these reports may not be representative of all STS [12,26].

2.3.1. T Cells

To explore the level of T cell infiltration in STS, two studies analyzed the expression profile of CD3E. The former suggested that T-cell infiltration could depend on the STS subtype and proposed that a highly mutated tumor type may have greater immunogenicity and a robust T-cell infiltrate [27]. In the latter, CD3E was highly expressed in some STS samples, such as rhabdomyosarcoma and alveolar soft part sarcoma, corroborating the idea that T-cell infiltration depends on the STS subtype [28].

CD8 T cells can mediate the lysis of neoplastic cells. For that reason, these cells are usually associated with a direct anti-tumor immune response. Furthermore, there is an influence of these cells on the clinical course of several types of tumors. However, the excessive and constant exposure of CD8 T cells to cancer antigens and inflammatory signals leads to a progressive loss of the T cell effector function; this is called "exhaustion". Exhausted T cells can be characterized by the presence of inhibitory receptors; PD-1 and LAG3 are among them [29]. The analysis of CD8 T cells in the TME, including their receptor repertoire, has been increasing, given the availability of new activating drugs [30].

CD4 T cells are also required for anti-tumor immunity. They comprise diverse subsets with different and sometimes opposing roles in TME, upregulating or downregulating the immune response. Regarding their anti-tumor activity, they are responsible for enhancing the cytotoxic function of CD8 T cells, increasing clonal expansion, functioning as antigen-presenting cells, for example [31,32]. Fresh tumors resected at surgery and analyzed by flow cytometry have shown a greater prevalence of CD4 than CD8 T cells in well differentiated and dedifferentiated retroperitoneal liposarcoma [30]. The majority of tumor-infiltrating lymphocytes were CD4 'helper' T cells, and most CD8 T cells expressed their programmed cell death protein 1 (PD-1). This information suggests that CD8 T cells have been triggered by tumor antigen but are suppressed.

On the contrary, D'Angelo et al. described a greater prevalence of CD8 than CD4 T cells in STS tumors [33]. Those tumors were more likely to express PD-L1 and PD-1, once more suggesting the inactivation of these cells. Another study analyzed the density of T cells in 28 tumors diagnosed as undifferentiated sarcoma [34]. They observed a positive correlation between the density of CD8 T cells and the density of macrophages. Since some studies have indicated that TAMs suppress the cytotoxic functions and chemotaxis of CD8

T cells in other tumors, it would be interesting to know whether TAMs also affect CD8 T cells in undifferentiated sarcomas [35,36].

Several studies have been trying to correlate the frequency of immune cells with the prognosis in STS (Figure 1). An association between CD8 T cells and improved outcomes has been observed [26,37,38]. However, conflicting studies have also observed an association with poor outcomes [39]. Moreover, there are also other studies that state that there is no statistical significance in this correlation [34,40]. Concerning CD4 T cells, the controversy remains. Although in some studies, CD4 T cells have been associated with a positive outcome [40,41], the opposite, an association with a poor prognosis, has also been observed [33,39]. In addition, some studies do not observe any significant prognostic value [38]. These discrepancies between studies may be due to the differences in methodology, antibody clones, and cutoff values used [39]. Furthermore, studies have indicated that these cell frequencies vary between STS subtypes and treatments [42,43]. For these reasons, the differences in sarcoma subtypes and the limited size of patient cohorts may also explain the discrepancies in the results.

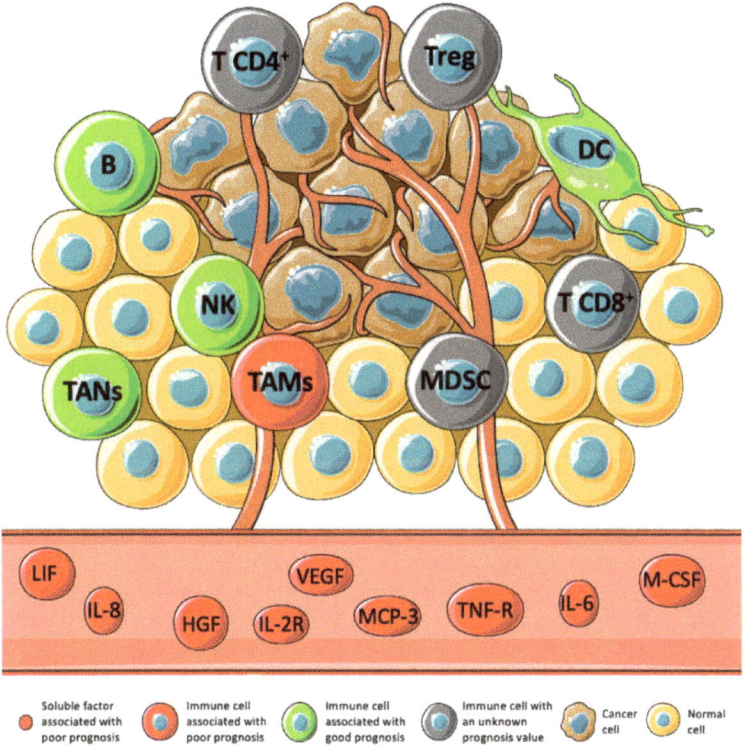

Figure 1. Expression levels of immune cell subtypes, cytokines, chemokines, growth factors, and soluble receptors and their prognostic value in STS. The TME has been associated with the prognosis in several tumors. However, in STS, this association is still underexplored. Immune cells such as B cell, DC, TANs, and NK have been associated with a positive prognosis (green). On the contrary, TAMs, and some soluble factors: LIF, IL-8, HGF, IL-2R, VEGF, MCP-3, TNF-R, IL-6, and M-CSF, have been associated with a negative prognosis (red). The prognostic value of MDSCs, Tregs, CD4 T cells, and CD8 T cells is not clear yet (gray) [11,22,24,26,40,42,44–47].

2.3.2. B Cells

Recent data have shown that B cells can shape immune responses in tumors [48]. However, the association of these cells with disease prognosis has been a reason for disagreement.

In several tumors, it described an association with a good prognosis. However, the opposite has been reported, too [16]. In well-differentiated and dedifferentiated retroperitoneal liposarcoma, B cells were found, generally with a low frequency, in some of the tumors analyzed [30]. In 2011, it was suggested that B cells could be an independent favorable prognostic factor in STS patients with wide resection margins [40]. Later, the association of B cells with a good prognosis was supported by Tsagozis et al. [16]. This study also observed an absence of B cells in many tumor areas, corroborating previous works.

Recently, Petitprez et al. published an integrative analysis dedicated to B cells and their influence on sarcoma survival and immunotherapy response [12]. They found that B cells are a key discriminative feature of a group of patients with improved survival and a better response to PD-1 blockade therapy, confirming their role as a positive prognostic factor. In addition, Helmink et al. found that B cell markers were the most differentially expressed genes in the tumors of STS responsive patients versus tumors of patients that did not respond to immunotherapy [49]. This data confirmed once more the potential of B cells as biomarkers.

2.3.3. Natural Killer Cells

Natural killer cells (NK) have the ability to lyse transformed cells [50]. Therefore, these cells play an important role in cancer immunosurveillance [51]. Studies of other tumors, such as clear cell renal cancer and non-small cell lung cancer, have evaluated the role of NK cells in the TME and the relationship between the infiltration of NK cells and the clinical outcome [52–54].

There have been a few studies of the NK cell function in STS. One of them used flow cytometry to detect infiltrating NK cells, generally in a low density, in some well-differentiated and dedifferentiated retroperitoneal liposarcoma tissues [30]. Another study analyzed the tumor immune microenvironment signatures of 206 STS patients [11]. Regarding NK cell infiltrate, they reported that these immune cells were the only cells to correlate significantly with better disease-specific survival (DSS) in several sarcoma types. Later, Judge et al. also correlated tumor-infiltrating NK cells with improved survival in STS [26].

Although NK cells display an even higher cytolytic activity compared to CD8 T cells, their cytolytic function may be drastically dependent on the balance of activating and inhibiting surface receptors [55]. One activating receptor, NKp30, was found to be particularly downregulated in peripheral and tumor-infiltrating NK cells in gastrointestinal sarcoma (GIST) when compared to the circulating NKp30+ NK cells of healthy volunteers [56]. Nevertheless, the levels of total NK cells were similar in GIST and healthy volunteers. These results highlight the importance of further studies focused on NK cell receptors, since they affect the functions of these cells without affecting their frequency.

2.4. Dendritic Cells

Dendritic cells (DCs) also play an essential role in the immunological environment. The TCGA analyzed the immune cell infiltrates based on tumor gene expression signatures and showed a correlation between the presence of tumor-infiltrating DCs and improved DSS in UPS and myxofibrosarcoma [11]. Although there is a lack of studies concerning DCs in STS, this conclusion suggests an important role of antigen presentation in immune responses against these tumors.

2.5. Suppressor Cells

2.5.1. Regulatory T Cells

Regulatory T cells (Tregs) are physiologically suppressive cells and play an important role in maintaining the homeostasis of the immune response. They can produce immunosuppressive cytokines such as interleukin 10 (IL-10) and tumor growth factor-β (TGF-β), they can express negative costimulatory molecules such as cytotoxic T-lymphocyte-associated protein 4 (CTLA-4), PD-1, or PD-L1, and they consume cytokine interleukin 2 (IL-2). These functions lead to an inhibition of T lymphocytes and the promotion of immune escape [57]. Studies of other tumors have associated high density of tumor-infiltrating Tregs with a poor outcome. However, the opposite has also been demonstrated [58]. In STS, D'Angelo et al., using immunohistochemistry, observed a high density of tumor-infiltrating Tregs in 75% of STS patients, most of them of GIST histology [33]. Later, another study evaluated tumor-infiltrating Tregs by immunohistochemistry and showed an association between the increased infiltration of these cells and a poor prognosis in STS [44]. However, an association has also been found between a greater percentage of Tregs, analyzed by multiplex immunofluorescence, and a better outcome [59]. The same study also correlated the increased tumor-infiltrating Tregs with a better response to pembrolizumab, anti-PD-1 monotherapy. Despite this, it has also been suggested that Tregs are not associated with STS prognosis [26,38]. Due to these controversial results and the limited number of studies, the prognostic significance of Tregs remains undefined.

2.5.2. Myeloid-Derived Suppressor Cells

Myeloid-derived suppressor cells (MDSCs) are another subset of suppressive cells that can facilitate tumor immune escape, impairing the function of T cells, NK cells, and DCs. These immature myeloid cells can be phenotypically divided into early-MDSCs (e-MDSCs), monocytic MDSCs (M-MDSCs), and polymorphonuclear MDSCs (PMN-MDSCs) [60,61].

A study performed by Highfill et al. sought to investigate whether there was an expansion of MDSCs in rhabdomyosarcoma, the most common soft tissue sarcoma of childhood [60]. They used mice bearing rhabdomyosarcoma and observed, by flow cytometry, an expansion of MDSCs, preferentially PMN-MDSCs, localized at the tumor site. It was demonstrated that PMN-MDSCs have an essential role in rhabdomyosarcoma immune escape. Preventing the trafficking of these cells to the tumor could also improve the efficacy of checkpoint blockade. The role of MDSCs in human STS tumors remains underexplored.

3. Soluble Factors: Cytokines, Chemokines, Growth Factors, and Others

The network of pro- and anti-inflammatory cytokines and chemokines orchestrates the immune cell signaling and function and, as such, largely contributes to the complexity of the TME. Cytokines have been studied in a broad range of tumors, and their involvement in cancer development, progression, and recurrence has been suggested. Moreover, the cytokine profile might be a prognostic factor for clinical outcome [62,63]. The prognostic value of cytokines, chemokines, growth factors, and soluble receptors in STS is summarized in Figure 1.

As well as cytokines, chemokines have multifaceted roles in tumor development and progression, promoting malignancy or restricting tumor growth [64]. Likewise, growth factors and soluble receptors also play a significant role in TME [65,66].

Preliminary studies have found an elevated serum level of some cytokines, growth factors, and immune-related soluble receptors in patients with STS. Higher serum levels of vascular endothelial growth factor (VEGF) and fibroblast growth factor (FGF) have been reported. They promote angiogenesis, facilitating the tumor's growth and increased metastatic spread. Furthermore, VEGF also promotes the proliferation of immunosuppressive cells and T cell exhaustion, contributing largely to immune escape and cancer development [67–69]. In addition, increased serum levels of interleukin 6 (IL-6), receptors for TNF (TNF-RI and TNF-RII), interleukin 2 receptor α (IL-2Rα), interleukin 10 (IL-10), macrophage-colony stimulating factor (M-CSF), and interleukin-8 (IL-8) were also found in STS patients [45,70,71].

Rutkowski et al. analyzed the serum levels of 13 cytokines and soluble receptors in STS patients before treatment [45]. The results confirmed the elevated levels of VEGF, FGF, IL-6, TNF RI, TNF RII, IL-2Rα, IL-10, M-CSF, and IL-8 stated above. Furthermore, they tried to correlate the serum levels of these cytokines with clinic-pathological features. IL-2Rα, TNF RI, M-CSF, and VEGF correlated with tumor size, IL-8 was associated with tumor grade, and IL-6 appeared to be correlated with tumor size, grade, and metastases. Additionally, it was proved that IL-6 and IL-8 were correlated with decreased survival [45].

In relation to IL-6, a few more studies have confirmed the association of its serum levels with survival. Hagi et al. observed high levels of IL-6 associated with the presence of STS and proposed that IL-6 could be used as a marker for the differential diagnosis [72]. Furthermore, they confirmed the correlation between elevated IL-6 serum levels and decreased survival [69].

Wysoczynski et al. proposed that leukemia inhibitory factor (LIF) promotes the progression and the metastatic behavior of rhabdomyosarcoma cells, contributing to the resistance of rhabdomyosarcoma to conventional treatment [46]. Later, Wysoczynski found that IL-8 was a pivotal pro-angiogenic factor in rhabdomyosarcoma cells during hypoxia [73]. Still, in rhabdomyosarcoma cells, another study showed that tumor cell progression seemed to be regulated by the interleukin-4 receptor (IL-4R)-dependent signaling pathway, highlighting the role of IL-4 in this common type of STS [74].

TNF was also found in high levels in STS patient serum [45]. Similar to IL-6, the correlation between TNF and tumor grade, size, metastases, or recurrence was investigated. However, there was no significant association between the serum levels of TNF and these clinic-pathological features. Similarly, no association between these features and serum levels of IL-10 and granulocyte colony-stimulating factor (G-CSF) was demonstrated in STS patients [45].

Regarding IL-2Rα, its higher level in STS patients has been correlated with tumor size. Another study performed in 2012 suggested that a low serum level of IL-2Rα was associated with prolonged overall survival (OS) [47]. In this same study, Sleijfer et al. also indicated that low monocyte chemotactic protein-3 (MCP3) and hepatocyte growth factor (HGF) levels were associated with extended progression-free survival (PFS). However, they mentioned that these associations might be false-positive ones, so these results should be interpreted with caution and confirmed by more studies.

4. Expression of Immune Checkpoints and Their Ligands in STS

Immune checkpoints are essential in regulating the immune response. In cancer, they can be dysregulated, working as an immune resistance mechanism [75].

In 2013, the impact of the immune checkpoints PD-1 and PD-L1 in STS (Figure 2) was evaluated for the first time [76]. The result from immunohistochemistry showed an intratumoral infiltration of PD-1 positive lymphocytes and the expression of PD-L1 in most STS samples. Additionally, PD-1 positivity, PD-L1 positivity, and the combined PD-1/PD-L1 pattern were independent prognostic indicators of OS and event-free survival. Furthermore, more studies have evaluated these immune checkpoints, the majority by immunohistochemistry, and confirmed the presence of PD-1 and PD-L1, and their association with a negative prognosis [77–86]. However, in some studies, PD-1 and PD-L1 expression appear to be low or absent, and the PD-L1 expression has not been associated with the outcome in STS [26,33,42,59,77,81,87]. Wunder et al. showed recently that the PD-1 and PD-L1 expression depended on the STS subtype and the prognostic value of PD-L1, justifying the discrepancies between studies with different subtypes of STS [88]. In addition, these discrepancies may also be due to the use of different methods of expression assessment, cutoff values, antibody clones, and tissue samples analyzed before and after therapeutical interventions [37,88].

PD-1 and PD-L1 expression levels have also been correlated in some studies with T-cell infiltration, and PD-L1 expression has been associated with more PD-1 positive TILs [27,79].

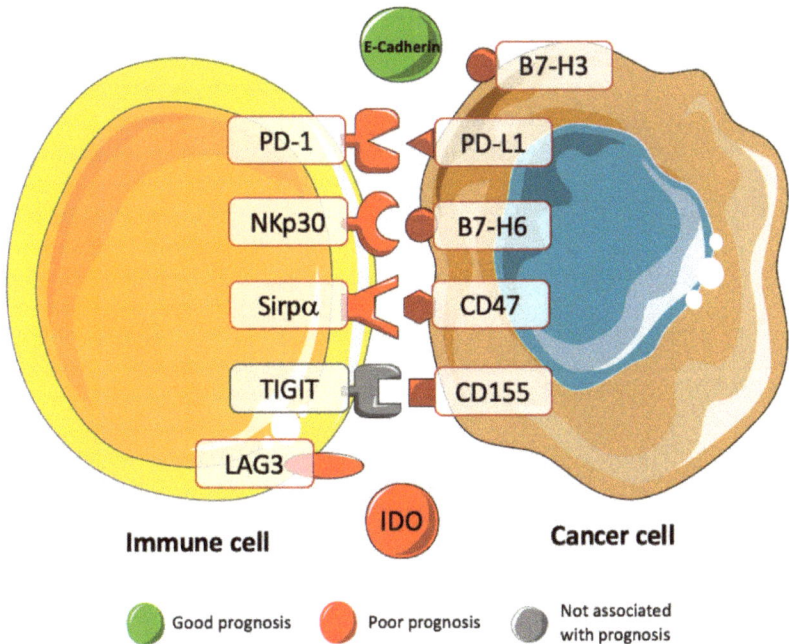

Figure 2. Prognostic value of immune checkpoints in STS. Several studies have been trying to correlate the presence of immune checkpoints with the prognosis of patients with STS. These studies have showed a negative prognostic value for B7-H3, PD-1, PD-L1, NKp30, B7-H6, Sirpα, CD47, CD155, LAG3, and IDO (red). A positive prognostic value was associated with the immune checkpoint E-Cadherin (green) [15,26,39,76–79,89–92].

Although the presence and prognostic value of these immune checkpoints has been controversial and underexplored in this type of tumor, they might still have a role in predicting the prognosis of STS patients. Furthermore, the expression of these immune checkpoints may also indicate the patients who will benefit from PD-1 therapies. In 2020, a study concluded that STS patients who responded to pembrolizumab, an anti-PD-1 monotherapy, exhibited more PD-L1-expressing macrophages than non-responders [59].

Other immune checkpoints have been studied in several tumors, but there are only a few reports for STS. A recent study analyzed the expression of the B- and T-lymphocyte attenuator (BTLA) in sarcoma and found a lower expression mainly in CD4 TIL [77]. The same study also showed a high expression of lymphocyte-activation gene 3 (LAG3) on CD8 TILs. Other studies analyzed the expression of LAG3 by immunohistochemistry [39]. They confirmed its overexpression on TILs and found a significant association of LAG3 expression with a poor clinical outcome. Ishihara et al. suggested that a lower expression of indoleamine-pyrrole 2,3-dioxygenase 1 (IDO-1) was associated with a better prognosis in UPS [89]. E-Cadherin has also been studied in STS. It has been suggested that E-Cadherin has a possible role in the maintenance of epithelial architecture [93]. Furthermore, it was observed that upregulated E-Cadherin expression was associated with a better prognosis in STS patients [90,94]. The expression of B7-H6 and B7-H3 has also been evaluated in metastatic gastrointestinal stromal tumors and rhabdomyosarcoma, respectively [91,92]. In both studies, the expression of these molecules was associated with a worse prognosis. Dancsok et al. evaluated the immune checkpoints CD47 and Sirpα expression in sarcomas for the first time [15]. Through immunohistochemistry, the expression of both macrophage-related immune checkpoints was correlated with an adverse prognostic factor. Recently, the expression of the exhaustion marker T cell immunoreceptor with Ig and ITIM domains

(TIGIT) was assessed in STS samples [26]. Although TIGIT expression was not associated with survival, the expression of its dominant ligand CD155 was associated with worse OS using the TCGA.

5. Immune-Related Gene Expression in STS

Studies of lung cancer, ovarian cancer, head and neck squamous cell carcinoma, and renal cancer have suggested that immune-related genes (IRGs) may be used as prognostic biomarkers [95–98]. The IRG expression is underexplored in STS, and its prognostic significance remains unclear (Figure 3).

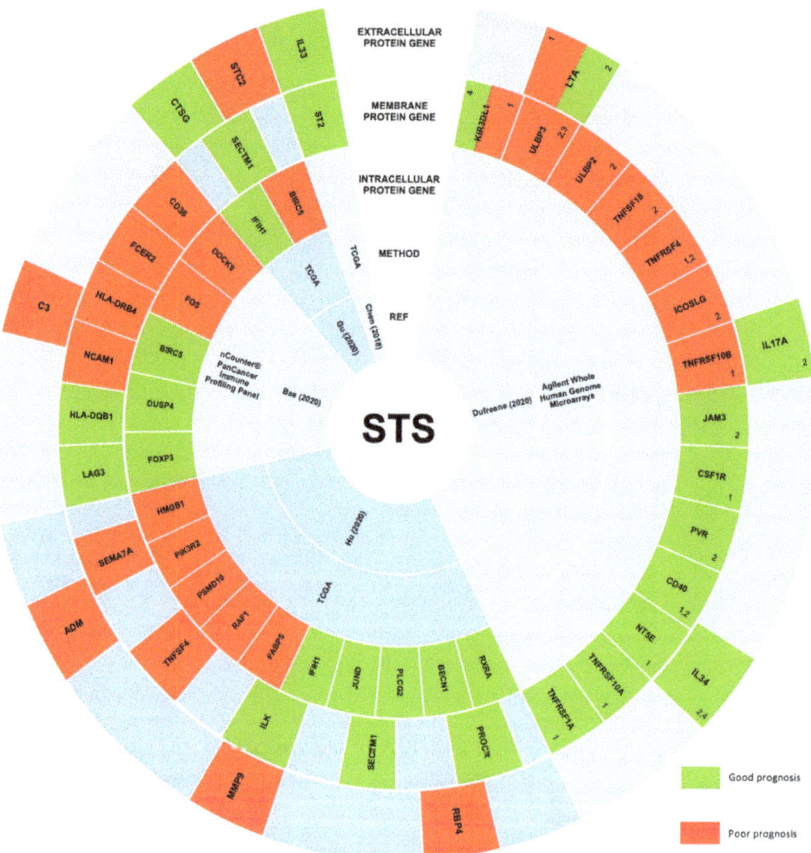

Figure 3. STS studies correlating the expression levels of immune-related genes and their prognostic significance. In STS, the expression of immune-related genes remains underexplored, and consequently, the prognostic value of these genes is still unclear. However, five main studies aimed at understanding this correlation, and their results are represented in this figure. Immune-related genes correlated with a good prognosis in STS are represented in green. On the other hand, immune-related genes associated with a bad prognosis are represented in red. From the peripheral to the center, circles represent genes encoding extracellular proteins, genes encoding transmembrane proteins, genes encoding intracellular proteins, the method used, and the respective study's first author and publication year [99–103]. [1] Prognostic value in synovial sarcomas; [2] Prognostic value in gastrointestinal stromal tumors; [3] Prognostic value in myxoid liposarcomas; [4] Prognostic value in sarcomas with complex genetics.

In STS, high and low transcription levels of IL33 and its receptor ST2 were associated with the recruitment of CD8 T cells and the recruitment of Tregs and MDSCs, respectively [99]. Moreover, in the same report, both IL33 and ST2 levels were associated with a better outcome.

Recently, the gene expression of 364 differentially expressed IRGs was analyzed [100]. It was established that 18 of these genes were significantly associated with overall OS or/and with PFS, validating their value as prognostic biomarkers. Likewise, Dufresne et al. analyzed the expression of 93 genes encoding for immune checkpoints and membrane proteins in 253 STS samples [101]. This analysis showed a correlation between the immune signature and each sarcoma subgroup, concluding that the prognostic value could depend on the group. Another study constructed an immune gene-related prognostic model using five immune-related prognostic genes: IFIH1, CTSG, STC2, SECTM1, and BIRC5 [102]. These five genes had an effective performance in risk stratification of patients, showing their potential as biomarkers for predicting the response of STS patients to immunotherapy. In addition, in 2020, the analysis of high-grade STS tissue samples, divided according to OS, identified seven genes (C3, CD36, DOCK9, FCER2, FOS, HLA-DRB4, and NCAM1) correlated with a poor prognosis, and six genes (BIRC5, DUSP4, FOXP3, HLA-DQA1, HLA-DQB1, and LAG3) correlated with a good prognosis [103].

6. Peripheral Blood Immune Status

The immunological status of peripheral blood in patients with STS remains unclear, just as its role as a prognostic indicator.

The circulating monocyte count has been studied recently as a marker of poor prognosis in several tumors [104]. In addition, the correlation between the increasing monocytes and decreasing lymphocytes with tumor growth and progression has already been proved in cancer populations [104,105]. In 2014, the lymphocyte/monocyte ratio (LMR) was studied for the first time in STS patients [106]. They concluded that the pre-treatment LMR ratio could act as a negative prognostic factor. Jiang et al. also analyzed the monocyte ratio in 124 STS patients [107]. Their analysis observed a significant association between poor prognosis for OS and PFS, and the presence of a monocyte ratio > 1, which is in line with studies concerning other tumors. In addition to being a poor prognosis factor, a low LMR indicates systemic inflammation in cancer, including STS. However, the association between inflammation indexes and the prognosis has been challenging and controversial. A study performed in 2019 evaluated 26 cases of STS and did not find significant differences in OS and PFS associated with the LMR [108].

Two meta-analyses aimed at evaluating the effect of neutrophil-to-lymphocyte ratio (NLR) in STS [109,110]. Both concluded that higher NLR was associated with poor OS, disease-free survival (DFS), and PFS. Although multiple studies have proved an association between different cellular ratios with the prognosis for several tumors, data for STS are still sparse [106]. The peripheral immunological status of STS was investigated by Kim et al. in 2021; they observed that a high level of M-MDSCs was associated with poor DFS and PFS [111]. In the same way, high levels of T-cell immunoglobulin and mucin-domain containing-3 (Tim-3) positive CD8 T cells were associated with lower DFS. On the contrary, high levels of NKG2D positive CD8 T cells were significantly associated with longer DFS times. The collection of tumor samples is usually difficult; therefore, more studies based on a minimally invasive method, such as collecting peripheral blood, are needed.

The aim of another study was to analyze the immune cells in both peripheral blood and tumor tissue [26]. The data showed that NK and T cells are both more activated and exhausted in tumor tissue than in circulation when comparing these two locations. Concerning NK cells, both $CD56^{bright}$ and $CD56^{dim}$ subsets were found in peripheral blood. However, in tumor tissues, $CD56^{bright}$, the less mature and cytotoxic subset, appears to be less prevalent. The activation marker CD69 was also evaluated, and it is more expressed in both NK subsets in the tumor, compared to the peripheral blood. Similarly, the expression of the receptor of NK and T cell exhaustion TIGIT was increased in the tumor.

Regarding NK cells from peripheral blood, Bücklein et al. analyzed this cell subset in two groups of STS patients: chemotherapy-naïve STS patients and STS patients with a progression or relapse after chemotherapeutical treatment [112]. In both, NK cells were found to be dysfunctional during a chromium release assay using K562 cells as targets. The CD56^{dim} NK cell subset frequency, studied using flow cytometry, was significantly lower in the blood from STS patients with a progression or relapse after therapy when compared to healthy donors. These conclusions could be specific to STS patients, since these alterations were not found in NK cells from renal cell carcinoma patients. In addition, a decreased expression of NKG2D, CD3ζ, and perforin was found and associated with the activation of NK cells in the second group of patients. On the contrary, Delahaye et al. did not find significant differences in the levels of peripheral NK cells nor in the NKG2D expression in GIST patients when compared to healthy volunteers [56]. However, they showed that a predominant expression of the immunosuppressive NKp30c isoform of the NKp30 receptor was associated with an unfavorable outcome.

7. Immunotherapy in STS

In 1891, William B. Coley injected streptococcal organisms into a patient with sarcoma. The injection stimulated the immune system, and the sarcoma disappeared. After this successful experiment, he treated hundreds of patients with sarcomas, including STS. Coley initiated the discipline of cancer immunotherapy and demonstrated the possible use of this type of therapy for this disease [113].

It is now clear that the immune microenvironment is highly variable in STS, and this variability is frequently justified by STS heterogenicity. Despite this heterogenicity, clinical trials continue to incorporate various sarcoma subtypes to obtain the minimum number of patients required. Although there have been hints of positive responses to immunotherapy trials for STS, most trials have been negative or are not representative of all STS subtypes. Currently (July 2021), there are 85 clinical trials focused on immunotherapy in STS. Phase II and phase III clinical trials that have been completed and targeting the immune system in STS are shown in Table 1.

As was mentioned before, the expression of PD-1 and PD-L1 were present in some studies and absent in others, which appears to depend on the STS subtype. The presence of these immune checkpoints in some subtypes offers a promise for immunotherapy based on checkpoint inhibitors in these specific subtypes. Unfortunately, clinical trials testing immune checkpoint inhibitors in STS have not showed the impressive results achieved for many other cancers. The intention of the first study was to analyze the efficacy of targeting the immune checkpoint CTLA-4 with ipilimumab in synovial sarcoma, but neither a clinical benefit nor immunological activity was demonstrated [114]. Similarly, uterine leiomyosarcoma patients did not respond to anti-PD-1 antibody nivolumab in a phase II study [115]. Later, the clinical trial SARC028 tested the anti-PD-1 therapy with pembrolizumab. Promising responses for specific subtypes were observed in this trial, such as UPS and dedifferentiated liposarcoma. Moreover, the response to pembrolizumab was correlated to higher tumor-infiltrating lymphocytes at the baseline. Based on these promising results for specific subtypes of STS and in specific immune microenvironments, further research and correlative studies are required to improve the selection of patients for future clinical trials with immune checkpoint blockade in STS.

Table 1. Completed phase II and III clinical trials for immunotherapy in soft tissue sarcomas.

	NCT Identifier	Phase	Enrollment	Title	Interventions
Adoptive Cell therapy	NCT02849366	I and II	30	Combination of Cryosurgery and NK Immunotherapy for Recurrent Sarcoma	Cryosurgery
					NK cell immunotherapy
	NCT00001566	II	42	A Pilot Study of Autologous T-Cell Transplantation With Vaccine Driven Expansion of Anti-Tumor Effectors After Cytoreductive Therapy in Metastatic Pediatric Sarcomas	Therapeutic autologous dendritic cells
					Indinavir sulfate
					Peripheral blood stem cell transplantation
	NCT00003887	II	Not	Lymphocyte Infusion in Treating Patients With Relapsed Cancer After Bone Marrow or Peripheral Stem Cell Transplantation	Peripheral blood lymphocyte therapy
Vaccine Therapy	NCT01347034	II	20	Radiation Therapy and Intratumoral Autologous Dendritic Cells in Soft Tissue Sarcomas (STS)	External Beam Radiation Therapy
					Autologous Dendritic Cells
	NCT02496520	I and II	6	Dendritic Cell-based Immunotherapy for Advanced Solid Tumours of Children and Young Adults	Dendritic Cells
					Surgery, chemotherapy, and radiation therapy as needed by the patient's tumor and stage
	NCT00365872	II	17	External Beam Radiation With Intratumoral Injection of Dendritic Cells As Neo-Adjuvant Treatment for Sarcoma	Dendritic Cell Injections
					Radiation therapy
					Complete Resection
	NCT00948961	I and II	70	A Study of CDX-1401 in Patients With Malignancies Known to Express NY-ESO-1	CDX-1401
					Resiquimod (TLR7/8 agonist)
					Hiltonol®(Poly-ICLC, TLR3 agonist)
	NCT03357315	I and II	30	Mix Vaccine for Metastatic Sarcoma Patients	Mix vaccine
	NCT00005628	II	35	Vaccine Therapy in Treating Patients With Recurrent Soft Tissue Sarcoma	Vitespen
	NCT00001564	II	30	A Pilot Study of Tumor-Specific Peptide Vaccination and IL-2 With or Without Autologous T Cell Transplantation in Recurrent Pediatric Sarcomas	EF-1, EF-2, PXFK, and E7 peptides
					IL-2, IL-4, GM-CSF, and CD40 Ligand
	NCT00003408	II	40	Biological Therapy Following Chemotherapy and Peripheral Stem Cell Transplantation in Treating Patients With Cancer	Aldesleukin (synthetic IL-2) Recombinant interferon alfa Sargramostim (recombinant GM-CSF)
	NCT00923351	I and II	44	Therapy to Treat Ewing's Sarcoma, Rhabdomyosarcoma or Neuroblastoma	Tumor Purged/CD25 Depleted Lymphocytes
					Tumor Purged/CD25 Depleted Lymphocytes with Tumor Lysate/KLH Pulsed Dendritic Cell Vaccine
					rhIL-7
					Tumor Lysate/KLH Pulsed Dendritic Cell Vaccine
	NCT02423863	II	26	In Situ, Autologous Therapeutic Vaccination Against Solid Cancers With Intratumoral Hiltonol®	Hiltonol®(Poly-ICLC, TLR3 agonist)

Adoptive cell therapy is based on the manipulation, modulation, and selection of immune cells to eliminate the tumor, overcoming the immune system's tolerance to cancer cells. As sarcomas appear to be one of the tumors most vulnerable to NK cell cytotoxicity, NK cell-based therapies seem to be a promising alternative treatment [116]. In 2010, it was demonstrated that rhabdomyosarcoma is sensitive to expanded NK cells [117], and phase I and II clinical trials of expanded haploidentical NK cells in rhabdomyosarcoma patients have begun (NCT02409576). The aim of another ongoing clinical trial is to combine cryosurgery and multiple NK immunotherapies (NCT02849366) (Table 1). Similar to NK cells, lymphocytes could also be harvested from the patient or a donor, expanded, and then reinfused into the patient. Although the use of TILs against STS is poorly investigated, two ongoing phase II clinical trials have started. One of them proposes a donor lymphocyte infusion in patients with relapsed malignancies, including sarcoma (NCT00003887). The other is trying to eradicate minimal residual disease in sarcomas, including alveolar rhabdomyosarcoma, with autologous T cell transplantation concomitant with the tumor-specific peptides vaccine (NCT00001566). Alternatively, genetically engineered T cells expressing receptors for specific recognition of the cancer testis antigen New York esophageal squamous cell carcinoma-1 (NY-ESO-1) could be a promising strategy, since the expression of NY-ESO-1 in some subtypes of STS has been demonstrated, especially in synovial sarcomas [118,119]. In this STS subtype, a T-cell receptor-based gene therapy against NY-ESO-1 demonstrated promising results [120]. In another pilot study, an autologous T-cell expressing T-cell receptor recognizing NY-ESO-1 confirmed previous results with an anti-tumor response in 50% of metastatic synovial sarcoma [121]. Considering all these previous promising results, the aim of an ongoing clinical trial is to create an immune response against NY-ESO-1 antigen with a CDX-1401 cancer vaccine (NCT00948961) (Table 1). Cancer vaccines are a strategy to treat tumors. These vaccines attempt to elicit an immune response against tumor cells through the active manipulation of DCs. However, in addition to other limited reports of DC-based vaccination in STS, a study performed in 2017 indicated that the treatment is effective only in a small number of patients [122]. Several current clinical trials use vaccination with autologous dendritic cells to try to strengthen the immune system against sarcomas, including STS (NCT01347034; NCT02496520; NCT00365872). Peptide vaccination could also be an approach to treat STS, and clinical trials are testing peptide vaccines to enhance the immune response in STS (Table 1).

Clinical trials concerning immunotherapy for STS have, so far, shown limited and inconclusive results, which is largely due to the lack of representativity of several STS histologic types in the studies. However, attempts are still ongoing to identify biomarkers for monitoring immunotherapy and predict clinical outcome [123,124].

8. Future Perspectives

Beyond the necessity of large-scale studies on tumor-infiltrating immune cells and their role in clinical features, it is also necessary to pair the analysis of tumor samples with peripheral blood samples to understand whether the information obtained about the circulating immune cells could be used to predict disease outcome or the response to treatment. The collection of peripheral blood is a minimally invasive procedure, which facilitates sample harvesting and consequently increases the number of patients who could undergo such a process and would allow patient monitoring during the treatment.

Regarding the soluble factors, there is still much to be learned about the array of these factors secreted by the tumor and their activity and interactions in TME. Given the pleiotropic and redundant nature of the soluble factors, the therapeutical target should be the balance between pro- and anti-inflammatory ones instead of the inhibition or activation of one in particular.

Treatments targeting immune checkpoints may represent a promising approach for other types of cancers as well. Nevertheless, it is necessary to select the patients who will benefit from this type of therapy carefully. Regarding IRGs, there are still only very few studies, so more research is required to understand the potential functional mechanisms of IRGs and their role in STS. The dual role of immunity in cancer leads us to believe that combination approaches that both stimulate protective host responses and inhibit immune subversion tactics might be more efficacious. The heterogenicity of STS implies that a "one size fits all" approach may be less successful. Furthermore, comprehensive immune profiling in combination with the evaluation of clinical features will be important to predict the response to therapy and survival. Lastly, the immune profiling of each patient might lead to personalized therapy.

The knowledge accumulated regarding tumor and peripheral immune status could be helpful in designing novel immunotherapeutic approaches for STS.

9. Conclusions

STS have been treated as "non-immunogenic" tumors until now. However, this current work has proved that this characterization did not apply to all of them, since elements of the immune system were highly expressed in some STS samples. These elements, including immune cells, soluble plasmatic factors, immune checkpoints, and the expression of immune-related genes have been correlated with STS prognosis. Furthermore, their role in predicting the response to therapy and their potential as therapeutical agents or targets has been proven in STS. The infiltration of B cells, NK cells, TANs, and DC in STS tumors were correlated with a better outcome. On the contrary, TAMs were associated with a negative prognostic value. Regarding infiltrating CD8 T, CD4 T, and Tregs, their role in the outcome of the disease remains controversial. Some soluble plasmatic factors such as LIF, IL-8, HGF, IL-2Ra, VEGF, MCP-3, TNF-RI, IL-6, and M-CSF were associated with a negative prognosis in STS. Nevertheless, only a few studies have tried to understand their role in this type of cancer. A favorable prognostic value was associated with the immune checkpoint E-Cadherin, and a negative prognostic value was associated with the presence of B7-H3, PD-1, PD-L1, NKp30, B7-H6, Sirpα, CD47, CD155, LAG3, and IDO. Likewise, immune-related genes such as IL-33, ST2, BIRC5, DUSP4, FOXP3, HLA-DQA1, HLA-DQB1, and LAG3 were associated with a better outcome, while C3, CD36, DOCK9, FCER2, FOS, HLA-DRB4, and NCAM1 were correlated with a worse outcome. In another study, an immune gene-related prognostic model using IFIH1, CTSG, STC2, SECTM1, and BIRC5 showed potential to predict the response of STS patients to immunotherapy. The immunological status of peripheral blood in STS is still largely unknown. Increased LMR and NLR ratios have been associated with a poor prognosis in some studies. Higher levels of M-MDSCs and Tim-3 positive CD8 T cells also appear to be negative prognostic markers. On the contrary, NKG2D-positive CD8 T cells were correlated with a better outcome.

The main limitations that concern the studies mentioned above are the small sample sizes, the short follow-up, and the use of restricted STS histology types. Taking this into account, the studies might not be representative of the whole. In addition, in most of these studies, the stage of STS and treatments were not considered and might have a significant impact on prognosis. For these reasons, a large-scale prospective study, investigation of each subtype, and studies that consider the STS stage and treatment are warranted to substantiate and validate the results discussed in this article.

Author Contributions: J.M.C. and P.R.-S.: manuscript outline. L.M.S., J.S.A., T.F.-A., M.S.-R., P.F.-T., J.M.C. and P.R.-S.: manuscript writing. All authors have read and agreed to the published version of the manuscript.

Funding: This work was supported by the European Regional Development Fund (ERDF), through the Centro 2020 Regional Operational Program and through the COMPETE 2020—Operational Programme for Competitiveness and Internationalisation and Portuguese national funds via FCT—Fundação para a Ciência e a Tecnologia, under the projects POCI-01-0145-FEDER-007440, UIDB/04539 /2020 and UIDP/04539/2020 (to P.R.-S. and M.S.-R.).

Institutional Review Board Statement: Not applicable.

Informed Consent Statement: Not applicable.

Data Availability Statement: Not applicable.

Acknowledgments: J.S.A. was supported by PhD Grant (SFRH/BD/148007/2019) from the Portuguese Science and Technology Foundation (FCT), through the European Social Fund from the European Union.

Conflicts of Interest: The authors declare no conflict of interest.

References

1. Mohindra, N.; Agulnik, M. Targeted Therapy and Promising Novel Agents for the Treatment of Advanced Soft Tissue Sarcomas. *Expert Opin. Investig. Drugs* **2015**, *24*, 1409–1418. [CrossRef]
2. Wisdom, A.J.; Mowery, Y.M.; Riedel, R.F.; Kirsch, D.G. Rationale and Emerging Strategies for Immune Checkpoint Blockade in Soft Tissue Sarcoma. *Cancer* **2018**, *124*, 3819–3829. [CrossRef]
3. Tseng, W.W.; Somaiah, N.; Engleman, E.G. Potential for Immunotherapy in Soft Tissue Sarcoma. *Hum. Vaccin. Immunother.* **2014**, *10*, 3117–3124. [CrossRef]
4. Yen, C.C.; Chen, T.W.W. Next Frontiers in Systemic Therapy for Soft Tissue Sarcoma. *Chin. Clin. Oncol.* **2018**, *7*, 43. [CrossRef]
5. Linch, M.; Miah, A.B.; Thway, K.; Judson, I.R.; Benson, C. Systemic Treatment of Soft-Tissue Sarcoma—Gold Standard and Novel Therapies. *Nat. Rev. Clin. Oncol.* **2014**, *11*, 187–202. [CrossRef]
6. Bourcier, K.; le Cesne, A.; Tselikas, L.; Adam, J.; Mir, O.; Honore, C.; de Baere, T. Basic Knowledge in Soft Tissue Sarcoma. *Cardiovasc. Intervent. Radiol.* **2019**, *42*, 1255–1261. [CrossRef]
7. Doyle, L.A. Sarcoma Classification: An Update Based on the 2013 World Health Organization Classification of Tumors of Soft Tissue and Bone. *Cancer* **2014**, *120*, 1763–1774. [CrossRef]
8. Jo, V.Y.; Doyle, L.A. Refinements in Sarcoma Classification in the Current 2013 World Health Organization Classification of Tumours of Soft Tissue and Bone. *Surg. Oncol. Clin. N. Am.* **2016**, *25*, 621–643. [CrossRef]
9. Ruiu, R.; Tarone, L.; Rolih, V.; Barutello, G.; Bolli, E.; Riccardo, F.; Cavallo, F.; Conti, L. Cancer stem cell immunology and immunotherapy: Harnessing the immune system against cancer's source. *Prog. Mol. Biol. Transl. Sci.* **2019**, *164*, 119–188. [CrossRef]
10. Bagaev, A.; Kotlov, N.; Nomie, K.; Svekolkin, V.; Gafurov, A.; Isaeva, O.; Osokin, N.; Kozlov, I.; Frenkel, F.; Gancharova, O.; et al. Conserved Pan-Cancer Microenvironment Subtypes Predict Response to Immunotherapy. *Cancer Cell* **2021**, *39*, 845–865. [CrossRef]
11. Abeshouse, A.; Adebamowo, C.; Adebamowo, S.N.; Akbani, R.; Akeredolu, T.; Ally, A.; Anderson, M.L.; Anur, P.; Appelbaum, E.L.; Armenia, J.; et al. Comprehensive and Integrated Genomic Characterization of Adult Soft Tissue Sarcomas. *Cell* **2017**, *171*, 950–965. [CrossRef] [PubMed]
12. Petitprez, F.; de Reyniès, A.; Keung, E.Z.; Chen, T.W.W.; Sun, C.M.; Calderaro, J.; Jeng, Y.M.; Hsiao, L.P.; Lacroix, L.; Bougoüin, A.; et al. B Cells Are Associated with Survival and Immunotherapy Response in Sarcoma. *Nature* **2020**, *577*, 556–560. [CrossRef] [PubMed]
13. Pollard, J.W. Tumour-Educated Macrophages Promote Tumour Progression and Metastasis. *Nat. Rev. Cancer* **2004**, *4*, 71–78. [CrossRef]
14. Lee, C.; Jeong, H.; Bae, Y.; Shin, K.; Kang, S.; Kim, H.; Oh, J.; Bae, H. Targeting of M2-like Tumor-Associated Macrophages with a Melittin-Based pro-Apoptotic Peptide. *J. Immunother. Cancer* **2019**, *7*, 147. [CrossRef]
15. Dancsok, A.R.; Gao, D.; Lee, A.F.; Steigen, S.E.; Blay, J.Y.; Thomas, D.M.; Maki, R.G.; Nielsen, T.O.; Demicco, E.G. Tumor-Associated Macrophages and Macrophage-Related Immune Checkpoint Expression in Sarcomas. *OncoImmunology* **2020**, *9*, 1747340. [CrossRef]
16. Tsagozis, P.; Augsten, M.; Zhang, Y.; Li, T.; Hesla, A.; Bergh, J.; Haglund, F.; Tobin, N.P.; Ehnman, M. An Immunosuppressive Macrophage Profile Attenuates the Prognostic Impact of CD20-Positive B Cells in Human Soft Tissue Sarcoma. *Cancer Immunol. Immunother.* **2019**, *68*, 927–936. [CrossRef]
17. Zhao, X.; Qu, J.; Sun, Y.; Wang, J.; Liu, X.; Wang, F.; Zhang, H.; Wang, W.; Ma, X.; Gao, X.; et al. Prognostic Significance of Tumor-Associated Macrophages in Breast Cancer: A Meta-Analysis of the Literature. *Oncotarget* **2017**, *8*, 30576–30586. [CrossRef]
18. Troiano, G.; Caponio, V.C.A.; Adipietro, I.; Tepedino, M.; Santoro, R.; Laino, L.; lo Russo, L.; Cirillo, N.; lo Muzio, L. Prognostic Significance of CD68+ and CD163+ Tumor Associated Macrophages in Head and Neck Squamous Cell Carcinoma: A Systematic Review and Meta-Analysis. *Oral Oncol.* **2019**, *93*, 66–75. [CrossRef]
19. Lee, C.-H.; Espinosa, I.; Vrijaldenhoven, S.; Subramanian, S.; Montgomery, K.D.; Zhu, S.; Marinelli, R.J.; Peterse, J.L.; Poulin, N.; Nielsen, T.O.; et al. Prognostic Significance of Macrophage Infiltration in Leiomyosarcomas. *Clin. Cancer Res.* **2008**, *14*, 1423–1430. [CrossRef]
20. Kostine, M.; Briaire-de Bruijn, I.H.; Cleven, A.H.G.; Vervat, C.; Corver, W.E.; Schilham, M.W.; van Beelen, E.; van Boven, H.; Haas, R.L.; Italiano, A.; et al. Increased Infiltration of M2-Macrophages, T-Cells and PD-L1 Expression in High Grade Leiomyosarcomas Supports Immunotherapeutic Strategies. *Oncoimmunology* **2017**, *7*, e1386828. [CrossRef]
21. Nabeshima, A.; Matsumoto, Y.; Fukushi, J.; Iura, K.; Matsunobu, T.; Endo, M.; Fujiwara, T.; Iida, K.; Fujiwara, Y.; Hatano, M.; et al. Tumour-Associated Macrophages Correlate with Poor Prognosis in Myxoid Liposarcoma and Promote Cell Motility and Invasion via the HB-EGF-EGFR-PI3K/Akt Pathways. *Br. J. Cancer* **2015**, *112*, 547–555. [CrossRef]
22. Smolle, M.A.; Herbsthofer, L.; Goda, M.; Granegger, B.; Brcic, I.; Bergovec, M.; Scheipl, S.; Prietl, B.; El-Heliebi, A.; Pichler, M.; et al. Influence of Tumor-Infiltrating Immune Cells on Local Control Rate, Distant Metastasis, and Survival in Patients with Soft Tissue Sarcoma. *Oncoimmunology* **2021**, *10*, 1896658. [CrossRef]
23. Shaul, M.E.; Fridlender, Z.G. Tumour-Associated Neutrophils in Patients with Cancer. *Nat. Rev. Clin. Oncol* **2019**, *16*, 601–620. [CrossRef]
24. Ponzetta, A.; Carriero, R.; Carnevale, S.; Barbagallo, M.; Molgora, M.; Perucchini, C.; Magrini, E.; Gianni, F.; Kunderfranco, P.; Polentarutti, N.; et al. Neutrophils Driving Unconventional T Cells Mediate Resistance against Murine Sarcomas and Selected Human Tumors. *Cell* **2019**, *178*, 346–360.e24. [CrossRef] [PubMed]

25. Bruno, T.C. New Predictors for Immunotherapy Responses Sharpen Our View of the Tumour Microenvironment. *Nature* **2020**, *577*, 474–476. [CrossRef]
26. Judge, S.J.; Darrow, M.A.; Thorpe, S.W.; Gingrich, A.A.; O'Donnell, E.F.; Bellini, A.R.; Sturgill, I.R.; Vick, L.V.; Dunai, C.; Stoffel, K.M.; et al. Analysis of Tumor-Infiltrating NK and T Cells Highlights IL-15 Stimulation and TIGIT Blockade as a Combination Immunotherapy Strategy for Soft Tissue Sarcomas. *J. ImmunoTher. Cancer* **2020**, *8*, e001355. [CrossRef] [PubMed]
27. Pollack, S.M.; He, Q.; Yearley, J.H.; Emerson, R.; Vignali, M.; Zhang, Y.; Redman, M.W.; Baker, K.K.; Cooper, S.; Donahue, B.; et al. T-Cell Infiltration and Clonality Correlate with Programmed Cell Death Protein 1 and Programmed Death-Ligand 1 Expression in Patients with Soft Tissue Sarcomas. *Cancer* **2017**, *123*, 3291–3304. [CrossRef] [PubMed]
28. Nakajima, K.; Raz, A. T-cell Infiltration Profile in Musculoskeletal Tumors. *J. Orthop. Res.* **2021**, *39*, 536–542. [CrossRef] [PubMed]
29. Ando, M.; Ito, M.; Srirat, T.; Kondo, T.; Yoshimura, A. Memory T Cell, Exhaustion, and Tumor Immunity. *Immunol. Med.* **2020**, *43*, 1–9. [CrossRef] [PubMed]
30. Tseng, W.W.; Malu, S.; Zhang, M.; Chen, J.; Sim, G.C.; Wei, W.; Ingram, D.; Somaiah, N.; Lev, D.C.; Pollock, R.E.; et al. Analysis of the Intratumoral Adaptive Immune Response in Well Differentiated and Dedifferentiated Retroperitoneal Liposarcoma. *Sarcoma* **2015**, *2015*. [CrossRef]
31. Kennedy, R.; Celis, E. Multiple Roles for CD4+ T Cells in Anti-Tumor Immune Responses. *Immunol. Rev.* **2008**, *222*, 129–144. [CrossRef]
32. Borst, J.; Ahrends, T.; Bąbała, N.; Melief, C.J.M.; Kastenmüller, W. CD4+ T Cell Help in Cancer Immunology and Immunotherapy. *Nat. Rev. Immunol.* **2018**, *18*, 635–647. [CrossRef] [PubMed]
33. D'Angelo, S.P.; Shoushtari, A.N.; Agaram, N.P.; Kuk, D.; Qin, L.X.; Carvajal, R.D.; Dickson, M.A.; Gounder, M.; Keohan, M.L.; Schwartz, G.K.; et al. Prevalence of Tumor-Infiltrating Lymphocytes and PD-L1 Expression in the Soft Tissue Sarcoma Microenvironment. *Hum. Pathol.* **2015**, *46*, 357–365. [CrossRef]
34. Komohara, Y.; Takeya, H.; Wakigami, N.; Kusada, N.; Bekki, H.; Ishihara, S.; Takeya, M.; Nakashima, Y.; Oda, Y. Positive Correlation between the Density of Macrophages and T-Cells in Undifferentiated Sarcoma. *Med. Mol. Morphol.* **2019**, *52*, 44–51. [CrossRef]
35. Peranzoni, E.; Lemoine, J.; Vimeux, L.; Feuillet, V.; Barrin, S.; Kantari-Mimoun, C.; Bercovici, N.; Guérin, M.; Biton, J.; Ouakrim, H.; et al. Macrophages Impede CD8 T Cells from Reaching Tumor Cells and Limit the Efficacy of Anti–PD-1 Treatment. *Proc. Natl. Acad. Sci. USA* **2018**, *115*, E4041–E4050. [CrossRef]
36. Mills, C.D.; Lenz, L.L.; Harris, R.A. A Breakthrough: Macrophage-Directed Cancer Immunotherapy. *Cancer Res.* **2016**, *76*, 513–516. [CrossRef] [PubMed]
37. Boxberg, M.; Steiger, K.; Lenze, U.; Rechl, H.; von Eisenhart-Rothe, R.; Wörtler, K.; Weichert, W.; Langer, R.; Specht, K. PD-L1 and PD-1 and Characterization of Tumor-Infiltrating Lymphocytes in High Grade Sarcomas of Soft Tissue—Prognostic Implications and Rationale for Immunotherapy. *Oncoimmunology* **2017**, *7*, e1389366. [CrossRef]
38. Fujii, H.; Arakawa, A.; Utsumi, D.; Sumiyoshi, S.; Yamamoto, Y.; Kitoh, A.; Ono, M.; Matsumura, Y.; Kato, M.; Konishi, K.; et al. CD8+ Tumor-Infiltrating Lymphocytes at Primary Sites as a Possible Prognostic Factor of Cutaneous Angiosarcoma. *Int. J. Cancer* **2014**, *134*, 2393–2402. [CrossRef]
39. Yi, Q.; Zhixin, F.; Yuanxiang, G.; Wei, X.; Bushu, X.; Jingjing, Z.; Huoying, C.; Xinke, Z.; Musheng, Z.; Yao, L.; et al. LAG-3 Expression on Tumor-Infiltrating T Cells in Soft Tissue Sarcoma Correlates with Poor Survival. *Cancer Biol. Med.* **2019**, *16*, 331–340. [CrossRef]
40. Sorbye, S.W.; Kilvaer, T.; Valkov, A.; Donnem, T.; Smeland, E.; Al-Shibli, K.; Bremnes, R.M.; Busund, L.T. Prognostic Impact of Lymphocytes in Soft Tissue Sarcomas. *PLoS ONE* **2011**, *6*, e14611. [CrossRef]
41. Bi, Q.; Liu, Y.; Yuan, T.; Wang, H.; Li, B.; Jiang, Y.; Mo, X.; Lei, Y.; Xiao, Y.; Dong, S.; et al. Predicted CD4 + T Cell Infiltration Levels Could Indicate Better Overall Survival in Sarcoma Patients. *J. Int Med. Res.* **2021**, *49*, 0300060520981539. [CrossRef]
42. Keung, E.Z.; Tsai, J.-W.; Ali, A.M.; Cormier, J.N.; Bishop, A.J.; Guadagnolo, B.A.; Torres, K.E.; Somaiah, N.; Hunt, K.K.; Wargo, J.A.; et al. Analysis of the Immune Infiltrate in Undifferentiated Pleomorphic Sarcoma of the Extremity and Trunk in Response to Radiotherapy: Rationale for Combination Neoadjuvant Immune Checkpoint Inhibition and Radiotherapy. *Oncoimmunology* **2017**, *7*, e1385689. [CrossRef] [PubMed]
43. Klaver, Y.; Rijnders, M.; Oostvogels, A.; Wijers, R.; Smid, M.; Grünhagen, D.; Verhoef, K.; Sleijfer, S.; Lamers, C.; Debets, R. Differential Quantities of Immune Checkpoint-Expressing CD8 T Cells in Soft Tissue Sarcoma Subtypes. *J. Immunother. Cancer* **2020**, *8*, e000271. [CrossRef]
44. Que, Y.; Xiao, W.; Guan, Y.X.; Liang, Y.; Yan, S.M.; Chen, H.Y.; Li, Q.Q.; Xu, B.S.; Zhou, Z.W.; Zhang, X. PD-L1 Expression Is Associated with FOXP3+ Regulatory T-Cell Infiltration of Soft Tissue Sarcoma and Poor Patient Prognosis. *J. Cancer* **2017**, *8*, 2018–2025. [CrossRef] [PubMed]
45. Rutkowski, P.; Kaminska, J.; Kowalska, M.; Ruka, W.; Steffen, J. Cytokine Serum Levels in Soft Tissue Sarcoma Patients: Correlations with Clinico-Pathological Features and Prognosis. *Int. J. Cancer* **2002**, *100*, 463–471. [CrossRef] [PubMed]
46. Wysoczynski, M.; Miekus, K.; Jankowski, K.; Wanzeck, J.; Bertolone, S.; Janowska-Wieczorek, A.; Ratajczak, J.; Ratajczak, M.Z. Leukemia Inhibitory Factor: A Newly Identified Metastatic Factor in Rhabdomyosarcomas. *Cancer Res.* **2007**, *67*, 2131–2140. [CrossRef] [PubMed]

47. Sleijfer, S.; Gorlia, T.; Lamers, C.; Burger, H.; Blay, J.Y.; le Cesne, A.; Scurr, M.; Collin, F.; Pandite, L.; Marreaud, S.; et al. Cytokine and Angiogenic Factors Associated with Efficacy and Toxicity of Pazopanib in Advanced Soft-Tissue Sarcoma: An EORTC-STBSG Study. *Br. J. Cancer* **2012**, *107*, 639–645. [CrossRef]
48. Sharonov, G.V.; Serebrovskaya, E.O.; Yuzhakova, D.V.; Britanova, O.V.; Chudakov, D.M. B Cells, Plasma Cells and Antibody Repertoires in the Tumour Microenvironment. *Nat. Rev. Immunol.* **2020**, *20*, 294–307. [CrossRef]
49. Helmink, B.A.; Reddy, S.M.; Gao, J.; Zhang, S.; Basar, R.; Thakur, R.; Yizhak, K.; Sade-Feldman, M.; Blando, J.; Han, G.; et al. B Cells and Tertiary Lymphoid Structures Promote Immunotherapy Response. *Nature* **2020**, *577*, 549–555. [CrossRef] [PubMed]
50. Herberman, R.B.; Nunn, M.E.; Holden, H.T.; Lavrin, D.H. Natural Cytotoxic Reactivity of Mouse Lymphoid Cells against Syngeneic and Allogeneic Tumors. II. Characterization of Effector Cells. *Int J. Cancer* **1975**, *16*, 230–239. [CrossRef]
51. Waldhauer, I.; Steinle, A. NK Cells and Cancer Immunosurveillance. *Oncogene* **2008**, *27*, 5932–5943. [CrossRef] [PubMed]
52. Chiossone, L.; Dumas, P.-Y.; Vienne, M.; Vivier, E. Natural Killer Cells and Other Innate Lymphoid Cells in Cancer. *Nat. Rev. Immunol.* **2018**, *18*, 671–688. [CrossRef]
53. Platonova, S.; Cherfils-Vicini, J.; Damotte, D.; Crozet, L.; Vieillard, V.; Validire, P.; André, P.; Dieu-Nosjean, M.-C.; Alifano, M.; Régnard, J.-F.; et al. Profound Coordinated Alterations of Intratumoral NK Cell Phenotype and Function in Lung Carcinoma. *Cancer Res.* **2011**, *71*, 5412–5422. [CrossRef] [PubMed]
54. Eckl, J.; Buchner, A.; Prinz, P.U.; Riesenberg, R.; Siegert, S.I.; Kammerer, R.; Nelson, P.J.; Noessner, E. Transcript Signature Predicts Tissue NK Cell Content and Defines Renal Cell Carcinoma Subgroups Independent of TNM Staging. *J. Mol. Med.* **2012**, *90*, 55–66. [CrossRef] [PubMed]
55. Moretta, L.; Pietra, G.; Vacca, P.; Pende, D.; Moretta, F.; Bertaina, A.; Mingari, M.C.; Locatelli, F.; Moretta, A. Human NK Cells: From Surface Receptors to Clinical Applications. *Immunol. Lett.* **2016**, *178*, 15–19. [CrossRef]
56. Delahaye, N.F.; Rusakiewicz, S.; Martins, I.; Ménard, C.; Roux, S.; Lyonnet, L.; Paul, P.; Sarabi, M.; Chaput, N.; Semeraro, M.; et al. Alternatively Spliced NKp30 Isoforms Affect the Prognosis of Gastrointestinal Stromal Tumors. *Nat. Med.* **2011**, *17*, 700–707. [CrossRef]
57. Liu, Y.; Cao, X. Immunosuppressive Cells in Tumor Immune Escape and Metastasis. *J. Mol. Med.* **2016**, *94*, 509–522. [CrossRef] [PubMed]
58. Salama, P.; Phillips, M.; Grieu, F.; Morris, M.; Zeps, N.; Joseph, D.; Platell, C.; Iacopetta, B. Tumor-Infiltrating FOXP3+ T Regulatory Cells Show Strong Prognostic Significance in Colorectal Cancer. *J. Clin. Oncol* **2009**, *27*, 186–192. [CrossRef]
59. Keung, E.Z.; Burgess, M.; Salazar, R.; Parra, E.R.; Rodrigues-Canales, J.; Bolejack, V.; van Tine, B.A.; Schuetze, S.M.; Attia, S.; Riedel, R.F.; et al. Correlative Analyses of the SARC028 Trial Reveal an Association Between Sarcoma-Associated Immune Infiltrate and Response to Pembrolizumab. *Clin. Cancer Res.* **2020**, *26*, 1258–1266. [CrossRef]
60. Highfill, S.L.; Cui, Y.; Giles, A.J.; Smith, J.P.; Zhang, H.; Morse, E.; Kaplan, R.N.; Mackall, C.L. Disruption of CXCR2-Mediated MDSC Tumor Trafficking Enhances Anti-PD1 Efficacy. *Sci. Transl. Med.* **2014**, *6*, 237ra67. [CrossRef]
61. Kiss, M.; van Gassen, S.; Movahedi, K.; Saeys, Y.; Laoui, D. Myeloid Cell Heterogeneity in Cancer: Not a Single Cell Alike. *Cell Immunol.* **2018**, *330*, 188–201. [CrossRef] [PubMed]
62. Segura, B.; Zhang, H.; Bernstein, L.J.; Tannock, I.F. Cytokines and Their Relationship to the Symptoms and outcome of Cancer. *Nat. Rev. Cancer* **2008**, *8*, 887–899. [CrossRef]
63. Dranoff, G. Cytokines in Cancer Pathogenesis and Cancer Therapy. *Nat. Rev. Cancer* **2004**, *4*, 11–22. [CrossRef]
64. Ben-Baruch, A. The Multifaceted Roles of Chemokines in Malignancy. *Cancer Metastasis Rev.* **2006**, *25*, 357–371. [CrossRef]
65. Witsch, E.; Sela, M.; Yarden, Y. Roles for Growth Factors in Cancer Progression. *Physiology* **2010**, *25*, 85–101. [CrossRef] [PubMed]
66. Heaney, M.L.; Golde, D.W. Soluble Receptors in Human Disease. *J. Leukoc. Biol.* **1998**, *64*, 135–146. [CrossRef] [PubMed]
67. Lapeyre-Prost, A.; Terme, M.; Pernot, S.; Pointet, A.-L.; Voron, T.; Tartour, E.; Taieb, J. Immunomodulatory Activity of VEGF in Cancer. *Int. Rev. Cell Mol. Biol.* **2017**, *330*, 295–342. [CrossRef]
68. Katoh, M.; Nakagama, H. FGF Receptors: Cancer Biology and Therapeutics. *Med. Res. Rev.* **2014**, *34*, 280–300. [CrossRef]
69. Claesson-Welsh, L.; Welsh, M. VEGFA and Tumour Angiogenesis. *J. Intern. Med.* **2013**, *273*, 114–127. [CrossRef]
70. Graeven, U.; Andre, N.; Achilles, E.; Zornig, C.; Schmiegel, W. Serum Levels of Vascular Endothelial Growth Factor and Basic Fibroblast Growth Factor in Patients with Soft-Tissue Sarcoma. *J. Cancer Res. Clin. Oncol.* **1999**, *125*, 577–581. [CrossRef]
71. Kusakabe, H.; Sakatani, S.; Yonebayashi, K.; Kiyokane, K. Establishment and Characterization of an Epithelioid Sarcoma Cell Line with an Autocrine Response to Interleukin-6. *Arch. Dermatol. Res.* **1997**, *289*, 224–233. [CrossRef] [PubMed]
72. Hagi, T.; Nakamura, T.; Iino, T.; Matsubara, T.; Asanuma, K.; Matsumine, A.; Sudo, A. The Diagnostic and Prognostic Value of Interleukin-6 in Patients with Soft Tissue Sarcomas. *Sci. Rep.* **2017**, *7*, 9640. [CrossRef]
73. Wysoczynski, M.; Shin, D.M.; Kucia, M.; Ratajczak, M.Z. Selective Upregulation of Interleukin-8 by Human Rhabdomyosarcomas in Response to Hypoxia: Therapeutic Implications. *Int. J. Cancer* **2010**, *126*, 371–381. [CrossRef]
74. Hosoyama, T.; Aslam, M.I.; Abraham, J.; Prajapati, S.I.; Nishijo, K.; Michalek, J.E.; Zarzabal, L.A.; Nelon, L.D.; Guttridge, D.C.; Rubin, B.P.; et al. IL-4R Drives Dedifferentiation, Mitogenesis, and Metastasis in Rhabdomyosarcoma. *Clin. Cancer Res.* **2011**, *17*, 2757–2766. [CrossRef] [PubMed]
75. Pardoll, D.M. The Blockade of Immune Checkpoints in Cancer Immunotherapy. *Nat. Rev. Cancer* **2012**, *12*, 252–264. [CrossRef]
76. Kim, J.R.; Moon, Y.J.; Kwon, K.S.; Bae, J.S.; Wagle, S.; Kim, K.M.; Park, H.S.; Lee, H.; Moon, W.S.; Chung, M.J.; et al. Tumor Infiltrating PD1-Positive Lymphocytes and the Expression of PD-L1 Predict Poor Prognosis of Soft Tissue Sarcomas. *PLoS ONE* **2013**, *8*, e82870. [CrossRef]

77. Dancsok, A.R.; Setsu, N.; Gao, D.; Blay, J.Y.; Thomas, D.; Maki, R.G.; Nielsen, T.O.; Demicco, E.G. Expression of Lymphocyte Immunoregulatory Biomarkers in Bone and Soft-Tissue Sarcomas. *Mod. Pathol.* **2019**, *32*, 1772–1785. [CrossRef]
78. Torabi, A.; Amaya, C.N.; Wians, F.H.; Bryan, B.A. PD-1 and PD-L1 Expression in Bone and Soft Tissue Sarcomas. *Pathology* **2017**, *49*, 506–513. [CrossRef]
79. Orth, M.F.; Buecklein, V.L.; Kampmann, E.; Subklewe, M.; Noessner, E.; Cidre-Aranaz, F.; Romero-Pérez, L.; Wehweck, F.S.; Lindner, L.; Issels, R.; et al. A Comparative View on the Expression Patterns of PD-L1 and PD-1 in Soft Tissue Sarcomas. *Cancer Immunol. Immunother.* **2020**, *69*, 1353–1362. [CrossRef] [PubMed]
80. Budczies, J.; Mechtersheimer, G.; Denkert, C.; Klauschen, F.; Mughal, S.S.; Chudasama, P.; Bockmayr, M.; Jöhrens, K.; Endris, V.; Lier, A.; et al. PD-L1 (CD274) Copy Number Gain, Expression, and Immune Cell Infiltration as Candidate Predictors for Response to Immune. *Oncoimmunology* **2017**, *6*, e1279777. [CrossRef]
81. Kim, C.; Kim, E.K.; Jung, H.; Chon, H.J.; Han, J.W.; Shin, K.H.; Hu, H.; Kim, K.S.; Choi, Y.D.; Kim, S.; et al. Prognostic Implications of PD-L1 Expression in Patients with Soft Tissue Sarcoma. *BMC Cancer* **2016**, *16*, 434. [CrossRef] [PubMed]
82. Movva, S.; Wen, W.; Chen, W.; Millis, S.Z.; Gatalica, Z.; Reddy, S.; von Mehren, M.; van Tine, B.A. Multi-Platform Profiling of over 2000 Sarcomas: Identification of Biomarkers and Novel Therapeutic Targets. *Oncotarget* **2015**, *6*, 12234–12247. [CrossRef]
83. Nowicki, T.S.; Akiyama, R.; Huang, R.R.; Shintaku, I.P.; Wang, X.; Tumeh, P.C.; Singh, A.; Chmielowski, B.; Denny, C.; Federman, N.; et al. Infiltration of CD8 T Cells and Expression of PD-1 and PD-L1 in Synovial Sarcoma. *Cancer Immunol. Res.* **2017**, *5*, 118–126. [CrossRef] [PubMed]
84. Cohen, J.E.; Eleyan, F.; Zick, A.; Peretz, T.; Katz, D. Intratumoral Immune-Biomarkers and Mismatch Repair Status in Leiyomyosarcoma -Potential Predictive Markers for Adjuvant Treatment: A Pilot Study. *Oncotarget* **2018**, *9*, 30847–30854. [CrossRef] [PubMed]
85. Paydas, S.; Bagir, E.K.; Deveci, M.A.; Gonlusen, G. Clinical and Prognostic Significance of PD-1 and PD-L1 Expression in Sarcomas. *Med. Oncol.* **2016**, *33*, 93. [CrossRef] [PubMed]
86. Yan, L.; Wang, Z.; Cui, C.; Guan, X.; Dong, B.; Zhao, M.; Wu, J.; Tian, X.; Hao, C. Comprehensive Immune Characterization and T-cell Receptor Repertoire Heterogeneity of Retroperitoneal Liposarcoma. *Cancer Sci.* **2019**, *110*, 3038–3048. [CrossRef] [PubMed]
87. Nielsen, M.; Krarup-Hansen, A.; Hovgaard, D.; Petersen, M.M.; Loya, A.C.; Westergaard, M.C.W.; Svane, I.M.; Junker, N. In Vitro 4-1BB Stimulation Promotes Expansion of CD8+ Tumor-Infiltrating Lymphocytes from Various Sarcoma Subtypes. *Cancer Immunol. Immunother.* **2020**, *69*, 2179–2191. [CrossRef]
88. Wunder, J.S.; Lee, M.J.; Nam, J.; Lau, B.Y.; Dickson, B.C.; Pinnaduwage, D.; Bull, S.B.; Ferguson, P.C.; Seto, A.; Gokgoz, N.; et al. Osteosarcoma and Soft-Tissue Sarcomas with an Immune Infiltrate Express PD-L1: Relation to Clinical Outcome and Th1 Pathway Activation. *Oncoimmunology* **2020**, *9*, 1737385. [CrossRef]
89. Ishihara, S.; Yamada, Y.; Iwasaki, T.; Yoshimoto, M.; Toda, Y.; Kohashi, K.; Yamamoto, H.; Matsumoto, Y.; Nakashima, Y.; Oda, Y. PD-L1 and IDO-1 Expression in Undifferentiated Pleomorphic Sarcoma: The Associations with Tumor Infiltrating Lymphocytes, DMMR and HLA Class I. *Oncol. Rep.* **2020**, *45*, 379–389. [CrossRef]
90. Wang, N.; He, Y.L.; Pang, L.J.; Zou, H.; Liu, C.X.; Zhao, J.; Hu, J.M.; Zhang, W.J.; Qi, Y.; Li, F. Down-Regulated E-Cadherin Expression Is Associated with Poor Five-Year Overall Survival in Bone and Soft Tissue Sarcoma: Results of a Meta-Analysis. *PLoS ONE* **2015**, *10*, e0121448. [CrossRef]
91. Rusakiewicz, S.; Perier, A.; Semeraro, M.; Pitt, J.M.; von Strandmann, E.P.; Reiners, K.S.; Aspeslagh, S.; Pipéroglou, C.; Vély, F.; Ivagnes, A.; et al. NKp30 Isoforms and NKp30 Ligands Are Predictive Biomarkers of Response to Imatinib Mesylate in Metastatic GIST Patients. *Oncoimmunology* **2016**, *6*, e1137418. [CrossRef] [PubMed]
92. Gregorio, A.; Corrias, M.V.; Castriconi, R.; Dondero, A.; Mosconi, M.; Gambini, C.; Moretta, A.; Moretta, L.; Bottino, C. Small Round Blue Cell Tumours: Diagnostic and Prognostic Usefulness of the Expression of B7-H3 Surface Molecule. *Histopathology* **2008**, *53*, 73–80. [CrossRef]
93. Sato, H.; Hasegawa, T.; Abe, Y.; Sakai, H.; Hirohashi, S. Expression of E-Cadherin in Bone and Soft Tissue Sarcomas: A Possible Role in Epithelial Differentiation. *Hum. Pathol.* **1999**, *30*, 1344–1349. [CrossRef]
94. Jolly, M.K.; Ware, K.E.; Xu, S.; Gilja, S.; Shetler, S.; Yang, Y.; Wang, X.; Austin, R.G.; Runyambo, D.; Hish, A.J.; et al. E-Cadherin Represses Anchorage-Independent Growth in Sarcomas through Both Signaling and Mechanical Mechanisms. *Mol. Cancer Res.* **2019**, *17*, 1391–1402. [CrossRef]
95. Zhang, F.; Liu, Y.; Yang, Y.; Yang, K. Development and Validation of a Fourteen- Innate Immunity-Related Gene Pairs Signature for Predicting Prognosis Head and Neck Squamous Cell Carcinoma. *BMC Cancer* **2020**, *20*, 1015. [CrossRef] [PubMed]
96. Shen, S.; Wang, G.; Zhang, R.; Zhao, Y.; Yu, H.; Wei, Y.; Chen, F. Development and Validation of an Immune Gene-Set Based Prognostic Signature in Ovarian Cancer. *EBioMedicine* **2019**, *40*, 318–326. [CrossRef] [PubMed]
97. Shen, C.; Liu, J.; Wang, J.; Zhong, X.; Dong, D.; Yang, X.; Wang, Y. Development and Validation of a Prognostic Immune-Associated Gene Signature in Clear Cell Renal Cell Carcinoma. *Int. Immunopharmacol.* **2020**, *81*, 106274. [CrossRef]
98. Shi, X.; Li, R.; Dong, X.; Chen, A.M.; Liu, X.; Lu, D.; Feng, S.; Wang, H.; Cai, K. IRGS: An Immune-Related Gene Classifier for Lung Adenocarcinoma Prognosis. *J. Transl. Med.* **2020**, *18*, 55. [CrossRef]
99. Chen, H.; Chen, Y.; Liu, H.; Que, Y.; Zhang, X.; Zheng, F. Integrated Expression Profiles Analysis Reveals Correlations between the IL-33/ST2 Axis and CD8+ T Cells, Regulatory T Cells, and Myeloid-Derived Suppressor Cells in Soft Tissue Sarcoma. *Front. Immunol.* **2018**, *9*, 1179. [CrossRef]

100. Hu, C.; Chen, B.; Huang, Z.; Liu, C.; Ye, L.; Wang, C.; Tong, Y.; Yang, J.; Zhao, C. Comprehensive Profiling of Immune-Related Genes in Soft Tissue Sarcoma Patients. *J. Transl. Med.* **2020**, *18*, 337. [CrossRef]
101. Dufresne, A.; Lesluyes, T.; Ménétrier-Caux, C.; Brahmi, M.; Darbo, E.; Toulmonde, M.; Italiano, A.; Mir, O.; le Cesne, A.; le Guellec, S.; et al. Specific Immune Landscapes and Immune Checkpoint Expressions in Histotypes and Molecular Subtypes of Sarcoma. *Oncoimmunology* **2020**, *9*, 1792036. [CrossRef]
102. Gu, H.Y.; Lin, L.L.; Zhang, C.; Yang, M.; Zhong, H.C.; Wei, R.X. The Potential of Five Immune-Related Prognostic Genes to Predict Survival and Response to Immune Checkpoint Inhibitors for Soft Tissue Sarcomas Based on Multi-Omic Study. *Front. Oncol.* **2020**, *10*, 1317. [CrossRef]
103. Bae, J.Y.; Choi, K.U.; Kim, A.; Lee, S.J.; Kim, K.; Kim, J.Y.; Lee, I.S.; Chung, S.H.; Kim, J.I. Evaluation of Immune-biomarker Expression in High-grade Soft-tissue Sarcoma: HLA-DQA1 Expression as a Prognostic Marker. *Exp. Ther. Med.* **2020**, *20*, 107. [CrossRef] [PubMed]
104. Sasaki, A.; Iwashita, Y.; Shibata, K.; Matsumoto, T.; Ohta, M.; Kitano, S. Prognostic Value of Preoperative Peripheral Blood Monocyte Count in Patients with Hepatocellular Carcinoma. *Surgery* **2006**, *139*, 755–764. [CrossRef]
105. Ma, J.Y.; Hu, G.; Liu, Q. Prognostic Significance of the Lymphocyte-to-Monocyte Ratio in Bladder Cancer Undergoing Radical Cystectomy: A Meta-Analysis of 5638 Individuals. *Dis. Markers* **2019**, *2019*, 7593560. [CrossRef] [PubMed]
106. Szkandera, J.; Gerger, A.; Liegl-Atzwanger, B.; Absenger, G.; Stotz, M.; Friesenbichler, J.; Trajanoski, S.; Stojakovic, T.; Eberhard, K.; Leithner, A.; et al. The Lymphocyte/Monocyte Ratio Predicts Poor Clinical Outcome and Improves the Predictive Accuracy in Patients with Soft Tissue Sarcomas. *Int. J. Cancer* **2014**, *135*, 362–370. [CrossRef] [PubMed]
107. Jiang, L.; Jiang, S.; Situ, D.; Lin, Y.; Yang, H.; Li, Y.; Long, H.; Zhou, Z. Prognostic Value of Monocyte and Neutrophils to Lymphocytes Ratio in Patients with Metastatic Soft Tissue Sarcoma. *Oncotarget* **2015**, *6*, 9542–9550. [CrossRef] [PubMed]
108. Mirili, C.; Paydas, S.; Guney, I.B.; Ogul, A.; Gokcay, S.; Buyuksimsek, M.; Yetisir, A.E.; Karaalioglu, B.; Tohumcuoglu, M.; Seydaoglu, G. Assessment of Potential Predictive Value of Peripheral Blood Inflammatory Indexes in 26 Cases with Soft Tissue Sarcoma Treated by Pazopanib: A Retrospective Study. *Cancer Manag. Res.* **2019**, *11*, 3445–3453. [CrossRef]
109. Liu, G.; Ke, L.; Sun, S. Prognostic Value of Pretreatment Neutrophil-to-Lymphocyte Ratio in Patients with Soft Tissue Sarcoma. *Medicine* **2018**, *97*, e12176. [CrossRef] [PubMed]
110. Li, L.-Q.; Bai, Z.-H.; Zhang, L.-H.; Zhang, Y.; Lu, X.-C.; Zhang, Y.; Liu, Y.-K.; Wen, J.; Li, J.-Z. Meta-Analysis of Hematological Biomarkers as Reliable Indicators of Soft Tissue Sarcoma Prognosis. *Front. Oncol.* **2020**, *10*, 30. [CrossRef]
111. Kim, Y.; Kobayashi, E.; Suehara, Y.; Ito, A.; Kubota, D.; Tanzawa, Y.; Endo, M.; Nakatani, F.; Nakatsura, T.; Kawai, A.; et al. Immunological Status of Peripheral Blood Is Associated with Prognosis in Patients with Bone and Soft-Tissue Sarcoma. *Oncol. Lett.* **2021**, *21*, 212. [CrossRef] [PubMed]
112. Bücklein, V.; Adunka, T.; Mendler, A.N.; Issels, R.; Subklewe, M.; Schmollinger, J.C.; Noessner, E. Progressive Natural Killer Cell Dysfunction Associated with Alterations in Subset Proportions and Receptor Expression in Soft-Tissue Sarcoma Patients. *Oncoimmunology* **2016**, *5*, e1178421. [CrossRef] [PubMed]
113. Coley, W.B. Contribution to the Knowledge of Sarcoma. *Ann. Surg.* **1891**, *14*, 199. [CrossRef]
114. Maki, R.G.; Jungbluth, A.A.; Gnjatic, S.; Schwartz, G.K.; D'Adamo, D.R.; Keohan, M.L.; Wagner, M.J.; Scheu, K.; Chiu, R.; Ritter, E.; et al. A Pilot Study of Anti-CTLA4 Antibody Ipilimumab in Patients with Synovial Sarcoma. *Sarcoma* **2013**, *2013*, 168145. [CrossRef] [PubMed]
115. Ben-Ami, E.; Barysauskas, C.M.; Solomon, S.; Tahlil, K.; Malley, R.; Hohos, M.; Polson, K.; Loucks, M.; Severgnini, M.; Patel, T.; et al. Immunotherapy with Single Agent Nivolumab for Advanced Leiomyosarcoma of the Uterus: Results of a Phase 2 Study. *Cancer* **2017**, *123*, 3285–3290. [CrossRef]
116. Lachota, M.; Vincenti, M.; Winiarska, M.; Boye, K.; Zagożdżon, R.; Malmberg, K.-J. Prospects for NK Cell Therapy of Sarcoma. *Cancers* **2020**, *12*, 3719. [CrossRef]
117. Cho, D.; Shook, D.R.; Shimasaki, N.; Chang, Y.-H.; Fujisaki, H.; Campana, D. Cytotoxicity of Activated Natural Killer Cells against Pediatric Solid Tumors. *Clin. Cancer Res.* **2010**, *16*, 3901–3909. [CrossRef]
118. Park, T.S.; Groh, E.M.; Patel, K.; Kerkar, S.P.; Lee, C.-C.R.; Rosenberg, S.A. Expression of MAGE-A and NY-ESO-1 in Primary and Metastatic Cancers. *J. Immunother.* **2016**, *39*. [CrossRef]
119. Endo, M.; de Graaff, M.A.; Ingram, D.R.; Lim, S.; Lev, D.C.; Briaire-de Bruijn, I.H.; Somaiah, N.; Bovée, J.V.; Lazar, A.J.; Nielsen, T.O. NY-ESO-1 (CTAG1B) Expression in Mesenchymal Tumors. *Mod. Pathol.* **2015**, *28*, 587–595. [CrossRef]
120. Robbins, P.F.; Morgan, R.A.; Feldman, S.A.; Yang, J.C.; Sherry, R.M.; Dudley, M.E.; Wunderlich, J.R.; Nahvi, A.V.; Helman, L.J.; Mackall, C.L.; et al. Tumor Regression in Patients with Metastatic Synovial Cell Sarcoma and Melanoma Using Genetically Engineered Lymphocytes Reactive with NY-ESO-1. *J. Clin. Oncol.* **2011**, *29*, 917–924. [CrossRef]
121. D'Angelo, S.P.; Melchiori, L.; Merchant, M.S.; Bernstein, D.; Glod, J.; Kaplan, R.; Grupp, S.; Tap, W.D.; Chagin, K.; Binder, G.K.; et al. Antitumor Activity Associated with Prolonged Persistence of Adoptively Transferred NY-ESO-1 c259 T Cells in Synovial Sarcoma. *Cancer Discov.* **2018**, *8*, 944–957. [CrossRef]
122. Miwa, S.; Nishida, H.; Tanzawa, Y.; Takeuchi, A.; Hayashi, K.; Yamamoto, N.; Mizukoshi, E.; Nakamoto, Y.; Kaneko, S.; Tsuchiya, H. Phase 1/2 Study of Immunotherapy with Dendritic Cells Pulsed with Autologous Tumor Lysate in Patients with Refractory Bone and Soft Tissue Sarcoma. *Cancer* **2017**, *123*, 1576–1584. [CrossRef] [PubMed]

123. Pagès, F.; Galon, J.; Dieu-Nosjean, M.C.; Tartour, E.; Sautès-Fridman, C.; Fridman, W.H. Immune Infiltration in Human Tumors: A Prognostic Factor That Should Not Be Ignored. *Oncogene* **2010**, *29*, 1093–1102. [CrossRef] [PubMed]
124. Grünewald, T.G.; Alonso, M.; Avnet, S.; Banito, A.; Burdach, S.; Cidre-Aranaz, F.; di Pompo, G.; Distel, M.; Dorado-Garcia, H.; Garcia-Castro, J.; et al. Sarcoma Treatment in the Era of Molecular Medicine. *EMBO Mol. Med.* **2020**, *12*, e11131. [CrossRef] [PubMed]

Review
Acid Microenvironment in Bone Sarcomas

Gemma Di Pompo [1], Margherita Cortini [1], Nicola Baldini [1,2] and Sofia Avnet [2,*]

1. Biomedical Science and Technologies Lab, IRCCS Istituto Ortopedico Rizzoli, 40136 Bologna, Italy; gemma.dipompo@ior.it (G.D.P.); margherita.cortini@ior.it (M.C.); nicola.baldini@ior.it (N.B.)
2. Department of Biomedical and Neuromotor Sciences, University of Bologna, 40126 Bologna, Italy
* Correspondence: sofia.avnet3@unibo.it

Simple Summary: Although rare, malignant bone sarcomas have devastating clinical implications for the health and survival of young adults and children. To date, efforts to identify the molecular drivers and targets have focused on cancer cells or on the interplay between cancer cells and stromal cells in the tumour microenvironment. On the contrary, in the current literature, the role of the chemical-physical conditions of the tumour microenvironment that may be implicated in sarcoma aggressiveness and progression are poorly reported and discussed. Among these, extracellular acidosis is a well-recognized hallmark of bone sarcomas and promotes cancer growth and dissemination but data presented on this topic are fragmented. Hence, we intended to provide a general and comprehensive overview of the causes and implications of acidosis in bone sarcoma.

Abstract: In bone sarcomas, extracellular proton accumulation is an intrinsic driver of malignancy. Extracellular acidosis increases stemness, invasion, angiogenesis, metastasis, and resistance to therapy of cancer cells. It reprograms tumour-associated stroma into a protumour phenotype through the release of inflammatory cytokines. It affects bone homeostasis, as extracellular proton accumulation is perceived by acid-sensing ion channels located at the cell membrane of normal bone cells. In bone, acidosis results from the altered glycolytic metabolism of bone cancer cells and the resorption activity of tumour-induced osteoclasts that share the same ecosystem. Proton extrusion activity is mediated by extruders and transporters located at the cell membrane of normal and transformed cells, including vacuolar ATPase and carbonic anhydrase IX, or by the release of highly acidic lysosomes by exocytosis. To date, a number of investigations have focused on the effects of acidosis and its inhibition in bone sarcomas, including studies evaluating the use of photodynamic therapy. In this review, we will discuss the current status of all findings on extracellular acidosis in bone sarcomas, with a specific focus on the characteristics of the bone microenvironment and the acid-targeting therapeutic approaches that are currently being evaluated.

Keywords: bone sarcoma; extracellular acidosis; tumour microenvironment; tumour-associated stroma; acid-sensing ion channels; vacuolar-ATP-ase; carbonic anhydrase IX; acridine orange

1. Introduction

1.1. Bone Sarcomas

Bone sarcomas comprise highly heterogeneous subtypes of mesenchymal tumours originating from the bone. The most common types of bone sarcoma are osteosarcoma, Ewing's sarcoma, and chondrosarcoma. Bone sarcomas account for <0.2% of malignant neoplasms registered in the EUROCARE (European Cancer Registry-based study on survival and care of cancer patients) database [1] and their incidence varies according to the different histotype. Osteosarcoma is the first primary cancer of bone (incidence: 0.3 per 100,000 per year), with a higher incidence in adolescents (0.8–1.1 per 100,000 per year at age 15–19 years) [2,3]. Ewing's sarcoma is the second most common primary malignant bone tumour. It occurs most frequently in children and adolescents, but adults can also be affected. Chondrosarcoma is the most frequent bone sarcoma of adulthood. The incidence is around 0.2 per 100,000 per year, with a median age at diagnosis between 30 and 60 years [2,3]. The survival rate after 5 years for patients with localised primary tumour is 60–70% and 50–60% for osteosarcoma and Ewing's sarcoma, respectively, with a dramatic drop to 30% for the former and to only around 20% for the latter, in metastatic patients. The survival rate of chondrosarcoma is 50–60% at 10 years according to the histological grade [4]. Current treatments for osteosarcoma and Ewing's sarcoma combine surgery (preoperative or neoadjuvant), followed by chemotherapy (postoperative or neoadjuvant), and long-term polychemotherapy [5,6]. However, most conventional chemotherapy commonly fails, leading to the cogent need for the identification of novel therapeutic targets and the development of more effective approaches. Among them, the employment of tyrosine kinase and cyclin-dependent kinase inhibitors, DNA repair or chemoresistance targeting, and immunotherapies are currently the most attractive [7].

1.2. Cancer-Associated Extracellular Acidosis

Extracellular acidosis is a well-established hallmark of malignancy in solid tumours [8]. Similarly to hypoxia [9–11], it influences tumour cell behaviour and clinical outcome by modulating cancer stemness, invasion, invadopodia formation, metastasis, anticancer immune reaction, and response to therapy [8,12].

Solid tumours, including sarcomas [12–14], are characterised by an extracellular pH (pHe) that ranges from 6.4 to 7.3, whereas in normal tissues, the range is 7.2 to 7.5 [15]. Tumour formation and progression are strongly influenced by biophysical factors including extracellular acidosis. Understanding how sarcoma cells cope and adapt to the microenvironmental stress that is promoted by an excess of extracellular protons will contribute to a better knowledge of sarcoma pathophysiology and the identification of novel anticancer strategies.

In this review, we will discuss the current status of knowledge on interstitial acidosis in bone sarcomas, taking also into consideration the unique characteristics of sarcoma cells in the bone microenvironment and the acidtargeting therapeutic approaches that are under investigation.

2. Source of Acidosis in the Microenvironment of Bone Sarcomas

Acidosis in bone sarcomas is mainly due to (1) the metabolic switch of cancer cells to glycolytic metabolism which, in turn, causes the efflux of lactic acid and protons in the extracellular space; (2) the active release of protons by normal bone cells, mainly osteoclasts, to resorb bone during the formation of osteolytic lesions that occurs with tumour expansion.

2.1. Altered Tumour Metabolism and Intratumoural Acidosis in Bone Sarcomas

High glycolytic activity is a common feature of many cancer types, including sarcomas [10,16–19]. Cancer cells switch to a glycolytic phenotype in a poorly perfused environment. However, as elegantly described by Otto Warburg in 1927 [20,21], glycolysis in cancer cells also occurs under conditions of normal oxygen tension.

In bone cancers, hypoxia results from increased proliferation of cancer cells in association with a high rate of oxygen consumption, and from the intrinsic hypoxia of the bone microenvironment. Indeed, hypoxia greatly influences bone biology and physiology [22]. As a demonstration, in the medullary cavity of animal models, pO_2 values range from 11.7 to 31.7 mm Hg (1.5–4.2%), with a mean of 20.4 mm Hg (2.7%) [23].

The switch to glycolysis, both under normoxic and hypoxic conditions, follows the activation of hypoxia-inducible factor-1 (HIF-1), which drives the transcription of crucial enzymes of the glycolytic pathway [24]. As an end result, the increased glycolytic rate leads to intracellular accumulation of protons in the cytoplasm, but also the release of protons into the extracellular space as a waste product along with lactate. To survive this harsh microenvironment, cancer cells develop adaptive mechanisms, including transcriptional, posttranslational, and morphological alterations, which eventually lead to profound changes in their phenotype and the metabolic profile [12]. Cancer-associated acidosis is attracting increasing interest in the field of cancer research. New in vivo imaging tools are being developed to assess the association between cancer metabolism and the acidic microenvironment [25]. For example, in a near future, it will be possible to combine ^{8}F-FDG PET, currently used for staging bone sarcomas [26,27], together with chemical exchange saturation transfer magnetic resonance imaging (CEST-MRI), to detect acidic regions of the tumour in order to determine its metastatic potential.

Finally, an additional metabolic trigger of tumour interstitial acidosis, in addition to glycolysis exacerbation, could be the hydration of excessive CO_2 production in the more oxidative areas of the tumour [28]. However, this mechanism has not been explored in bone sarcoma.

In this context, although not thoroughly explored, it is noteworthy that acidosis, conversely, may lead to HIF-1 regulation. In order to maintain energy homeostasis, highly glycolytic cancer cells lead to glucose deprivation in the extracellular space by consuming large amounts of glucose (and glutamine). Low-glucose conditions in the tumour microenvironment, in turn, can cause a loss of stromal caveolin-1, yielding oxidative stress which mimics hypoxia ('pseudohypoxia') through activation of HIF-1 and NF-kB [29]. NF-kB has been shown to be a direct modulator of HIF-1 expression in inflammation and hypoxia [30,31], and in osteosarcoma, NF-kB upregulation has been demonstrated to be induced by acidosis [32], supporting the idea that acidosis and hypoxia can reciprocally modulate each other's behaviour.

2.2. Proton Extruders in Bone Sarcomas

Cytosolic acidification is extremely toxic to both normal and cancer cells, eventually leading to apoptosis [33]. Sarcoma cells get rid of excessive intracellular proton accumulation through extruders and transporters located on the plasma membrane or lysosomal membrane, which strongly acidify the extracellular space via direct pumping/transport or by exocytosis, respectively [34].

Previous reports on extracellular acidification in bone sarcomas have made use of preclinical in vitro models and various techniques to measure pHe, such as the use of macro- or microelectrodes or the measurement of extracellular acidification rate (EACR) values by Seahorse technology. These techniques have shown that the activity of these extruders/transporters is responsible for strong acidification of the medium, both in the extracellular space and near the cell membrane [16]. Additionally, the enhanced acidification ability in stem cells derived from a soft tissue sarcoma has been demonstrated using acridine orange and lysosensor staining [16,34,35].

Among the most studied proton exchangers and transporters, sarcomas express certain subunits of vacuolar H^+-ATPase (V-ATPase), such as V_1B_2 and V_0c V-ATPase subunits, the Na^+/H^+ exchanger isoform 1 (NHEs, mainly NHE1), the monocarboxylate transporters (MCTs, mainly MCT1, also known as lactate–proton symporter), the Na^+-dependent $Cl^-/HCO3^-$ exchanger, and carbonic anhydrases (CAs) isozymes, mainly CAII, CAIX and CAXII [36]. Studies describing the expression and the role of these molecules in the extracellular acidification and behaviour of bone sarcomas are reported in Tables 1–4.

Table 1. V-ATPase expression and targeting in bone sarcomas.

Type of Cancer	Expression of the Ion Extruders /Transporters	Inhibitors	Targeted Biological Function of Clinical Outcome	Biological Samples and/or Cell Lines Used	Refs.
Ewing Sarcoma	V_0c, V_1B_2, and V_0a_1 V-ATPase	Bafilomycin A1, omeprazole, V_0c V-ATPase siRNA	Cell viability and growth	A-673, SK-N-MC, RD-ES, SK-ES-1	[16]
Chondrosarcoma, osteosarcoma	V_0c, V_1B_2, and V_0a_1 V-ATPase	Esomeprazole alone or combined with sulphasalazine, omeprazole	Cell viability and motility, chemoresistance to doxorubicin, in vivo tumour growth, stemness	Primary cell cultures obtained from tumour biopsies, and Saos-2, SW1353, MG63, HOS, 143B, and RD cells and, 143B-mouse xenograft, frozen samples from human sarcoma and 3-methylcholanthrene (3-MCA)-induced sarcoma model.	[34,35,37,38]

Table 2. CA expression and targeting in bone sarcomas.

Types of Cancers	Expression of the Ion Extruders	Inhibitors Used	CA-Related Studied Biological Function or Clinical Outcome	Biological Samples and/or Cell Lines Used	Refs.
Chondrosarcoma, osteosarcoma	CAII and CAIX	CAIX, sulphonamide-derived inhibitors (and anti-HIF-1α inhibitors)	Cell viability, proliferation and motility, chemoresistance to doxorubicin, in vivo tumour growth, stemness	Primary cell cultures obtained from tumour biopsies, and Saos-2, SW1353, and MG63, HOS cells.	[34,39–41]
Osteosarcoma	CAVIII	None	Drug resistance, cell invasion, tumour growth, aerobic glycolysis	143b, HOS, MG63, U2-OS cells, and 143b xenografts	[42]
Fibrosarcoma	CAIX	None specific to CAIX (only HIF-1α inhibitors)	Hypoxia-modulated survival w/o and after irradiation	HT 1080 human fibrosarcoma cells and xenograft	[43,44]
Chondrosarcoma	CAIX	None	metastasis-free survival of patients	tumour biopsies	[45]

Table 3. MCT expression and targeting in bone sarcomas.

Types of Cancers	Expression of the Ion Extruders	Inhibitors Used	MCT-Related Studied Biological Function or Clinical Outcome	Biological Samples and/or Cell Lines Used	Refs.
Chondrosarcoma, osteosarcoma	MCT1	[alpha]-Cyano-4-hydroxycinnamate (CHC), shRNA anti MCT1	Cell viability and motility, chemoresistance to doxorubicin, in vivo tumour growth, stemness	Primary cell cultures obtained from tumour biopsies, and Saos-2, SW1353, MG63, MNNG/HOS, HOS, and 143B cells, and xenograft	[34,46,47]
Osteosarcoma	MCT4	none	Overall survival	Tumour biopsies	[48]

Table 4. NHE expression and targeting in bone sarcomas.

Types of Cancers	Expression of the Ion Extruders	Inhibitors Used	Targeted Biological Function	Biological Samples and/or Cell Lines Used	Refs.
Chondrosarcoma, osteosarcoma	NHE1	None	Cell viability and motility, chemoresistance to doxorubicin, in vivo tumour growth, stemness	Primary cell cultures obtained from tumour biopsies, and Saos-2, SW1353, and MG63, and HOS	[34]

Several drugs have been tested to target these ion extruders/transporters as anticancer therapy. For a more extensive discussion, see Section 5.1.

The most studied ion/proton extruders/transporter is the V-ATPase, followed by the CAIX enzyme. V-ATPases are ubiquitous proton pumps that are found either on the intracellular membranes, such as lysosomes, or, for specialised cells, at the plasma membrane. V-ATPases use the energy of ATP to transport protons from the cytosol to intracellular compartments or to the extracellular space. The V-ATPase consists of an ATP-hydrolytic domain (V_1) and a proton-translocation domain (V_0) [49]. Its energy-consuming activity requires the close association of all the components of the complex, which is provided by the C-loop [50]. Studies on V-ATPase expression and activity in bone sarcomas are mainly related to the analysis of preclinical models and, less frequently, of tissue samples.

CAIX is one of the 15 carbonic anhydrase isoforms present in humans, among which 12 are functional [51]. Carbonic anhydrases are a large family of dimeric zinc metalloenzymes with an extracellular active site that catalyses the reversible hydration of carbon dioxide to carbonic acid and are involved in respiration and acid–base balance, facilitating acid secretion in different cell types [52]. Evidence for CAIX expression in bone sarcomas has been largely based on the analysis of human tissue samples.

A less considered but important acid extruder is the voltage-gated proton channel (Hv1). This has been found to be expressed in the cells of origin of bone sarcoma, the mesenchymal stromal cells (MSC). Its pharmacological inhibition in MSC significantly decreases cell differentiation and mineral matrix deposition [53]. However, although Hv1 expression has been demonstrated in different cancers that frequently colonise bone, including breast and colorectal carcinomas [54,55], no data have been reported in bone sarcomas. In this context, it might be interesting to compare the ability of bone sarcomas to acidify the extracellular space with respect to other types of cancers that are able to expand in bone, such as bone metastases (BM) (see ref. [50]); carcinoma cells metastasizing to the bone share with bone sarcoma cells different mechanisms of proton extrusion, including the expression of V_1B_2 and V_0c V-ATPase subunits, CAIX, MCT1, and MCT4. As an example, we have recently found mRNA expression of CAIX in breast and renal carcinoma cell lines, with a significant increase under reduced oxygen conditions with respect to normoxia [50,56]. Additionally, different isoforms of V-ATPase, including the V_1C_1 [57] and the V_1B_2 and V_1G_1 subunits [58], are expressed by breast carcinoma cells with a specific tropism for bone. Finally, it has been demonstrated that the expression of MCT4 in tumour cells is responsible for a metabolic coupling with bone-resorbing osteoclasts, thereby inducing a higher osteolytic activity in BM from breast carcinoma [18].

In summary, several lines of evidence suggest that an increased glycolytic rate and subsequent activation of several ion extruders and transporters in different cancer cells that grow in bone are the main causes of tumour interstitial acidosis.

2.3. Bone Resorption as a Source of Extracellular Acidification

In the bone soil, to expand and invade the surrounding normal tissue, sarcoma cells degrade the hard extracellular matrix by directly or indirectly stimulating the activity of osteoclasts, the highly specialised bone-resorbing cells. The bone microenvironment is a fertile ground for tumour growth. Under physiological conditions, the process of bone remodelling couples osteoclast-mediated bone resorption and osteoblast-promoted bone formation to maintain bone homeostasis. However, the development and progression of primary bone tumours, including osteosarcoma, severely disrupt this balance and induces a 'vicious cycle' between osteoclasts, osteoblasts, stromal cells, and cancer cells. In the bone soil, in order to expand and invade the surrounding normal tissue, sarcoma cells degrade the hard extracellular matrix by directly or indirectly stimulating the activity of osteoclasts that resorb bone, as well as directly eroding bone through the secretion of metalloproteinases (MMPs). The induction of osteoclast activity can be triggered by a plethora of growth factors that also commonly regulate physiological bone remodelling and can be secreted by cancer cells, or by tumour-stimulated osteoblasts. Of these, the most important is the receptor activator of nuclear factor-kappa B ligand (RANKL). Other factors, such as interleukin 1 (IL-1), interleukin 6 (IL-6), tumour necrosis factor-alpha (TNFa), parathyroid hormone-related protein (PTHrP), or transforming growth factor-beta (TGFb), mediate RANKL receptor (RANK) expression on the surface of osteoclasts, thereby favouring osteoclast maturation and activation [59]. Furthermore, we have recently demonstrated that a low pH further induces osteoclast activity, both directly and indirectly, by stimulating osteoblasts to secrete pro-osteoclastogenic paracrine mediators such as IL-8 and IL-6 [56].

Once stimulated, mature osteoclasts can resorb bone through a multistep dynamic process. First, osteoclasts migrate and attach to the bone surface that is to be degraded and removed, thus forming a tight 'sealing zone'. Then, the plasma membrane polarises to form the resorption organelle, the ruffled border, a unique folded highly permeable membrane facing to the bone surface to be resorbed [60]. Subsequently, to dissolve the mineralised component of bone, osteoclasts secrete hydrochloric acid into the resorption lacunae (Howship's lacunae) mainly via plasma membrane V-ATPase (a3 isoform) [61]. Proton pumping performed by osteoclasts during bone resorption activity is an energy-consuming intensive process that relies primarily on the glycolytic metabolism of osteoclasts [62]. It is noteworthy that the expression of a3 is 100-fold higher in osteoclasts than in other cell types [63]. The activity of V-ATPase is also coupled with the activity of the chloride ion–proton channel antiporter ClC-7 [64], and both proteins are clustered in the ruffled border domain.

Finally, as an additional player in the acidification activity of osteoclasts, it has been demonstrated the expression of Hv1 that helps proton release and bone mineral dissolution, thereby promoting bone resorption [65–67].

As a consequence of the proton extrusion activity, in Howship's lacunae, the pH reaches very low values, around 4.5 [60]. At the end of the resorption process, protons pumped into Howship's lacunae diffuse in the extracellular space, thus causing further acidification of the tumour microenvironment. Adversely, proteinaceous component of the matrix, mainly type I collagen, is degraded through the activity of the osteoclast-derived cysteine proteinase cathepsin K, which is responsible for the breakdown of collagen I, osteopontin, and osteonectin [68].

Osteoclast differentiation and activity result in dysregulated bone lysis and release of bone matrix growth factors such as TGFb, insulin-like growth factor 1 (IGF1), fibroblast growth factor (FGF), or bone morphogenetic protein (BMP), which, in turn, can promote tumour cell proliferation and further bone destruction [69,70]. This 'vicious cycle' between cancer cells and the bone microenvironment was first described in bone metastasis, but in fact, there is evidence supporting the notion that osteosarcoma cells, for example, mediate bone destruction by stimulating osteoclast differentiation and activity as bone metastasis [71,72]. In addition to osteoclasts, acid-mediated resorption of the bone mineralised matrix can also be performed by osteocytes. Osteocytes are the final fully differentiated form of osteoblasts that are trapped in the hard matrix and directly remodel the bone walls of their lacunar–canalicular systems in a process known as perilacunar/canalicular osteocytic remodelling. As with osteoclasts, this process relies on the combined activity of MMPs, vacuolar acid-secreting H^+-ATPases [73,74], and other enzymes, such as cathepsin

K and carbonic anhydrases [75]. However, the interaction between sarcoma cells and osteocytes is completely unexplored, and it is still unknown whether perilacunar remodelling can be induced by invading cancer cells.

Finally, in the context of the acid extracellular tumour microenvironment, it should be noted that an excess of extracellular protons may also modulate the activity of cation channels, including calcium receptors [76,77]. Calcium (Ca^{2+}) signalling is crucial, both for bone physiology and sarcoma progression. Indeed, both osteoblasts and osteoclasts, as well as osteosarcoma cells, express calcium-sensing receptors on the cell membrane [78,79], and Ca^{2+} is an essential mediator for cell differentiation, bone resorption, and gene transcription in osteoclasts, and for the aggressiveness of tumour cells [80,81]. However, the interference of extracellular acidosis in Ca^{2+} signalling in bone sarcoma is an unexplored field of research. For a more detailed discussion of the potential effect of high H^+ extracellular concentration on cation channels that are expressed by bone sarcomas, see Section 4.1.

In conclusion, these findings demonstrate that, in addition to tumour cells, tumour-induced bone-resorbing cells of the bone microenvironment contribute to acidify the microenvironment of sarcomas.

3. Effect of Acidosis on Sarcoma Cells

The extracellular acidification derived from cancer cells and from the tumour-associated stroma is responsible for the modulation of bone colonisation by sarcoma cells. Indeed, an acidic pHe promotes cancer invasion, survival, and angiogenesis, and alters the cell permeability to anticancer drugs by many different mechanisms, thereby preventing their effective targeting.

Extracellular acidosis has also been described to influence anticancer immune response and autophagy in a number of solid tumours. However, the role of autophagy in mediating survival to acidosis has not been confirmed in osteosarcoma, where the autophagic flux seems to be unchanged between pH conditions (7.4 and 6.8) [37,82], and the impact of acidosis on the infiltration of inflammatory or immune cells has not been explored thus far. Furthermore, the system by which tumour cells can sense extracellular acidosis has not been deeply investigated yet, but few specific sensors have been identified. Finally, it is important to bear in mind that preclinical studies that investigated on sarcoma acidic microenvironment and based on cell culture medium acidification have high heterogeneity of pH values: in most cases, the studies were carried out with a pH range between 6.5 and 6.8 [22,24–26], but in other cases, harsher experimental conditions were used (pH 5.8 in [9]). On the other hand, the development of a 3D model has led to the development of physiological pH culture values by using an unbuffered culture medium, thus allowing 3D spheroids to adapt the pH value to their own metabolism [54]. Thus, these different experimental systems and different pH values might have led to different outcomes.

3.1. pH Sensors in Sarcoma Cells

In the TME, different ion channels behave not only similar to ion transporters but also similar to sensors and transducers of altered pH as they can be affected by both extracellular and intracellular pH [83]. Furthermore, they greatly contribute to cancer progression [84–87]. As an example, in osteosarcoma, the voltage-gated potassium channel Kv1.3, transient receptor potential cation channel subfamily M member 8 (TRPM8), and piezo type mechanosensitive ion channel component 1 (Piezo1) are among the most expressed pH-sensitive ion channels and correlate with tumour progression [88–90].

On the other hand, the high concentration of protons in TME may also strongly affect the biological functions of these pH-sensitive proteins and receptors, since it may induce Kv1.3 potassium channel inactivation, and the alteration of the signalling pathway mediated by the Ca^{2+}-permeable channels, TRPM8 and Piezo1 [91–93], ultimately altering their proaptoptotic signalling. However, the acid-mediated effect on these ion channels and the downstream signalling has never been explored in sarcoma.

3.2. Effect of Extracellular Acidosis on Tumour Invasion, Survival, and Metabolism

Invasion occurs through invadopodia, dynamic actin-rich membrane protrusions that penetrate within the extracellular matrix and degrade it through the spatial and temporal release of proteases and protons [94]. The protonation of the matrix metalloproteinases is dependent on the activation of the proteinases and requires the redistribution and activation of V-ATPases and NHE1 to the tip of the invadopodia. Thus, local invasion is strongly modulated by the acidification activity of these proton/ion transporters and by the presence of an acidic pHe.

In sarcomas, the acidic microenvironment activates survival pathways and increases migration and invasive potential [16,37]. However, further molecular mechanisms are responsible for the acidosis-mediated progression of sarcomas. In osteosarcoma, we demonstrated the pH-dependent activation (at a pH of 6.5) of a stress-regulated switch that promotes the recruitment of the TNF-receptor-associated factors/cellular inhibitor of apoptosis protein 1 (TRAF/cIAP) complexes, and nuclear factor kappa-light-chain-enhancer of activated B cells (NF-κB) pathway [95]. This activation ultimately leads to an increase in cancer cell survival, suggesting a role for TRAF/cIAP proteins as promising targets for anticancer therapy. As an in vivo confirmation of the intimate association between acidosis and cancer cell survival, we found a significant correlation between V-ATPase and TRAF1 or NF-κB1 expression in tissues from osteosarcoma xenografts.

More recently, evidence has shown that extracellular acidosis, obtained in unbuffered conditions, is also responsible for prominent metabolic plasticity that leads to the accumulation of intracellular lipids, specifically sphingolipids and sphingosine 1-phosphate (S1P). Impairing S1P levels by means of Fingolimod, an FDA-approved drug for the treatment of multiple sclerosis, was of predominant importance to decrease the migration potential of acid-resistant cells, to increase apoptosis, and to impair xenograft growth [82]. This suggests, for the first time, the use of an anticancer drug that has the potential to specifically target the acid-resistant subpopulation in osteosarcoma.

Finally, by studying both standard monolayer cultures and cancer stem cells and by extensive metabolomic analysis, we demonstrated that extracellular acidosis completely remodels cancer cell metabolism by inducing glycolysis repression and by increasing the amino acid catabolism and the urea cycle [96].

3.3. Effect of Extracellular Acidosis on Tumour Sensitivity to Anticancer Drugs

Tumour acidosis is also a major cause of drug resistance and therapeutic failure. First of all, a low pHe (pH 6.5) significantly decreases the growth rate of cancer cells, thereby affecting the IC50 values of drugs that target actively proliferating cells [37]. However, an acidic pHe may also impact the response to therapeutics through additional complex mechanisms. The pH gradient across cellular membranes is crucial for determining the passive diffusion of small molecules. 'Ion trapping' (or pH partitioning) is the physiological process regulating passive permeability through the cellular membrane of negatively or positively charged compounds, such as ionisable compounds containing weak bases or weak acids. The lysosomal and the cytoplasmic membranes can compartmentalise drugs and, as a consequence of the pH partitioning, drugs can be hindered from reaching their molecular target because they become trapped on the wrong side of cellular membranes. The extent of ionisation for a molecule depends both on its intrinsic pKa values(s) and the pH of the solution. In an acidic extracellular microenvironment, weak bases will be positively charged to a larger extent, thus influencing the diffusion of the drug inside the target cells [14].

The cellular membranes that can compartmentalise drugs are both the cytoplasmic membrane and the lysosomal membrane. Acidic lysosomes can sequester weakly basic molecules from the cytosol to an extent that is directly related to the level of lysosomal acidosis, thereby preventing the drug targeting [97]. In this context, it is noteworthy that a high extracellular concentration of protons increased both the number and the acidification of lysosomes in osteosarcoma cells [37].

Additionally, the cytoplasmic membrane contributes to the 'ion-trapping effect'. In the presence of an acidic extracellular microenvironment, weakly basic drugs are forced to stay outside the cell. We confirmed this mechanism for doxorubicin in osteosarcoma cells [37]. Conversely, the presence of a low extracellular pHe allows for the permeability of weakly acidic drugs. In such a case, the neutral form of a weakly acidic compound may be favoured, and the uncharged species can freely diffuse across the plasma membrane. Since the cytosolic pH is slightly alkaline, once the acidic drug has crossed the plasma membrane and entered the cell, it is ionised and trapped within the cell. In this case, the cytotoxic activity may be enhanced by extracellular acidosis. Known examples of anticancer drugs containing weak acids are 5-fluorouracil and cyclophosphamide [14]. However, preclinical studies on the comparison of cytotoxicity at different pH values of these drugs in inhibiting bone sarcomas have never been performed.

3.4. Effect of Extracellular Acidosis on Tumour Angiogenesis and Others

The anarchic formation of new vessels that provide O_2 and nutrients needed by actively proliferating cells is induced by tumour cells through the release of pro-angiogenic factors, such as vascular endothelial growth factor (VEGF) and interleukin 8 (IL-8) [98], or through the stabilisation of HIF-1 that are promoted by extracellular acidosis [99,100]. Interestingly, in osteosarcoma cells under acidic conditions, we observed increased release of extracellular nanovesicles with proangiogenic activity, including urokinase-type plasminogen activator (uPA), angiopoietin-2 (Ang-2), and VEGF, as well as the presence of miRNAs related to angiogenesis, as demonstrated by the formation of tubule branches in the chorioallantoic membrane (CAM) [101], suggesting that local acidosis might be responsible for promoting neoangiogenesis.

4. Effect of Acidosis on Different Cells and Elements of Sarcoma Microenvironment

Cancer cells are not solely responsible for the growth of cancer and the spread to distant organs. A complex structure, formed of cancer cells that directly interact with stromal cells under different microenvironmental conditions, constitutes the bulk of the tumour. Among stromal cells, the microenvironment of bone sarcomas includes MSC, osteoblasts and osteoclasts, cancer-associated fibroblasts, and immune cells: all these different cell types coexist and infiltrate the tumour [102,103]. In particular, similar to physiological wound healing, MSCs are recruited from the bloodstream to the site of the tumour lesion, where they contribute to the rapid tumour expansion [68]. MSCs are crucial for the initiation [104], as well as the progression of the lesion [105]. However, in the context of mesenchymal tumours, MSCs are hardly distinguishable from tumour cells.

Importantly, cancer cells are not the only population being affected by extracellular acidosis. The effects of a low pHe are observed also on stromal cells of the bone microenvironment, and these may, in turn, indirectly modulate the behaviour and the aggressiveness of tumour cells (Figure 1).

4.1. Bone Cells Sense and React to Extracellular Acidification

It is widely recognised that local variations of pHe greatly impact osteoblast and osteoclast differentiation and activity. Thus, as in other pathological conditions (i.e., inflammation), in the altered tumour microenvironment, bone cells can perceive acidosis and react to such stress signals by modulating their activities, as well as through paracrine communication by stimulating cancer progression.

Cells of the osteogenic lineage react to a high extracellular concentration of protons by impairing their osteogenic activities, namely, osteoblast differentiation, matrix deposition, and mineralisation [106,107]. Adversely, in osteoclasts, a low pHe increases the formation of resorption pits (maximal stimulus at pH < 6.9 [108]) and upregulates the activity of cathepsin K, tartrate-resistant acid phosphatase (TRACP), and TNF-receptor-associated factor 6 (TRAF6) [109–111].

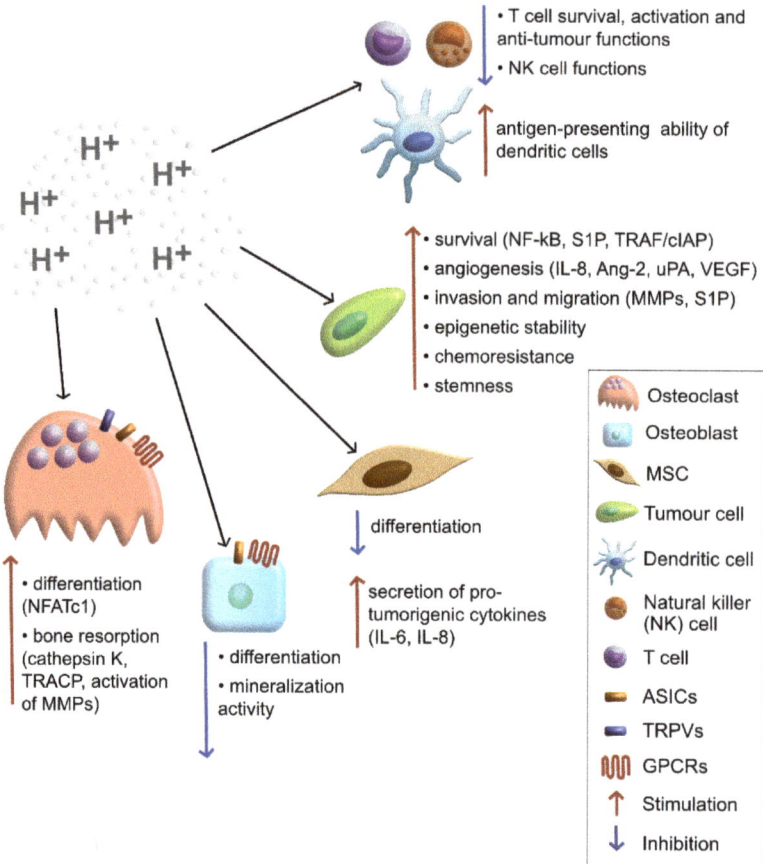

Figure 1. Graphical summary of the effects of extracellular acidosis on cells of the bone sarcoma microenvironment.

Bone cells sense pH changes through specific proton sensors and channels that are typically expressed by sensory neurons. Among them, the acid-sensing ion channels ASIC2, also known as amiloride-sensitive cation channel 1, neuronal (ACCN1), and ASIC3/ACCN3 are mostly abundant in bone. Specifically, previous reports have shown the expression of ASIC1/ACCN2, ASIC2/ACCN1, and ASIC3/ACCN3 mRNAs [112] in human osteoblasts. Besides ASICs, metabotropic proton-sensing G protein-coupled receptors (GPCRs) have also been recently identified as proton-sensing machinery in osteoblasts [113–115]. Similarly, we recently found that MSC, osteoblasts, and CAF express ASIC4/ACCN4, ASIC3/ACCN3, G protein-coupled receptor (GPR)-65, and GPR4 at levels comparable to or even higher than those expressed by cells of neuronal origin and that in MSC, the incubation with an acidic medium increases the expression of ASIC4/ACCN4 and GPR65 [58].

Regarding the osteoclastic lineage, human monocytic osteoclast precursors express ASIC1/ACCN2, ASIC2/ACCN1, and ASIC3/ACCN3. This expression persists also after the induction of osteoclast differentiation, albeit at a lower level. Likewise, transient receptor potential vanilloid (TRPV) channels, which are typically expressed by sensory neurons, and the ovarian cancer G protein-coupled receptor 1 (OGR1) which belongs to the GPCR family are proton sensors and have been involved in osteoclast differentiation and survival [50]. In particular, TRPV1, TRPV2, and TRPV4 channels are crucial for osteoclast biology [80,116,117]. Notably, TRPVs are activated also by severe acidosis (pH 5.4) [118] and TRPV4 seems to be the major mediator of the acidosis-induced osteoclast formation as its antagonist, RN1734, partially inhibited the pH-dependent osteoclastogenesis, while its agonist 4-α PDD enhanced osteoclast formation under mild acidosis [117].

Under this context, it is noteworthy that both ASICs and TRPVs are also permeable to cations other than H^+, like Ca^{2+} and the reciprocal interactions between H^+ and Ca^{2+}, and the competition of H^+ for the same binding-site of Ca^{2+} may modulate the activity of these pH sensors and, thus, the downstream biological effects. Specifically, for ASICs, due to the binding competition, Ca^{2+} binding favours the closed state, and H^+ binding leads to the open state [119]. Furthermore, increased extracellular Ca^{2+} concentration can significantly decrease the pH sensitivity of ASIC1 and ASIC3 [120]. Thus, this strong interplay between H^+ and Ca^{2+} may occurs also in normal bone cells in the sarcoma microenvironment: it is already well known that TRPVs mediate Ca^{2+} signalling and are produced in mature osteoclast differentiation to sustain the intracellular Ca^{2+} level for the maintenance of active NFATc1 that regulates terminal cell differentiation [121], and the presence of an excess of protons in the sarcoma TME may interfere with Ca^{2+} signalling mediated by TRPVs in osteoclasts and may directly alter the osteoclast physiology and activity.

Overall, these data indicate that normal bone cells perceive and react to the acidification of the bone sarcoma microenvironment. The ultimate result is an unbalance of bone remodelling. In conclusion, a low pHe appears to be an essential requirement for the initiation of the osteolytic process, but it may also be involved in altered bone formation as it occurs in osteogenic sarcomas such as osteosarcoma.

4.2. The Acid-Stimulated Secretome

Tumour-derived acidosis may favour tumour expansion by reprogramming stromal cells to the secretion of proinflammatory cytokines. Decrease of local pH is per se an inflammatory stimulus that causes the release of various enzymes during phagocytosis, the damage of vasculature and other surrounding tissues, and the prolonging of the healing process by stimulating new inflammatory reactions [29]. We have recently shown that extracellular acidosis directly activates the NF-kB inflammatory family of transcription factors and thus the secretion of NF-kB-related cytokines, chemokines, and growth factors by the osteosarcoma-associated stromal compartment formed by osteoblasts, MSC, and CAF [32,58]. Regardless of the source of acidosis, after a few hours, incubation with a pHe 6.8 activates RelA, RelB, or NF-kB that, in turn, induce the expression of the inflammatory cytokines IL-8 and IL-6 and enhances cancer stemness (formation of spheroids and expression of the stemness-related markers oct4 or Nanog [32]). In the same study, by using a blocking antibody against the IL-6 receptor, we demonstrated that acid-induced release of IL-6 by normal mesenchymal cells was directly responsible for bone cancer migration and invasion [32]. Intriguingly, IL-6 secretion seems to be directly dependent on the acid-stimulated MSC, whereas the tumour cells contribute little to the release of paracrine tumour-stimulating factors under acidic pH conditions. This is of note because it highlights the importance of the stromal subpopulation in enhancing cancer progression. Furthermore, the exposure of osteosarcoma cells to the secretome of acid-stimulated MSC reduced the toxicity of doxorubicin and thus promoted the development of a chemoresistant phenotype [32].

Altogether, these observations warrant the role of local acidosis in promoting a pro-tumourigenic phenotype in bone sarcomas also by inducing a proinflammatory and a pro-osteolytic secretome by cells of the osteogenic lineage.

4.3. Matrix Remodelling/Degradation

Another important feature of the sarcoma microenvironment is the composition and organisation of the ECM, whose mechanical properties affect cancer cell behaviour and that may be, in turn, influenced by tumour-derived extracellular acidosis. ECM is mainly secreted by stromal cells, and it is composed of various macromolecules, including collagens, glycoproteins (fibronectin and laminins), proteoglycans, and polysaccharides [122]. ECM is also secreted from tumour cells, especially from osteogenic sarcoma. However, how low extracellular pH affects the synthesis and secretion of proteins of ECM is an almost uncovered field of investigation. During cancer progression, an excessive ECM remodelling occurs by proteinase activity, such as MMP-2 and MMP-9, and small ECM fragments are released into the circulation [123]. In melanoma cells, it has been reported that acidic culture conditions induce the increase of 103-kDa gelatinase/type IV collagenase secretion [124]. Furthermore, the membrane-bound MMP-14 has an acidic pH optimum and has been observed to be in close association with CAIX in invadopodia [125]. Additionally, in sarcoma, with particular regard to Ewing sarcoma, we previously found an increase of MMPs activity when tumour cells were cultured at low pH, as evaluated by gelatine-quenching assay and an increase of the ability to degrade type I collagen [16]. However, with the exception of the mentioned report, no other data have been published about the correlation between acidosis and ECM remodelling/degradation in bone sarcomas.

4.4. Effect of Extracellular Acidosis on Immune Reactivity to Cancer Cells

In the sarcoma microenvironment, different cells and cytokines of the immune system may be included, such as tumour infiltrating lymphocytes (TILs) and associated macrophages, expression of immune checkpoint inhibitors such as cytotoxic T-lymphocyte-associated protein 4 (CTLA-4), programmed cell death-1 (PD-1), and programmed death-ligand 1 (PD-L1), and major histocompatibility complex (MHC) antigen expression [126]. All of these components may be important for prognosis and responses of tumours to immunologically targeted therapies and are potential therapeutics or therapeutic targets. However, although significant progress in the field of immunotherapy, particularly as regards the clinical use of immune checkpoint inhibitors, has been made [127], durable response rates remain low [128], and current sarcoma immunotherapies still fails to induce an antitumoural response [129] implying that other immunosuppressive activities or effects are possibly present. Among these, tumour-derived extracellular acidosis may have an unexplored role. Indeed, in other types of cancer, the formation of an acidic microenvironment represents an efficient tumour strategy and forms such as an immune sanctuary to overcome immune surveillance since it profoundly alters the functions of cells of the immune system, including T cells, neutrophils, macrophages and dendritic cells (DCs) [130,131]. In particular, both cancer and immune cells are highly dependent on the glycolytic pathway for survival, proliferation, and activity. An increased rate of glycolysis, as it occurs in cancer environment, leads to a significant decrease in glucose availability and, although cancer cells can enter quiescence in the absence of glucose, activated T cells are not able to survive without glucose when attempting to expand into an acidic environment [132]. Notably, a high extracellular concentration of protons impairs glycolysis per se [96,133]. Furthermore, an acidic pH blocks the activation and antitumour functions of T cells in vitro through sequestration of interferon-gamma (IFN-γ) [134]. Tumour acidity also promotes tumour progression by negatively affecting the maturation and function of Th1 lymphocytes while stimulating the progression of tumour-promoting Th2 lymphocytes by inactivation of IFN-γ and suppression of tumour necrosis factor-α [132]. Finally, several lines of evidence have suggested that the contribution of extracellular acidosis to cancer growth is related to both the suppression of T cell function and to modulatory effects on additional cells of the immune system. In particular, Husain et al. demonstrated that tumour-derived lactate inhibits natural killer (NK) cell function, both directly and indirectly, i.e., by increasing the numbers of myeloid-derived suppressor cells (MDSCs) that, in turn, inhibit NK cytotoxicity [135]. A low pH also reprogrammes tumour-associated macrophages (TAMs) into a proangiogenic phenotype [136], activates neutrophils [137,138], and improves the antigen-presenting capacity of DCs derived from murine bone marrow [139]. However, no investigations have been performed thus far on sarcomas in this regard. Future studies will help find possible novel approaches to improve the outcomes of immunotherapy in sarcoma patients.

5. Targeting Acidosis in Bone Sarcomas

The use of preclinical models that can mimic the extracellular acidic sarcoma microenvironment and the selection of assays that are not technically affected by the presence of an acidic pH have been fundamental for the identification of novel targets and the development of effective therapeutic strategies against acidosis in cancer. In vitro, monolayer models have to face the caveat of acidic pH being adjusted by a buffer solution that cannot be regulated throughout the experiment. In 3D experiments, spheroids or organoids grown in unbuffered media can, instead, adjust the pH to their own metabolic features and to the intrinsic acidification processes. The latter method has the advantage of resembling the physiological pH regulations seen in vivo. Additionally, the expression and the activity of reporter or housekeeping genes that are commonly used to study the induction or the inhibition of specific targets or proteins, such as b-actin or the green fluorescent protein (GFP), can be strongly affected by an acidic microenvironment. A recent paper has highlighted that among the most commonly used housekeeping genes, only YWHAZ, GAPDH, GUSB, and 18S rRNA are stable throughout pH modifications [140]. Furthermore, scientists working in this field of research should be aware that the fluorescence of wild-type GFP is stable from pH 6 to 10 but decreases at pH < 6 and increases from pH 10 to 12 [141]. The pH stability of GFP can also be exploited for specific purposes: for example, the superecliptic pHluorin (SEP) is a mutant GFP widely used in vitro as a pH reporter, as it is nearly nonfluorescent at pH 6 but brightly green at pH 7.4 [142].

Additionally, in vivo, the assessment of pH imaging methods is invasive, costly, or requires long acquisition times, and in some cases may not be suitable for high-throughput preclinical animal studies. Imaging methods include CEST-MRI, a quantitative method that accurately recapitulates tumour pH maps [143], or pH-sensitive ratiometric reporters such as pHLuc [142]. Despite the limitations, these imaging methods are of crucial importance in the assessment of therapeutics based on targeting cancer acidosis.

The therapeutic strategies that have been developed to target cancer acidosis are based on several approaches, namely, (1) hampering of proton extruders/ion transporters; (2) targeting cancer cell lysosomes through the use of photodynamic therapy; (3) use of inhibitors of acid-sensing ion channels that can possibly hinder the activation of the tumour-associated stroma (see Section 4.1). However, the last class of drugs has been extensively studied only as analgesic and anxiolytic drugs, and as drugs for the treatment of ischemic stroke [144], but has never been considered thus far for the treatment of sarcomas. Finally, recent evidence has highlighted molecular pathways that are selectively activated in acidic-treated cells. These pathways can regulate oncogenes or oncometabolites or be involved in the generation of bioactive lipids. In the former case, the RAB39A-RXRB axis has been shown to have a prominent role in the development of osteosarcoma stemness and aggressiveness at a pH of 6.5 [145], while in the latter case, the pH-dependent accumulation of S1P seems to be of paramount importance in the survival and growth potential of osteosarcoma xenografts [82].

5.1. Hampering Proton Extruders/Ion Transporters

Several drugs have been developed to target ion extruders/transporters as anticancer therapy. Inhibitors of the V-ATPase and CAIX have been the most explored for treating sarcomas. Studies considering these two approaches are listed in Tables 1 and 2.

To specifically target the V-ATPase, siRNA or Bafilomycin have been taken into account; nonetheless, their use can be hardly translated to the clinic for their instability or high toxicity, respectively. On the contrary, the use of proton pump inhibitors (PPIs), such as omeprazole or esomeprazole, has been extensively investigated. PPIs are acid-activated pro-drugs that reduce gastric acid production by inhibiting the H^+/K^+-ATPase pump and have been successfully used for the treatment of peptic disease [146]. Intriguingly, when used at high concentrations, PPIs can also effectively inhibit the activity of V-ATPase [147,148]. In preclinical models of bone sarcomas, although tumour growth was unaffected, treatment with a high concentration of PPI significantly increases the sensitivity to doxorubicin [16,37,95] Finally, in a multicentre trial on human patients, pretreatment with omeprazole increased the local cytotoxicity of standard chemotherapy, as expressed by the increased percentage of tumour necrosis. This was particularly evident in chondroblastic osteosarcoma, an histological subtype that normally shows poor histological response [149].

CAIX targeting has shown successful results with the use of sulphonamide-derived inhibitors. Among them, a compound obtained starting from benzenesulphonamide derivatives (covered by patent) has been successfully used to inhibit tumour growth in a xenograft model of osteosarcoma. Although not well investigated yet, the use of this compound is quite promising, since, among the different CA isoforms, CAIX appears to be highly and selectively expressed in cancer cells, concomitantly implying less toxicity and an increased selective anticancer effect [40]. In a recent paper, Tauro et al. have developed a dual CA/matrix metalloproteinase inhibitor incorporating a bisphosphonic acid, which increases selective anticancer targeting [150]; this drug possibly and directly targets tumour-induced osteolysis by combining a cargo molecule of bisphosphonate that delivers a blocker of MMP-mediated invasion and an inhibitor of CAIX-mediated acidification to the site of osteolysis.

Regarding the use of MCT1 and NHEs inhibitors for the treatment of bone cancers, very few in vitro data have been reported (see Tables 3 and 4), with the exception of the use of [alpha]-Cyano-4-hydroxycinnamate (CHC) that, in an orthotopic model of osteosarcoma, strongly impaired both chemoresistance and tumour growth [46].

5.2. Targeting of Cancer Cell Lysosomes by Photodynamic Therapy

Photodynamic therapy (PDT) is defined as the photo-induced irreversible destruction of abnormal cells and is based on the uptake of a photosensitiser molecule which, upon being excited by visible or near-infrared light, reacts with oxygen and generates reactive oxygen species (ROS) in target tissues, leading to cell death. PDT is therefore a minimally invasive anticancer modality with low-power light energy. ROS comprise singlet oxygen, superoxide anion, and radicals that generate from the conversion of molecular oxygen that reacts with the triplet state of the photosensitiser that is formed via photoexcitation. The generated free ROS oxidise biological substances, including nucleic acids, lipids, and proteins, leading to severe alterations in cell signalling cascades or in gene expression regulation and to activation of death-promoting physiological responses.

As discussed in Section 2.2, to avoid intracellular acidification, the excess of protons in the cytosol of tumour cells may be pumped into the lumen of the lysosomes, thereby decreasing the intra-organelle pH [16,151,152]. Acridine orange is a fluorescent cationic dye originally known as a detector of bacteria and parasites and an antimalarial drug. More recently, it has been described as an anticancer agent [153]. Since it has a low molecular weight, acridine orange easily diffuses into interstitial tissues and the cytoplasm and, due to protonation, accumulates into intracellular acid vesicles, leading to the formation of membrane-impermeable monomeric, dimeric, or oligomeric aggregates [16,151,152]. Acridine orange has thus a strong and selective tropism for tumour cells, as tumour cells have more acidic vesicles than normal cells because of their specific ability to effectively reduce the excess of protons in the cytoplasm by active transport across the plasma membrane and storage within the lysosomal compartment [154]. Furthermore, when photo-activated by blue light (466.5 nm) [155], or exposed to low-dose (1–5 Gy) X-ray irradiation [156], it generates singlet oxygen (1O2) thereby acting as an acid-targeting photosensitiser. The formed reactive species oxidise the fatty acids of the lysosomal membrane, causing the leakage of lysosomal enzymes and protons, followed by cell death [157].

To date, several data have demonstrated that acridine orange exerts selective cytocidal effects on tumour cells, showing no toxicity on normal cells. Furthermore, in the last 20 years, a combined technique of PDT and radioactivation (RDT) of acridine orange has been successfully developed and applied to clinical cases, demonstrating excellent outcomes in terms of inhibition of local recurrence and preservation of limb function after intra- or marginal tumour resection. These studies include humans affected by bone sarcomas, although the same type of approach has been tested in companion animals with spontaneous fibrosarcoma [158–162]. Specifically, following marginal or even intralesional gross removal of the tumour, it was possible to selectively target residual sarcoma and spare the surrounding normal tissues, with a satisfactory functional result. The procedure is safe without local or systemic complications. This technique proved to be particularly advantageous in sarcomas arising around the forearm and a valid alternative to wide surgical resection followed by limb reconstruction, without increasing the local recurrence rate [163]. Systemic administration of acridine orange with low-dose radiation therapy is also under evaluation for nonresectable bone sarcomas. The procedure appears to be safe and preliminary results are encouraging.

Talaporfin, also known as aspartyl chlorin, mono-L-aspartyl chlorin e6, NPe6, or LS11, is another photosensitiser that can target lysosomes and has been proposed for the treatment of bone sarcoma in addition to acridine orange [164–166]. Talaporfirin is uptaken by sarcoma cells through a KRAS-dependent endocytotic process. However, the correlation between its selective targeting and the degree of lysosomal acidification has not been unveiled yet.

6. Conclusions

After over 10 years of research, the crucial role of acidosis in bone sarcoma growth and progression has been clearly established. However, the development of acid-targeted drugs for the treatment of bone sarcomas is still in its infancy. To date, most of the drugs targeting ion/proton extruders and transporters have failed to be translated to clinical trials. One possible explanation is the redundancy of cellular systems controlling pHe. Thus, their targeting is quite challenging: it can easily turn to be ineffective, or when it works, extremely toxic. Nevertheless, given the relevance of intratumoural acidosis in bone cancers, the use of CAIX inhibitors, acid-targeted PDT strategies, or novel drugs that can safely and selectively impair the protumourigenic pathways that are selectively induced by extracellular acidosis may hold, for the future, helpful results to improve patient survival.

Author Contributions: Conceptualisation and writing—original draft preparation, S.A.; writing—review and editing, G.D.P., M.C., N.B. and S.A.; funding acquisition, N.B. All authors have read and agreed to the published version of the manuscript.

Funding: Funded by AIRC under IG 2018, grant number 21403 (to. N.B.), and by the financial support for Scientific Research 5xMille (to N.B.).

Conflicts of Interest: The authors declare no conflict of interest.

References

1. Stiller, C.A.; Trama, A.; Serraino, D.; Rossi, S.; Navarro, C.; Chirlaque, M.D.; Casali, P.G.; The Rare Care Working Group. Descriptive epidemiology of sarcomas in Europe: Report from the RARE CARE project. *Eur. J. Cancer* **2013**, *49*, 684–695. [CrossRef]
2. Whelan, J.; McTiernan, A.; Cooper, N.; Wong, Y.K.; Francis, M.; Vernon, S.; Strauss, S.J. Incidence and survival of malignant bone sarcomas in England 1979–2007. *Int. J. Cancer* **2012**, *131*, E508–E517. [CrossRef]
3. Valery, P.C.; Laversanne, M.; Bray, F. Bone cancer incidence by morphological subtype: A global assessment. *Cancer Causes Control* **2015**, *26*, 1127–1139. [CrossRef] [PubMed]
4. Brown, H.K.; Schiavone, K.; Gouin, F.; Heymann, M.F.; Heymann, D. Biology of bone sarcomas and new therapeutic developments. *Calcif. Tissue Int.* **2018**, *102*, 174–195. [CrossRef]
5. Heymann, M.F.; Brown, H.K.; Heymann, D. Drugs in early clinical development for the treatment of osteosarcoma. *Expert Opin. Investig. Drugs* **2016**, *25*, 1265–1280. [CrossRef]
6. Redini, F.; Odri, G.A.; Picarda, G.; Gaspar, N.; Heymann, M.F.; Corradini, N.; Heymann, D. Drugs targeting the bone microenvironment: New therapeutic tools in Ewing's sarcoma? *Expert Opin. Emerg. Drugs* **2013**, *18*, 339–352. [CrossRef] [PubMed]
7. Grunewald, T.G.; Alonso, M.; Avnet, S.; Banito, A.; Burdach, S.; Cidre-Aranaz, F.; Di Pompo, G.; Distel, M.; Dorado-Garcia, H.; Garcia-Castro, J.; et al. Sarcoma treatment in the era of molecular medicine. *EMBO Mol. Med.* **2020**, *12*, e11131. [CrossRef] [PubMed]

8. Pillai, S.R.; Damaghi, M.; Marunaka, Y.; Spugnini, E.P.; Fais, S.; Gillies, R.J. Causes, consequences and therapy of tumors acidosis. *Cancer Metastasis Rev.* **2019**, *38*, 205–222. [CrossRef]
9. Ouyang, Y.; Li, H.; Bu, J.; Li, X.; Chen, Z.; Xiao, T. Hypoxia-inducible factor-1 expression predicts osteosarcoma patients' survival: A meta-analysis. *Int. J. Biol. Markers* **2016**, *31*, e229–e234. [CrossRef]
10. Yang, C.; Tian, Y.; Zhao, F.; Chen, Z.; Su, P.; Li, Y.; Qian, A. Bone microenvironment and osteosarcoma metastasis. *Int. J. Mol. Sci.* **2020**, *21*, 6985. [CrossRef]
11. Hiraga, T. Hypoxic microenvironment and metastatic bone disease. *Int. J. Mol. Sci.* **2018**, *19*, 3523. [CrossRef] [PubMed]
12. Kolosenko, I.; Avnet, S.; Baldini, N.; Viklund, J.; De Milito, A. Therapeutic implications of tumor interstitial acidification. *Semin. Cancer Biol.* **2017**, *43*, 119–133. [CrossRef] [PubMed]
13. Spugnini, E.P.; Sonveaux, P.; Stock, C.; Perez-Sayans, M.; De Milito, A.; Avnet, S.; Garcia, A.G.; Harguindey, S.; Fais, S. Proton channels and exchangers in cancer. *Biochim. Biophys. Acta* **2015**, *1848*, 2715–2726. [CrossRef]
14. Viklund, J.; Avnet, S.; De Milito, A. Pathobiology and therapeutic implications of tumor acidosis. *Curr. Med. Chem.* **2017**, *24*, 2827–2845. [CrossRef]
15. Engin, K.; Leeper, D.B.; Cater, J.R.; Thistlethwaite, A.J.; Tupchong, L.; McFarlane, J.D. Extracellular pH distribution in human tumours. *Int. J. Hyperth.* **1995**, *11*, 211–216. [CrossRef] [PubMed]
16. Avnet, S.; Di Pompo, G.; Lemma, S.; Salerno, M.; Perut, F.; Bonuccelli, G.; Granchi, D.; Zini, N.; Baldini, N. V-ATPase is a candidate therapeutic target for Ewing sarcoma. *Biochim. Biophys. Acta* **2013**, *1832*, 1105–1116. [CrossRef]
17. Tiedemann, K.; Hussein, O.; Komarova, S.V. Role of altered metabolic microenvironment in osteolytic metastasis. *Front. Cell Dev. Biol.* **2020**, *8*, 435. [CrossRef] [PubMed]
18. Lemma, S.; Di Pompo, G.; Porporato, P.E.; Sboarina, M.; Russell, S.; Gillies, R.J.; Baldini, N.; Sonveaux, P.; Avnet, S. MDA-MB-231 breast cancer cells fuel osteoclast metabolism and activity: A new rationale for the pathogenesis of osteolytic bone metastases. *Biochim. Biophys. Acta Mol. Basis Dis.* **2017**, *1863*, 3254–3264. [CrossRef] [PubMed]
19. Li, Y.J.; Dai, Y.L.; Cheng, Y.S.; Zhang, W.B.; Tu, C.Q. Positron emission tomography (18)F-fluorodeoxyglucose uptake and prognosis in patients with bone and soft tissue sarcoma: A meta-analysis. *Eur. J. Surg. Oncol.* **2016**, *42*, 1103–1114. [CrossRef]
20. Warburg, O.; Wind, F.; Negelein, E. The metabolism of tumors in the body. *J. Gen. Physiol.* **1927**, *8*, 519–530. [CrossRef]
21. Warburg, O. On the origin of cancer cells. *Science* **1956**, *123*, 309–314. [CrossRef] [PubMed]
22. Hannah, S.S.; McFadden, S.; McNeilly, A.; McClean, C. "Take My Bone Away?" hypoxia and bone: A narrative review. *J. Cell Physiol.* **2021**, *236*, 721–740. [CrossRef]
23. Spencer, J.A.; Ferraro, F.; Roussakis, E.; Klein, A.; Wu, J.; Runnels, J.M.; Zaher, W.; Mortensen, L.J.; Alt, C.; Turcotte, R.; et al. Direct measurement of local oxygen concentration in the bone marrow of live animals. *Nature* **2014**, *508*, 269–273. [CrossRef] [PubMed]
24. Hayashi, Y.; Yokota, A.; Harada, H.; Huang, G. Hypoxia/pseudohypoxia-mediated activation of hypoxia-inducible factor-1alpha in cancer. *Cancer Sci.* **2019**, *110*, 1510–1517. [CrossRef]
25. Longo, D.L.; Bartoli, A.; Consolino, L.; Bardini, P.; Arena, F.; Schwaiger, M.; Aime, S. In vivo imaging of tumor metabolism and acidosis by combining PET and MRI-CEST pH imaging. *Cancer Res.* **2016**, *76*, 6463–6470. [CrossRef]
26. Eary, J.F.; Conrad, E.U.; Bruckner, J.D.; Folpe, A.; Hunt, K.J.; Mankoff, D.A.; Howlett, A.T. Quantitative [F-18] fluorodeoxyglucose positron emission tomography in pretreatment and grading of sarcoma. *Clin. Cancer Res.* **1998**, *4*, 1215–1220.
27. Sigal, I.R.; Sebro, R. Preclinical PET tracers for the evaluation of sarcomas: Understanding tumor biology. *Am. J. Nucl. Med. Mol. Imaging* **2018**, *8*, 428–440.
28. Corbet, C.; Feron, O. Tumour acidosis: From the passenger to the driver's seat. *Nat. Rev. Cancer* **2017**, *17*, 577–593. [CrossRef] [PubMed]
29. Vaupel, P.; Multhoff, G. Revisiting the Warburg effect: Historical dogma versus current understanding. *J. Physiol.* **2021**, *599*, 1745–1757. [CrossRef]
30. Van Uden, P.; Kenneth, N.S.; Webster, R.; Muller, H.A.; Mudie, S.; Rocha, S. Evolutionary conserved regulation of HIF-1β by NF-kB. *PLoS Genet.* **2011**, *7*, e1001285. [CrossRef]
31. Van Uden, P.; Kenneth, N.S.; Rocha, S. Regulation of hypoxia-inducible factor-1alpha by NF-kappaB. *Biochem. J.* **2008**, *412*, 477–484. [CrossRef] [PubMed]
32. Avnet, S.; Di Pompo, G.; Chano, T.; Errani, C.; Ibrahim-Hashim, A.; Gillies, R.J.; Donati, D.M.; Baldini, N. Cancer-associated mesenchymal stroma fosters the stemness of osteosarcoma cells in response to intratumoral acidosis via NF-kB activation. *Int. J. Cancer* **2017**, *140*, 1331–1345. [CrossRef] [PubMed]
33. Lagadic-Gossmann, D.; Huc, L.; Lecureur, V. Alterations of intracellular pH homeostasis in apoptosis: Origins and roles. *Cell Death Differ.* **2004**, *11*, 953–961. [CrossRef]
34. Perut, F.; Avnet, S.; Fotia, C.; Baglio, S.R.; Salerno, M.; Hosogi, S.; Kusuzaki, K.; Baldini, N. V-ATPase as an effective therapeutic target for sarcomas. *Exp. Cell Res.* **2014**, *320*, 21–32. [CrossRef] [PubMed]
35. Salerno, M.; Avnet, S.; Bonuccelli, G.; Hosogi, S.; Granchi, D.; Baldini, N. Impairment of lysosomal activity as a therapeutic modality targeting cancer stem cells of embryonal rhabdomyosarcoma cell line RD. *PLoS ONE* **2014**, *9*, e110340. [CrossRef] [PubMed]
36. Mboge, M.Y.; Mahon, B.P.; McKenna, R.; Frost, S.C. Carbonic anhydrases: Role in pH control and cancer. *Metabolites* **2018**, *8*, 19. [CrossRef]

37. Avnet, S.; Lemma, S.; Cortini, M.; Pellegrini, P.; Perut, F.; Zini, N.; Kusuzaki, K.; Chano, T.; Grisendi, G.; Dominici, M.; et al. Altered pH gradient at the plasma membrane of osteosarcoma cells is a key mechanism of drug resistance. *Oncotarget* **2016**, *7*, 63408–63423. [CrossRef]
38. Balza, E.; Castellani, P.; Moreno, P.S.; Piccioli, P.; Medrano-Fernandez, I.; Semino, C.; Rubartelli, A. Restoring microenvironmental redox and pH homeostasis inhibits neoplastic cell growth and migration: Therapeutic efficacy of esomeprazole plus sulfasalazine on 3-MCA-induced sarcoma. *Oncotarget* **2017**, *8*, 67482–67496. [CrossRef]
39. Jin, Z.; Aixi, Y.; Baiwen, Q.; Zonghuan, L.; Xiang, H. Inhibition of hypoxia-inducible factor-1 alpha radiosensitized MG-63 human osteosarcoma cells in vitro. *Tumori* **2015**, *101*, 578–584. [CrossRef]
40. Perut, F.; Carta, F.; Bonuccelli, G.; Grisendi, G.; Di Pompo, G.; Avnet, S.; Sbrana, F.V.; Hosogi, S.; Dominici, M.; Kusuzaki, K.; et al. Carbonic anhydrase IX inhibition is an effective strategy for osteosarcoma treatment. *Expert Opin. Ther. Targets* **2015**, *19*, 1593–1605. [CrossRef]
41. Zhang, D.; Cui, G.; Sun, C.; Lei, L.; Lei, L.; Williamson, R.A.; Wang, Y.; Zhang, J.; Chen, P.; Wang, A.; et al. Hypoxia promotes osteosarcoma cell proliferation and migration through enhancing platelet-derived growth factor-BB/platelet-derived growth factor receptor-beta axis. *Biochem. Biophys. Res. Commun.* **2019**, *512*, 360–366. [CrossRef]
42. Wang, T.K.; Lin, Y.M.; Lo, C.M.; Tang, C.H.; Teng, C.L.; Chao, W.T.; Wu, M.H.; Liu, C.S.; Hsieh, M. Oncogenic roles of carbonic anhydrase 8 in human osteosarcoma cells. *Tumor Biol.* **2016**, *37*, 7989–8005. [CrossRef] [PubMed]
43. Staab, A.; Loeffler, J.; Said, H.M.; Diehlmann, D.; Katzer, A.; Beyer, M.; Fleischer, M.; Schwab, F.; Baier, K.; Einsele, H.; et al. Effects of HIF-1 inhibition by chetomin on hypoxia-related transcription and radiosensitivity in HT 1080 human fibrosarcoma cells. *BMC Cancer* **2007**, *7*, 213. [CrossRef] [PubMed]
44. Yasuda, Y.; Arakawa, T.; Nawata, Y.; Shimada, S.; Oishi, S.; Fujii, N.; Nishimura, S.; Hattori, A.; Kakeya, H. Design, synthesis, and structure-activity relationships of 1-ethylpyrazole-3-carboxamide compounds as novel hypoxia-inducible factor (HIF)-1 inhibitors. *Bioorg. Med. Chem.* **2015**, *23*, 1776–1787. [CrossRef]
45. Boeuf, S.; Bovee, J.V.; Lehner, B.; Hogendoorn, P.C.; Richter, W. Correlation of hypoxic signalling to histological grade and outcome in cartilage tumours. *Histopathology* **2010**, *56*, 641–651. [CrossRef]
46. Zhao, Z.; Wu, M.S.; Zou, C.; Tang, Q.; Lu, J.; Liu, D.; Wu, Y.; Yin, J.; Xie, X.; Shen, J.; et al. Downregulation of MCT1 inhibits tumor growth, metastasis and enhances chemotherapeutic efficacy in osteosarcoma through regulation of the NF-kappaB pathway. *Cancer Lett.* **2014**, *342*, 150–158. [CrossRef] [PubMed]
47. Bonuccelli, G.; Avnet, S.; Grisendi, G.; Salerno, M.; Granchi, D.; Dominici, M.; Kusuzaki, K.; Baldini, N. Role of mesenchymal stem cells in osteosarcoma and metabolic reprogramming of tumor cells. *Oncotarget* **2014**, *5*, 7575–7588. [CrossRef]
48. Liu, Y.; Sun, X.; Huo, C.; Sun, C.; Zhu, J. Monocarboxylate transporter 4 (MCT4) overexpression is correlated with poor prognosis of osteosarcoma. *Med. Sci. Monit.* **2019**, *25*, 4278–4284. [CrossRef] [PubMed]
49. Mazhab-Jafari, M.T.; Rohou, A.; Schmidt, C.; Bueler, S.A.; Benlekbir, S.; Robinson, C.V.; Rubinstein, J.L. Atomic model for the membrane-embedded VO motor of a eukaryotic V-ATPase. *Nature* **2016**, *539*, 118–122. [CrossRef]
50. Avnet, S.; Di Pompo, G.; Lemma, S.; Baldini, N. Cause and effect of microenvironmental acidosis on bone metastases. *Cancer Metastasis Rev.* **2019**, *38*, 133–147. [CrossRef]
51. Nocentini, A.; Donald, W.A.; Supuran, C.T. Chapter 8—Human carbonic anhydrases: Tissue distribution, physiological role, and druggability. In *Carbonic Anhydrases*; Supuran, C.T., Nocentini, A., Eds.; Academic Press: Cambridge, MA, USA, 2019; pp. 151–185, ISBN 978-0-12-816476-1.
52. Supuran, C.T. Carbonic anhydrases as drug targets—An overview. *Curr. Top. Med. Chem.* **2007**, *7*, 825–833. [CrossRef]
53. Meszaros, B.; Papp, F.; Mocsar, G.; Kokai, E.; Kovacs, K.; Tajti, G.; Panyi, G. The voltage-gated proton channel hHv1 is functionally expressed in human chorion-derived mesenchymal stem cells. *Sci. Rep.* **2020**, *10*, 7100. [CrossRef] [PubMed]
54. Wang, Y.; Li, S.J.; Pan, J.; Che, Y.; Yin, J.; Zhao, Q. Specific expression of the human voltage-gated proton channel Hv1 in highly metastatic breast cancer cells, promotes tumor progression and metastasis. *Biochem. Biophys. Res. Commun.* **2011**, *412*, 353–359. [CrossRef] [PubMed]
55. Wang, Y.; Wu, X.; Li, Q.; Zhang, S.; Li, S.J. Human voltage-gated proton channel hv1: A new potential biomarker for diagnosis and prognosis of colorectal cancer. *PLoS ONE* **2013**, *8*, e70550. [CrossRef] [PubMed]
56. Di Pompo, G.; Errani, C.; Gillies, R.; Mercatali, L.; Ibrahim, T.; Tamanti, J.; Baldini, N.; Avnet, S. Acid-Induced Inflammatory Cytokines in Osteoblasts: A Guided Path to Osteolysis in Bone Metastasis. *Front. Cell Dev. Biol.* **2021**, *9*, 678532. [CrossRef] [PubMed]
57. McConnell, M.; Feng, S.; Chen, W.; Zhu, G.; Shen, D.; Ponnazhagan, S.; Deng, L.; Li, Y.P. Osteoclast proton pump regulator Atp6v1c1 enhances breast cancer growth by activating the mTORC1 pathway and bone metastasis by increasing V-ATPase activity. *Oncotarget* **2017**, *8*, 47675–47690. [CrossRef]
58. Di Pompo, G.; Lemma, S.; Canti, L.; Rucci, N.; Ponzetti, M.; Errani, C.; Donati, D.M.; Russell, S.; Gillies, R.; Chano, T.; et al. Intratumoral acidosis fosters cancer-induced bone pain through the activation of the mesenchymal tumor-associated stroma in bone metastasis from breast carcinoma. *Oncotarget* **2017**, *8*, 54478–54496. [CrossRef] [PubMed]
59. Dougall, W.C. Molecular pathways: Osteoclast-dependent and osteoclast-independent roles of the RANKL/RANK/OPG pathway in tumorigenesis and metastasis. *Clin. Cancer Res.* **2012**, *18*, 326–335. [CrossRef]
60. Teitelbaum, S.L. Bone resorption by osteoclasts. *Science* **2000**, *289*, 1504–1508. [CrossRef] [PubMed]

61. Blair, H.C.; Teitelbaum, S.L.; Ghiselli, R.; Gluck, S. Osteoclastic bone resorption by a polarized vacuolar proton pump. *Science* **1989**, *245*, 855–857. [CrossRef]
62. Lemma, S.; Sboarina, M.; Porporato, P.E.; Zini, N.; Sonveaux, P.; Di Pompo, G.; Baldini, N.; Avnet, S. Energy metabolism in osteoclast formation and activity. *Int. J. Biochem. Cell Biol.* **2016**, *79*, 168–180. [CrossRef] [PubMed]
63. Qin, A.; Cheng, T.S.; Pavlos, N.J.; Lin, Z.; Dai, K.R.; Zheng, M.H. V-ATPases in osteoclasts: Structure, function and potential inhibitors of bone resorption. *Int. J. Biochem. Cell Biol.* **2012**, *44*, 1422–1435. [CrossRef] [PubMed]
64. Blair, H.C.; Schlesinger, P.H.; Ross, F.P.; Teitelbaum, S.L. Recent advances toward understanding osteoclast physiology. *Clin. Orthop. Relat. Res.* **1993**, *294*, 7–22. [CrossRef]
65. Nordstrom, T.; Rotstein, O.D.; Romanek, R.; Asotra, S.; Heersche, J.N.; Manolson, M.F.; Brisseau, G.F.; Grinstein, S. Regulation of cytoplasmic pH in osteoclasts. Contribution of proton pumps and a proton-selective conductance. *J. Biol. Chem.* **1995**, *270*, 2203–2212. [CrossRef] [PubMed]
66. Li, G.; Miura, K.; Kuno, M. Extracellular phosphates enhance activities of voltage-gated proton channels and production of reactive oxygen species in murine osteoclast-like cells. *Pflugers Arch. Eur. J. Physiol.* **2017**, *469*, 279–292. [CrossRef]
67. Kuno, M.; Li, G.; Moriura, Y.; Hino, Y.; Kawawaki, J.; Sakai, H. Acid-inducible proton influx currents in the plasma membrane of murine osteoclast-like cells. *Pflugers Arch. Eur. J. Physiol.* **2016**, *468*, 837–847. [CrossRef]
68. Stoch, S.A.; Wagner, J.A. Cathepsin K inhibitors: A novel target for osteoporosis therapy. *Clin. Pharmacol. Ther.* **2008**, *83*, 172–176. [CrossRef]
69. Levallois, P.; Gauvin, D. Management in the context of incomplete evidence. *Can. J. Public Health* **1995**, *86*, 169.
70. Zeng, W.; Wan, R.; Zheng, Y.; Singh, S.R.; Wei, Y. Hypoxia, stem cells and bone tumor. *Cancer Lett.* **2011**, *313*, 129–136. [CrossRef]
71. Avnet, S.; Longhi, A.; Salerno, M.; Halleen, J.M.; Perut, F.; Granchi, D.; Ferrari, S.; Bertoni, F.; Giunti, A.; Baldini, N. Increased osteoclast activity is associated with aggressiveness of osteosarcoma. *Int. J. Oncol.* **2008**, *33*, 1231–1238. [CrossRef] [PubMed]
72. Miyamoto, N.; Higuchi, Y.; Mori, K.; Ito, M.; Tsurudome, M.; Nishio, M.; Yamada, H.; Sudo, A.; Kato, K.; Uchida, A.; et al. Human osteosarcoma-derived cell lines produce soluble factor(s) that induces differentiation of blood monocytes to osteoclast-like cells. *Int. Immunopharmacol.* **2002**, *2*, 25–38. [CrossRef]
73. Sano, H.; Kikuta, J.; Furuya, M.; Kondo, N.; Endo, N.; Ishii, M. Intravital bone imaging by two-photon excitation microscopy to identify osteocytic osteolysis in vivo. *Bone* **2015**, *74*, 134–139. [CrossRef]
74. Jahn, K.; Kelkar, S.; Zhao, H.; Xie, Y.; Tiede-Lewis, L.M.; Dusevich, V.; Dallas, S.L.; Bonewald, L.F. Osteocytes acidify their microenvironment in response to PTHrP in vitro and in lactating mice in vivo. *J. Bone Miner. Res.* **2017**, *32*, 1761–1772. [CrossRef]
75. Yee, C.S.; Schurman, C.A.; White, C.R.; Alliston, T. Investigating osteocytic perilacunar/canalicular remodeling. *Curr. Osteoporos. Rep.* **2019**, *17*, 157–168. [CrossRef]
76. Petho, Z.; Najder, K.; Carvalho, T.; McMorrow, R.; Todesca, L.M.; Rugi, M.; Bulk, E.; Chan, A.; Lowik, C.; Reshkin, S.J.; et al. pH-Channeling in cancer: How ph-dependence of cation channels shapes cancer pathophysiology. *Cancers* **2020**, *12*, 2484. [CrossRef]
77. Doroszewicz, J.; Waldegger, P.; Jeck, N.; Seyberth, H.; Waldegger, S. pH dependence of extracellular calcium sensing receptor activity determined by a novel technique. *Kidney Int.* **2005**, *67*, 187–192. [CrossRef]
78. Yang, Z.; Yue, Z.; Ma, X.; Xu, Z. Calcium Homeostasis: A potential vicious cycle of bone metastasis in breast cancers. *Front. Oncol.* **2020**, *10*, 293. [CrossRef] [PubMed]
79. Yamaguchi, T.; Chattopadhyay, N.; Kifor, O.; Ye, C.; Vassilev, P.M.; Sanders, J.L.; Brown, E.M. Expression of extracellular calcium-sensing receptor in human osteoblastic MG-63 cell line. *Am. J. Physiol. Cell Physiol.* **2001**, *280*, C382–C393. [CrossRef] [PubMed]
80. Kajiya, H. Calcium signaling in osteoclast differentiation and bone resorption. *Adv. Exp. Med. Biol.* **2012**, *740*, 917–932. [CrossRef]
81. Stewart, T.A.; Yapa, K.T.; Monteith, G.R. Altered calcium signaling in cancer cells. *Biochim. Biophys. Acta* **2015**, *1848*, 2502–2511. [CrossRef] [PubMed]
82. Cortini, M.; Armirotti, A.; Columbaro, M.; Longo, D.L.; Di Pompo, G.; Cannas, E.; Maresca, A.; Errani, C.; Longhi, A.; Righi, A.; et al. Exploring metabolic adaptations to the acidic microenvironment of osteosarcoma cells unveils sphingosine 1-phosphate as a valuable therapeutic target. *Cancers* **2021**, *13*, 311. [CrossRef] [PubMed]
83. Holzer, P. Acid-sensitive ion channels and receptors. In *Sensory Nerves*; Springer: New York, NY, USA, 2009; pp. 283–332, ISBN 978-3-540-79090-7.
84. Prevarskaya, N.; Skryma, R.; Shuba, Y. Ion channels and the hallmarks of cancer. *Trends Mol. Med.* **2010**, *16*, 107–121. [CrossRef]
85. Prevarskaya, N.; Skryma, R.; Shuba, Y. Ion Channels in cancer: Are cancer hallmarks oncochannelopathies? *Physiol. Rev.* **2018**, *98*, 559–621. [CrossRef] [PubMed]
86. Litan, A.; Langhans, S.A. Cancer as a channelopathy: Ion channels and pumps in tumor development and progression. *Front. Cell Neurosci.* **2015**, *9*, 86. [CrossRef]
87. Andersen, A.P.; Moreira, J.M.; Pedersen, S.F. Interactions of ion transporters and channels with cancer cell metabolism and the tumour microenvironment. *Philos. Trans. R. Soc. B Biol. Sci.* **2014**, *369*, 20130098. [CrossRef] [PubMed]
88. Wu, J.; Zhong, D.; Wu, X.; Sha, M.; Kang, L.; Ding, Z. Voltage-gated potassium channel Kv1.3 is highly expressed in human osteosarcoma and promotes osteosarcoma growth. *Int. J. Mol. Sci.* **2013**, *14*, 19245–19256. [CrossRef]
89. Zhao, W.; Xu, H. High expression of TRPM8 predicts poor prognosis in patients with osteosarcoma. *Oncol. Lett.* **2016**, *12*, 1373–1379. [CrossRef] [PubMed]

90. Jiang, L.; Zhao, Y.D.; Chen, W.X. The function of the novel mechanical activated ion channel piezo1 in the human osteosarcoma cells. *Med. Sci. Monit.* **2017**, *23*, 5070–5082. [CrossRef]
91. Teisseyre, A.; Mozrzymas, J.W. The influence of protons and zinc ions on the steady-state inactivation of Kv1.3 potassium channels. *Cell. Mol. Biol. Lett.* **2007**, *12*, 220–230. [CrossRef] [PubMed]
92. Behrendt, H.J.; Germann, T.; Gillen, C.; Hatt, H.; Jostock, R. Characterization of the mouse cold-menthol receptor TRPM8 and vanilloid receptor type-1 VR1 using a fluorometric imaging plate reader (FLIPR) assay. *Br. J. Pharmacol.* **2004**, *141*, 737–745. [CrossRef] [PubMed]
93. Bae, C.; Sachs, F.; Gottlieb, P.A. Protonation of the human PIEZO1 ion channel stabilizes inactivation. *J. Biol. Chem.* **2015**, *290*, 5167–5173. [CrossRef]
94. Ayala, I.; Baldassarre, M.; Giacchetti, G.; Caldieri, G.; Tete, S.; Luini, A.; Buccione, R. Multiple regulatory inputs converge on cortactin to control invadopodia biogenesis and extracellular matrix degradation. *J. Cell Sci.* **2008**, *121*, 369–378. [CrossRef] [PubMed]
95. Avnet, S.; Chano, T.; Massa, A.; Bonuccelli, G.; Lemma, S.; Falzetti, L.; Grisendi, G.; Dominici, M.; Baldini, N. Acid microenvironment promotes cell survival of human bone sarcoma through the activation of cIAP proteins and NF-kB pathway. *Am. J. Cancer Res.* **2019**, *9*, 1127–1144.
96. Chano, T.; Avnet, S.; Kusuzaki, K.; Bonuccelli, G.; Sonveaux, P.; Rotili, D.; Mai, A.; Baldini, N. Tumour-Specific metabolic adaptation to acidosis is coupled to epigenetic stability in osteosarcoma cells. *Am. J. Cancer Res.* **2016**, *6*, 859–875. [PubMed]
97. Raghunand, N.; Martinez-Zaguilan, R.; Wright, S.H.; Gillies, R.J. pH and drug resistance. II. Turnover of acidic vesicles and resistance to weakly basic chemotherapeutic drugs. *Biochem. Pharmacol.* **1999**, *57*, 1047–1058. [CrossRef]
98. Shi, Q.; Le, X.; Wang, B.; Abbruzzese, J.L.; Xiong, Q.; He, Y.; Xie, K. Regulation of vascular endothelial growth factor expression by acidosis in human cancer cells. *Oncogene* **2001**, *20*, 3751–3756. [CrossRef]
99. Mekhail, K.; Gunaratnam, L.; Bonicalzi, M.E.; Lee, S. HIF activation by pH-dependent nucleolar sequestration of VHL. *Nat. Cell Biol.* **2004**, *6*, 642–647. [CrossRef]
100. Nadtochiy, S.M.; Schafer, X.; Fu, D.; Nehrke, K.; Munger, J.; Brookes, P.S. Acidic pH Is a Metabolic Switch for 2-Hydroxyglutarate Generation and Signaling. *J. Biol. Chem.* **2016**, *291*, 20188–20197. [CrossRef]
101. Perut, F.; Roncuzzi, L.; Zini, N.; Massa, A.; Baldini, N. Extracellular nanovesicles secreted by human osteosarcoma cells promote angiogenesis. *Cancers* **2019**, *11*, 779. [CrossRef]
102. Barcellos-de-Souza, P.; Gori, V.; Bambi, F.; Chiarugi, P. Tumor microenvironment: Bone marrow-mesenchymal stem cells as key players. *Biochim. Biophys. Acta* **2013**, *1836*, 321–335. [CrossRef] [PubMed]
103. Bremnes, R.M.; Donnem, T.; Al-Saad, S.; Al-Shibli, K.; Andersen, S.; Sirera, R.; Camps, C.; Marinez, I.; Busund, L.T. The role of tumor stroma in cancer progression and prognosis: Emphasis on carcinoma-associated fibroblasts and non-small cell lung cancer. *J. Thorac. Oncol.* **2011**, *6*, 209–217. [CrossRef] [PubMed]
104. Xu, W.T.; Bian, Z.Y.; Fan, Q.M.; Li, G.; Tang, T.T. Human mesenchymal stem cells (hMSCs) target osteosarcoma and promote its growth and pulmonary metastasis. *Cancer Lett.* **2009**, *281*, 32–41. [CrossRef] [PubMed]
105. Perrot, P.; Rousseau, J.; Bouffaut, A.L.; Redini, F.; Cassagnau, E.; Deschaseaux, F.; Heymann, M.F.; Heymann, D.; Duteille, F.; Trichet, V.; et al. Safety concern between autologous fat graft, mesenchymal stem cell and osteosarcoma recurrence. *PLoS ONE* **2010**, *5*, e10999. [CrossRef] [PubMed]
106. Brandao-Burch, A.; Utting, J.C.; Orriss, I.R.; Arnett, T.R. Acidosis inhibits bone formation by osteoblasts in vitro by preventing mineralization. *Calcif. Tissue Int.* **2005**, *77*, 167–174. [CrossRef] [PubMed]
107. Massa, A.; Perut, F.; Chano, T.; Woloszyk, A.; Mitsiadis, T.A.; Avnet, S.; Baldini, N. The effect of extracellular acidosis on the behaviour of mesenchymal stem cells in vitro. *Eur. Cells Mater.* **2017**, *33*, 252–267. [CrossRef]
108. Granchi, D.; Torreggiani, E.; Massa, A.; Caudarella, R.; Di Pompo, G.; Baldini, N. Potassium citrate prevents increased osteoclastogenesis resulting from acidic conditions: Implication for the treatment of postmenopausal bone loss. *PLoS ONE* **2017**, *12*, e0181230. [CrossRef]
109. Arnett, T.R. Acidosis, hypoxia and bone. *Arch. Biochem. Biophys.* **2010**, *503*, 103–109. [CrossRef] [PubMed]
110. Shibutani, T.; Heersche, J.N. Effect of medium pH on osteoclast activity and osteoclast formation in cultures of dispersed rabbit osteoclasts. *J. Bone Miner. Res.* **1993**, *8*, 331–336. [CrossRef] [PubMed]
111. Yuan, F.L.; Xu, M.H.; Li, X.; Xinlong, H.; Fang, W.; Dong, J. The Roles of acidosis in osteoclast biology. *Front. Physiol.* **2016**, *7*, 222. [CrossRef] [PubMed]
112. Jahr, H.; van Driel, M.; van Osch, G.J.; Weinans, H.; van Leeuwen, J.P. Identification of acid-sensing ion channels in bone. *Biochem. Biophys. Res. Commun.* **2005**, *337*, 349–354. [CrossRef]
113. Ludwig, M.G.; Vanek, M.; Guerini, D.; Gasser, J.A.; Jones, C.E.; Junker, U.; Hofstetter, H.; Wolf, R.M.; Seuwen, K. Proton-Sensing G-protein-coupled receptors. *Nature* **2003**, *425*, 93–98. [CrossRef]
114. Tomura, H.; Wang, J.Q.; Liu, J.P.; Komachi, M.; Damirin, A.; Mogi, C.; Tobo, M.; Nochi, H.; Tamoto, K.; Im, D.S.; et al. Cyclooxygenase-2 expression and prostaglandin E2 production in response to acidic pH through OGR1 in a human osteoblastic cell line. *J. Bone Miner. Res.* **2008**, *23*, 1129–1139. [CrossRef]
115. Okito, A.; Nakahama, K.; Akiyama, M.; Ono, T.; Morita, I. Involvement of the G-protein-coupled receptor 4 in RANKL expression by osteoblasts in an acidic environment. *Biochem. Biophys. Res. Commun.* **2015**, *458*, 435–440. [CrossRef]

116. Lieben, L.; Carmeliet, G. The involvement of TRP channels in bone homeostasis. *Front. Endocrinol.* **2012**, *3*, 99. [CrossRef] [PubMed]
117. Kato, K.; Morita, I. Promotion of osteoclast differentiation and activation in spite of impeded osteoblast-lineage differentiation under acidosis: Effects of acidosis on bone metabolism. *Biosci. Trends* **2013**, *7*, 33–41. [CrossRef]
118. Tominaga, M.; Tominaga, T. Structure and function of TRPV1. *Pflugers Arch.* **2005**, *451*, 143–150. [CrossRef] [PubMed]
119. Sherwood, T.W.; Frey, E.N.; Askwith, C.C. Structure and activity of the acid-sensing ion channels. *Am. J. Physiol. Cell Physiol.* **2012**, *303*, C699–C710. [CrossRef]
120. Immke, D.C.; McCleskey, E.W. Protons open acid-sensing ion channels by catalyzing relief of Ca^{2+} blockade. *Neuron* **2003**, *37*, 75–84. [CrossRef]
121. Masuyama, R.; Vriens, J.; Voets, T.; Karashima, Y.; Owsianik, G.; Vennekens, R.; Lieben, L.; Torrekens, S.; Moermans, K.; Vanden Bosch, A.; et al. TRPV4-mediated calcium influx regulates terminal differentiation of osteoclasts. *Cell Metab.* **2008**, *8*, 257–265. [CrossRef] [PubMed]
122. Brassart-Pasco, S.; Brezillon, S.; Brassart, B.; Ramont, L.; Oudart, J.B.; Monboisse, J.C. Tumor microenvironment: Extracellular matrix alterations influence tumor progression. *Front. Oncol.* **2020**, *10*, 397. [CrossRef]
123. Kehlet, S.N.; Sanz-Pamplona, R.; Brix, S.; Leeming, D.J.; Karsdal, M.A.; Moreno, V. Excessive collagen turnover products are released during colorectal cancer progression and elevated in serum from metastatic colorectal cancer patients. *Sci. Rep.* **2016**, *6*, 30599. [CrossRef]
124. Kato, Y.; Nakayama, Y.; Umeda, M.; Miyazaki, K. Induction of 103-kDa gelatinase/type IV collagenase by acidic culture conditions in mouse metastatic melanoma cell lines. *J. Biol. Chem.* **1992**, *267*, 11424–11430. [CrossRef]
125. Swayampakula, M.; McDonald, P.C.; Vallejo, M.; Coyaud, E.; Chafe, S.C.; Westerback, A.; Venkateswaran, G.; Shankar, J.; Gao, G.; Laurent, E.M.N.; et al. The interactome of metabolic enzyme carbonic anhydrase IX reveals novel roles in tumor cell migration and invadopodia/MMP14-mediated invasion. *Oncogene* **2017**, *36*, 6244–6261. [CrossRef] [PubMed]
126. Li, X.; Wang, G.; Cai, Z.; Sun, W. Immunotherapeutic strategies for sarcoma: Current perspectives. *Am. J. Transl. Res.* **2020**, *12*, 7693–7701. [PubMed]
127. Dufresne, A.; Brahmi, M. Immunotherapy in sarcoma: Combinations or single agents? In whom? *Curr. Opin. Oncol.* **2020**, *32*, 339–343. [CrossRef]
128. Tawbi, H.A.; Burgess, M.; Bolejack, V.; Van Tine, B.A.; Schuetze, S.M.; Hu, J.; D'Angelo, S.; Attia, S.; Riedel, R.F.; Priebat, D.A.; et al. Pembrolizumab in advanced soft-tissue sarcoma and bone sarcoma (SARC028): A multicentre, two-cohort, single-arm, open-label, phase 2 trial. *Lancet Oncol.* **2017**, *18*, 1493–1501. [CrossRef]
129. Nathenson, M.J.; Conley, A.P.; Sausville, E. Immunotherapy: A new (and old) approach to treatment of soft tissue and bone sarcomas. *Oncologist* **2018**, *23*, 71–83. [CrossRef] [PubMed]
130. Draghiciu, O.; Nijman, H.W.; Daemen, T. From tumor immunosuppression to eradication: Targeting homing and activity of immune effector cells to tumors. *Clin. Dev. Immunol.* **2011**, *2011*, 439053. [CrossRef]
131. Pardoll, D.M. Immunology beats cancer: A blueprint for successful translation. *Nat. Immunol.* **2012**, *13*, 1129–1132. [CrossRef] [PubMed]
132. Kareva, I.; Hahnfeldt, P. The emerging "hallmarks" of metabolic reprogramming and immune evasion: Distinct or linked? *Cancer Res.* **2013**, *73*, 2737–2742. [CrossRef]
133. Lamonte, G.; Tang, X.; Chen, J.L.; Wu, J.; Ding, C.K.; Keenan, M.M.; Sangokoya, C.; Kung, H.N.; Ilkayeva, O.; Boros, L.G.; et al. Acidosis induces reprogramming of cellular metabolism to mitigate oxidative stress. *Cancer Metab.* **2013**, *1*, 23. [CrossRef] [PubMed]
134. Pilon-Thomas, S.; Kodumudi, K.N.; El-Kenawi, A.E.; Russell, S.; Weber, A.M.; Luddy, K.; Damaghi, M.; Wojtkowiak, J.W.; Mule, J.J.; Ibrahim-Hashim, A.; et al. Neutralization of tumor acidity improves antitumor responses to immunotherapy. *Cancer Res.* **2016**, *76*, 1381–1390. [CrossRef]
135. Husain, Z.; Huang, Y.; Seth, P.; Sukhatme, V.P. Tumor-derived lactate modifies antitumor immune response: Effect on myeloid-derived suppressor cells and NK cells. *J. Immunol.* **2013**, *191*, 1486–1495. [CrossRef]
136. Crowther, M.; Brown, N.J.; Bishop, E.T.; Lewis, C.E. Microenvironmental influence on macrophage regulation of angiogenesis in wounds and malignant tumors. *J. Leukoc. Biol.* **2001**, *70*, 478–490. [PubMed]
137. Trevani, A.S.; Andonegui, G.; Giordano, M.; Lopez, D.H.; Gamberale, R.; Minucci, F.; Geffner, J.R. Extracellular acidification induces human neutrophil activation. *J. Immunol.* **1999**, *162*, 4849–4857. [PubMed]
138. Martinez, D.; Vermeulen, M.; Trevani, A.; Ceballos, A.; Sabatte, J.; Gamberale, R.; Alvarez, M.E.; Salamone, G.; Tanos, T.; Coso, O.A.; et al. Extracellular acidosis induces neutrophil activation by a mechanism dependent on activation of phosphatidylinositol 3-kinase/Akt and ERK pathways. *J. Immunol.* **2006**, *176*, 1163–1171. [CrossRef] [PubMed]
139. Vermeulen, M.; Giordano, M.; Trevani, A.S.; Sedlik, C.; Gamberale, R.; Fernandez-Calotti, P.; Salamone, G.; Raiden, S.; Sanjurjo, J.; Geffner, J.R. Acidosis improves uptake of antigens and MHC class I-restricted presentation by dendritic cells. *J. Immunol.* **2004**, *172*, 3196–3204. [CrossRef]
140. Lemma, S.; Avnet, S.; Meade, M.J.; Chano, T.; Baldini, N. Validation of suitable housekeeping genes for the normalization of mRNA expression for studying tumor acidosis. *Int. J. Mol. Sci.* **2018**, *19*, 2930. [CrossRef] [PubMed]
141. Shinoda, H.; Shannon, M.; Nagai, T. Fluorescent proteins for investigating biological events in acidic environments. *Int. J. Mol. Sci.* **2018**, *19*, 1548. [CrossRef]

142. Ong, T.T.; Ang, Z.; Verma, R.; Koean, R.; Tam, J.K.C.; Ding, J.L. phLuc, a ratiometric luminescent reporter for in vivo monitoring of tumor acidosis. *Front. Bioeng. Biotechnol.* **2020**, *8*, 412. [CrossRef]
143. Romdhane, F.; Villano, D.; Irrera, P.; Consolino, L.; Longo, D.L. Evaluation of a similarity anisotropic diffusion denoising approach for improving in vivo CEST-MRI tumor pH imaging. *Magn. Reson. Med.* **2021**, *85*, 3479–3496. [CrossRef] [PubMed]
144. Vullo, S.; Kellenberger, S. A molecular view of the function and pharmacology of acid-sensing ion channels. *Pharmacol. Res.* **2020**, *154*, 104166. [CrossRef] [PubMed]
145. Chano, T.; Kita, H.; Avnet, S.; Lemma, S.; Baldini, N. Prominent role of RAB39A-RXRB axis in cancer development and stemness. *Oncotarget* **2018**, *9*, 9852–9866. [CrossRef]
146. Shi, S.; Klotz, U. Proton pump inhibitors: An update of their clinical use and pharmacokinetics. *Eur. J. Clin. Pharmacol.* **2008**, *64*, 935–951. [CrossRef] [PubMed]
147. Moriyama, Y.; Patel, V.; Ueda, I.; Futai, M. Evidence for a common binding site for omeprazole and N-ethylmaleimide in subunit A of chromaffin granule vacuolar-type H^+-ATPase. *Biochem. Biophys. Res. Commun.* **1993**, *196*, 699–706. [CrossRef]
148. Mattsson, J.P.; Vaananen, K.; Wallmark, B.; Lorentzon, P. Omeprazole and bafilomycin, two proton pump inhibitors: Differentiation of their effects on gastric, kidney and bone H^+-translocating ATPases. *Biochim. Biophys. Acta* **1991**, *1065*, 261–268. [CrossRef]
149. Ferrari, S.; Perut, F.; Fagioli, F.; Brach Del Prever, A.; Meazza, C.; Parafioriti, A.; Picci, P.; Gambarotti, M.; Avnet, S.; Baldini, N.; et al. Proton pump inhibitor chemosensitization in human osteosarcoma: From the bench to the patients' bed. *J. Transl. Med.* **2013**, *11*, 268. [CrossRef] [PubMed]
150. Tauro, M.; Loiodice, F.; Ceruso, M.; Supuran, C.T.; Tortorella, P. Dual carbonic anhydrase/matrix metalloproteinase inhibitors incorporating bisphosphonic acid moieties targeting bone tumors. *Bioorg. Med. Chem. Lett.* **2014**, *24*, 2617–2620. [CrossRef]
151. Kusuzaki, K.; Murata, H.; Takeshita, H.; Hashiguchi, S.; Nozaki, T.; Emoto, K.; Ashihara, T.; Hirasawa, Y. Intracellular binding sites of acridine orange in living osteosarcoma cells. *Anticancer Res.* **2000**, *20*, 971–975.
152. Cools, A.A.; Janssen, L.H. Fluorescence response of acridine orange to changes in pH gradients across liposome membranes. *Experientia* **1986**, *42*, 954–956. [CrossRef]
153. Hiruma, H.; Katakura, T.; Takenami, T.; Igawa, S.; Kanoh, M.; Fujimura, T.; Kawakami, T. Vesicle disruption, plasma membrane bleb formation, and acute cell death caused by illumination with blue light in acridine orange-loaded malignant melanoma cells. *J. Photochem. Photobiol. B* **2007**, *86*, 1–8. [CrossRef] [PubMed]
154. Damaghi, M.; Wojtkowiak, J.W.; Gillies, R.J. pH sensing and regulation in cancer. *Front. Physiol.* **2013**, *4*, 370. [CrossRef] [PubMed]
155. Zdolsek, J.M. Acridine orange-mediated photodamage to cultured cells. *APMIS* **1993**, *101*, 127–132. [CrossRef]
156. Hashiguchi, S.; Kusuzaki, K.; Murata, H.; Takeshita, H.; Hashiba, M.; Nishimura, T.; Ashihara, T.; Hirasawa, Y. Acridine orange excited by low-dose radiation has a strong cytocidal effect on mouse osteosarcoma. *Oncology* **2002**, *62*, 85–93. [CrossRef] [PubMed]
157. Brunk, U.T.; Dalen, H.; Roberg, K.; Hellquist, H.B. Photo-oxidative disruption of lysosomal membranes causes apoptosis of cultured human fibroblasts. *Free Radic. Biol. Med.* **1997**, *23*, 616–626. [CrossRef]
158. Kusuzaki, K.; Murata, H.; Matsubara, T.; Miyazaki, S.; Okamura, A.; Seto, M.; Matsumine, A.; Hosoi, H.; Sugimoto, T.; Uchida, A. Clinical trial of photodynamic therapy using acridine orange with/without low dose radiation as new limb salvage modality in musculoskeletal sarcomas. *Anticancer Res.* **2005**, *25*, 1225–1235.
159. Kusuzaki, K.; Murata, H.; Matsubara, T.; Miyazaki, S.; Shintani, K.; Seto, M.; Matsumine, A.; Hosoi, H.; Sugimoto, T.; Uchida, A. Clinical outcome of a novel photodynamic therapy technique using acridine orange for synovial sarcomas. *Photochem. Photobiol.* **2005**, *81*, 705–709. [CrossRef]
160. Yoshida, K.; Kusuzaki, K.; Matsubara, T.; Matsumine, A.; Kumamoto, T.; Komada, Y.; Naka, N.; Uchida, A. Periosteal Ewing's sarcoma treated by photodynamic therapy with acridine orange. *Oncol. Rep.* **2005**, *13*, 279–282. [PubMed]
161. Martano, M.; Morello, E.; Avnet, S.; Costa, F.; Sammartano, F.; Kusuzaki, K.; Baldini, N. Photodynamic Surgery for Feline Injection-Site Sarcoma. *Biomed. Res. Int.* **2019**, *2019*, 8275935. [CrossRef] [PubMed]
162. Matsubara, T.; Kusuzaki, K.; Matsumine, A.; Murata, H.; Marunaka, Y.; Hosogi, S.; Uchida, A.; Sudo, A. Photodynamic therapy with acridine orange in musculoskeletal sarcomas. *J. Bone Joint Surg.* **2010**, *92*, 760–762. [CrossRef]
163. Matsubara, T.; Kusuzaki, K.; Matsumine, A.; Murata, H.; Nakamura, T.; Uchida, A.; Sudo, A. Clinical outcomes of minimally invasive surgery using acridine orange for musculoskeletal sarcomas around the forearm, compared with conventional limb salvage surgery after wide resection. *J. Surg. Oncol.* **2010**, *102*, 271–275. [CrossRef] [PubMed]
164. Saito, T.; Tsukahara, T.; Suzuki, T.; Nojima, I.; Tadano, H.; Kawai, N.; Kubo, T.; Hirohashi, Y.; Kanaseki, T.; Torigoe, T.; et al. Spatiotemporal metabolic dynamics of the photosensitizer talaporfin sodium in carcinoma and sarcoma. *Cancer Sci.* **2020**. [CrossRef] [PubMed]
165. McMahon, K.S.; Wieman, T.J.; Moore, P.H.; Fingar, V.H. Effects of photodynamic therapy using mono-L-aspartyl chlorin e6 on vessel constriction, vessel leakage, and tumor response. *Cancer Res.* **1994**, *54*, 5374–5379. [PubMed]
166. Tsai, S.R.; Yin, R.; Huang, Y.Y.; Sheu, B.C.; Lee, S.C.; Hamblin, M.R. Low-Level light therapy potentiates NPe6-mediated photodynamic therapy in a human osteosarcoma cell line via increased ATP. *Photodiagn. Photodyn. Ther.* **2015**, *12*, 123–130. [CrossRef] [PubMed]

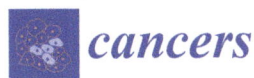

Article

Autophagic Markers in Chordomas: Immunohistochemical Analysis and Comparison with the Immune Microenvironment of Chordoma Tissues

Georgia Karpathiou [1,*], Maroa Dridi [1], Lila Krebs-Drouot [2], François Vassal [3], Emmanuel Jouanneau [4,5,6], Timothée Jacquesson [4,7], Cédric Barrey [6,8], Jean Michel Prades [9], Jean Marc Dumollard [1], David Meyronet [6,10,11], Jean Boutonnat [2] and Michel Péoc'h [1]

1. Pathology Department, University Hospital of Saint-Etienne, 42055 Saint-Etienne, France; maroa.dridi@etu.univ-st-etienne.fr (M.D.); j.marc.dumollard@chu-st-etienne.fr (J.M.D.); michel.peoch@chu-st-etienne.fr (M.P.)
2. Pathology Department, University Hospital of Grenoble, 38700 Grenoble, France; lkrebsdrouot@chu-grenoble.fr (L.K.-D.); jboutonnat@chu-grenoble.fr (J.B.)
3. Neurosurgery Department, University Hospital of Saint-Etienne, 42055 Saint-Etienne, France; francois.vassal@chu-st-etienne.fr
4. Department of Neurosurgery B, Neurological Hospital Pierre Wertheimer, 69500 Lyon, France; emmanuel.jouanneau@chu-lyon.fr (E.J.); timothee.jacquesson@neurochirurgie.fr (T.J.)
5. Inserm U1052, CNRS UMR5286, «Signaling, Metabolism and Tumor Progression» The Cancer Research Center of Lyon, 69373 Lyon, France
6. Claude Bernard University, Lyon 1, 69100 Lyon, France; c.barrey@wanadoo.fr (C.B.); david.meyronet@chu-lyon.fr (D.M.)
7. Department of Anatomy, Faculté de Médecine Lyon-Est, Université de Lyon, Université Claude Bernard Lyon 1, 69100 Lyon, France
8. Department of Spine and Spinal Cord Surgery, Neurological Hospital Pierre Wertheimer, 69500 Lyon, France
9. Head and Neck Surgery Department, University Hospital of Saint-Etienne, 42055 Saint-Etienne, France; jean.michel.prades@univ-st-etienne.fr
10. East Pathology Institute, Hospices Civils de Lyon, 69677 Lyon, France
11. Cancer Research Center of Lyon, Cancer Cell Plasticity Department, 69373 Lyon, France
* Correspondence: georgia.karpathiou@chu-st-etienne.fr

Simple Summary: In contrast to normal notochords, autophagic factors are often present in chordomas. Furthermore, PD-L1+ immune cells also express LC3B, suggesting the need for further investigations between autophagy and the immune microenvironment.

Abstract: Chordomas are notably resistant to chemotherapy. One of the cytoprotective mechanisms implicated in chemoresistance is autophagy. There are indirect data that autophagy could be implicated in chordomas, but its presence has not been studied in chordoma tissues. Sixty-one (61) chordomas were immunohistochemically studied for autophagic markers and their expression was compared with the expression in notochords, clinicopathological data, as well as the tumor immune microenvironment. All chordomas strongly and diffusely expressed cytoplasmic p62 (sequestosome 1, SQSTM1/p62), whereas 16 (26.2%) tumors also showed nuclear p62 expression. LC3B (Microtubule-associated protein 1A/1B-light chain 3B) tumor cell expression was found in 44 (72.1%) tumors. Autophagy-related 16-like 1 (ATG16L1) was also expressed by most tumors. All tumors expressed mannose-6-phosphate/insulin-like growth factor 2 receptor (M6PR/IGF2R). LC3B tumor cell expression was negatively associated with tumor size, while no other parameters, such as age, sex, localization, or survival, were associated with the immunohistochemical factors studied. LC3B immune cell expression showed a significant positive association with programmed death-ligand 1 (PD-L1)+ immune cells and with a higher vascular density. ATG16L1 expression was also positively associated with higher vascular density. Notochords ($n = 5$) showed different immunostaining with a very weak LC3B and M6PR expression, and no p62 expression. In contrast to normal notochords, autophagic factors such as LC3B and ATG16L1 are often present in chordomas, associated with a strong and diffuse expression of p62, suggesting a blocked autophagic flow. Furthermore, PD-L1+

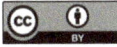

immune cells also express LC3B, suggesting the need for further investigations between autophagy and the immune microenvironment.

Keywords: LC3B; ATG16L1; p62; M6PR; PD-L1; CD8; notochord

1. Introduction

Chordomas are rare bone tumors, accounting for 1.4% of primary bone malignancies and showing a median overall survival of 7 years; they are assumed to derive from notochordal remnants probably driven by brachyury activation [1]. These malignant tumors, primarily treated with surgery and/or radiotherapy, are notably resistant to chemotherapy [2]. The reason for their chemoresistance is unknown. One mechanism that tumor cells use to survive during adverse conditions is autophagy [3], the discovery of which led to a 2016 Nobel Prize award for Yoshinori Ohsumi [4]. It is a process characterized by the formation of vesicles, autophagosomes, engulfing cellular constituents and leading them to degradation and recycling by fusion with the lysosomes [3]. It is one of the first responses in tumor cells exposed to chemotherapy, as it removes damaged proteins and organelles and generates energy [5]. Thus, autophagy often acts as a cytoprotective mechanism, and therefore chemotherapeutic drugs are used in combination with autophagy inhibitors in clinical trials [5]. Furthermore, lysosomes, that receive extracellular/cell surface molecules by endocytosis and intracellular components by autophagy, are important in drug resistance as they isolate chemotherapeutic drugs [6]. The principal morphologic feature of chordomas, already described by Virchow, is their cytoplasmic vacuoles, accounting for their bubbled cytoplasm and explaining the description Virchow gave to chordoma cells: "physaliphorous" (from the Greek words physalis = bubble and phorous = bearing) [2]. The exact nature of these vacuoles remains unknown, but they are considered lysosome-related organelles [7]. Furthermore, brachyury, the main gene implicated in chordomas pathology [2], has been shown to induce autophagy in glioblastoma cell lines [8]. Despite this indirect evidence of chordomas association with autophagy, to the best of our knowledge, the presence of this mechanism has never been studied in chordoma tissues.

Furthermore, the immune microenvironment is important for all tumors, even for sarcomas, with recent studies suggesting prognostic significance of immune cells, notably B cells, in soft tissue sarcomas [9]. Still, controversial findings as to the role of the immune microenvironment of chordomas [10–12], despite immunotherapy, could be considered a possible option for chordoma patients [13]. Moreover, there is recent evidence suggesting that the autophagic machinery of the tumor-associated lymphocytes, controls their own phenotype [14], implying an association of the autophagy with the immune microenvironment as well. This association has not been previously studied in chordomas.

Thus, the aim of this study is to investigate the possible presence of autophagic markers in a large series of chordomas and to correlate them with the immune microenvironment of these tumors.

2. Materials and Methods

This is a multicenter retrospective study of 61 patients diagnosed with chordoma of the conventional subtype, between 2000 and 2020, based on clinicoradiological data, typical morphological features and S100/cytokeratins expression, and confirmed in reassessment by a specialized soft-tissue pathologist (MP) and by brachyury expression. The local ethics committee approved the study (IRBN702020/CHUSTE). Tumor localization and size, treatment type, tumor recurrence and overall and progression-free survival were retrieved from medical records.

Immunohistochemistry was performed in formalin-fixed paraffin-embedded 4-µm thick full tumor sections using an automated staining system (OMNIS, Dako-Agilent, Santa Clara, CA, USA). Primary antibodies used were: LC3B (Rabbit monoclonal, ab192890, abcam, dilution 1/1000, pH 6, 20 min), SQSTM1 (sequestosome1)/p62 (Rabbit monoclonal, ab109012, abcam, dilution 1/2000, pH 6, 20 min), ATG16L1 (Rabbit monoclonal, ab195242, abcam, dilution 1/1000, pH 9, 20 min) and M6PR (cation independent) (Rabbit monoclonal, ab124767, abcam, dilution 1/2000, pH 6, 20 min). Positive immunoreactions were visualized using 3,3′-diaminobenzidine as the chromogenic substrate. The antibodies had been initially tested in a large variety of normal and neoplastic tissues to decide the best immunohistochemical protocol, giving no background staining and a range of staining intensities. Thereafter, nerve fiber and normal tonsillar tissue were used as positive controls for LC3B and p62/M6PR, respectively, while omission of the primary antibody was used as negative control. Given the histogenetic association of chordomas to notochord, 5 normal notochords (Figure 1) were also immunohistochemically studied for LC3B, p62 and M6PR, for comparison with the presumed tissue of origin of chordomas.

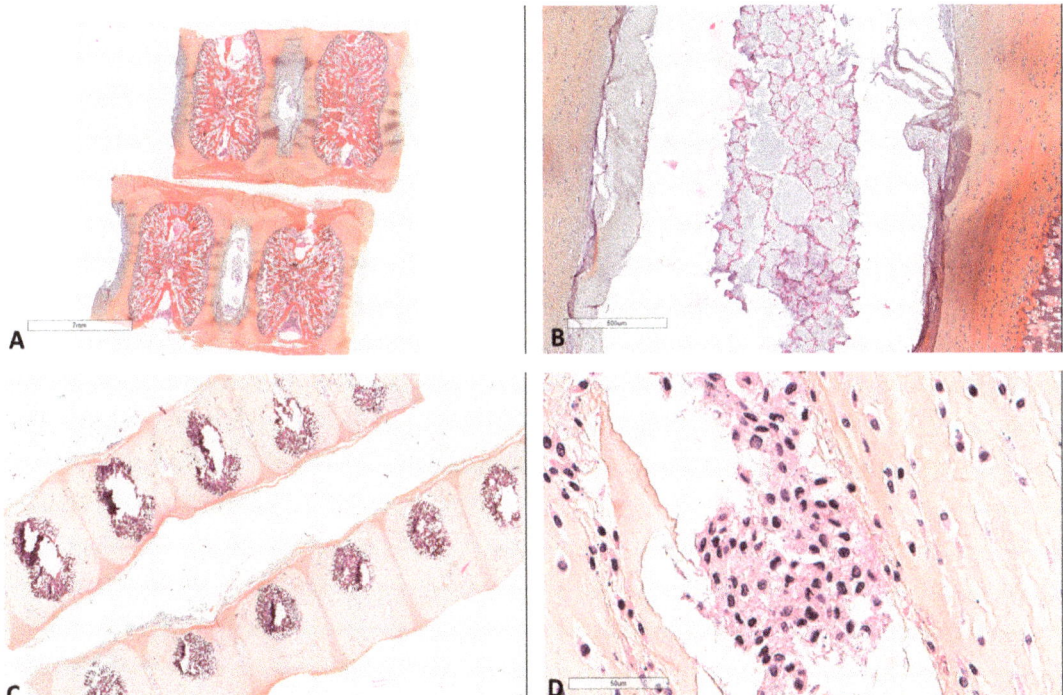

Figure 1. Morphology of fetal notochords. (**A**) Low magnification highlighting their intervertebral location (39 weeks of gestation, Hematoxylin, Eosin, Safran (HES) ×3). (**B**) Intermediate magnification showing their typical morphological resemblance to chordomas (39 weeks of gestation, HES ×40). (**C**) Low magnification highlighting their intervertebral location of another case (17 weeks of gestation, HES ×8). (**D**) High magnification showing their typical morphological resemblance to chordomas (17 weeks of gestation, HES ×400).

LC3B and M6PR staining was presented as cytoplasmic punctae and according to the density of dots per cell. This was recorded as negative (intensity score 0, no staining or ≤10 dots per cell); mild (intensity score 1, 11–20 dots per cell); moderate (intensity score 2, >20 dots per cell without clusters), and strong (intensity score 3, >20 dots per cell with clusters) [15]. The intensity of p62 and ATG16L1 staining was recorded as negative (intensity score 0), weak (intensity score 1), moderate (intensity score 2), and strong (intensity score 3). The percentage of positive cells was recorded from 0 to 100% and presented as the H score (percentage of positive cells × intensity). P62 can also show nuclear expression and tumors with at least 5% p62 nuclear staining were considered positive for nuclear expression, as previously suggested [16].

The tumors were also studied for the immunohistochemical expression of (work under submission): PD-L1 (22C3, Dako Agilent, 1/40), CD8 (C8/144B, Dako Agilent, 1/100), CD20 (L26, Dako Agilent, 1/200), CD163 (10D6, Novocastra, 1/200), CD34 (QBEnd10, Dako Agilent, 1/800) and MECA-79 (MECA-79, Santa Cruz Biotechnology, 1/750). MECA-79 is a factor detecting high endothelial venules; vessels specialized in the transport of lymphocytes [9]. We evaluated the immune cells in a semiquantitative manner (0: no cells, 1: few cells (<10%), 2: moderate number of positive cells ($\geq$10% and <40%), and 3: abundant cells ($\geq$40%). This resulted in low (scores 0 and 1) and high (scores 2 and 3) groups for CD8, CD20 and CD163; and present (score 0) or absent (score 1–3) for PD-L1+ immune cells [17,18]. Quantification of the number of CD34+ and MECA-79+ blood vessels (vascular density) was performed on 5 high power 20× (1 mm^2) fields per section, and these were counted and averaged, as previously proposed [19] while their median value was used as a cut-off for the classification into two groups.

Data were analyzed using StatView software (Abacus Concepts, Berkley, CA, USA). We used the χ^2 test to explore any relationship between two groups for categorical data, and factorial analysis of variances (ANOVAs) to consider the effect of at least one factor on a continuous parameter studied. Simple regression analysis was used to explore a possible relationship between two continuous parameters. Survival probability was estimated by Kaplan–Meier analysis with log-rank product limit estimation. For all analyses, statistical significance was indicated at a p value of <0.05.

3. Results

The cohort (n = 61), which is part of our previous study (work under submission), included 37 (60.7%) male and 24 female (39.3%) patients with a mean age at diagnosis of 56.5 ($\pm$16.8) and a median of 61 years. Tumors were more often skull chordomas (n = 23, 37.7%), followed by sacral (n = 21, 34.4%) and mobile spine (n = 17, 27.9%) tumors. Patients had been treated with surgery in most cases (n = 59, 96.7%), followed by adjuvant therapy in almost half of the cases. Follow up ranged from 2 to 264 months (median 64, mean 92.3$\pm$71.7). Recurrences were noted in 46 patients (75.4%). Thirteen patients (n = 13, 21.3%) died of disease. The 5-year and 10-year overall survival (log-rank) was 80% and 70% respectively.

The immunohistochemical study (Table 1 and Table S1) showed that all chordomas strongly expressed (Figure 2) cytoplasmic p62 (n = 61, median H score 300); thus, no further statistical correlations were performed for this factor.

Sixteen (n = 16, 26.2%) tumors also showed nuclear p62 expression. Similarly, all tumors (n = 61) expressed M6PR (Figure 2), and expression was homogenous in each tumor, thus, three groups of intensity score 1 (n = 23, 37.7%), 2 (n = 21, 34.4%), or 3 (n = 17, 27.9%) were used for further analyses. LC3B tumor cell expression (n = 61) was found in 44 (72.1%) tumors (Figure 3).

H score ranged from 0 to 100, with a median of 10 and a mean of 16.2 ($\pm$22.5). The median H score was used as a cut-off value to classify tumors into low ($\leq$10) or high (>10) expression. LC3B expression by immune cells (n = 61) inside tumor stroma (Figure 4) was found in 18 (29.5%) tumors, with the H score ranging from 0 to 50 (median 0 and mean 10.7 $\pm$ 23.4).

ATG16L1 (n = 55, due to technical issues) was also expressed (Figure 3) by most tumors (n = 42, 76.4%) with a median H score of 100 (0–300) and a mean of 106.7 $\pm$ 85.2. The median cut-off was used to classify tumors into low ($\leq$100) or high (>100) expression.

Table 1. Immunohistochemical analysis.

Parameter	Values
LC3B tumor cell expression H score	
Range	0–100
Median	10
Mean ± SD	16.2 ± 22.5
LC3B immune cell expression H score	
Range	0–100
Median	0
Mean ± SD	10.7 ± 23.4
P62 cytoplasmic tumor cell expression H score	
Range	0–300
Median	300
Mean ± SD	231.8 ± 89.4
P62 nuclear tumor cell expression	
Yes	16, 26.2%
No	45, 73.8%
ATG16L1 tumor cell expression H score	
Range	0–300
Median	100
Mean ± SD	106.7 ± 85.2
M6PR tumor cell intensity score	
1 (mild)	23, 37.7%
2 (moderate)	21, 34.4%
3 (strong)	17, 27.9%

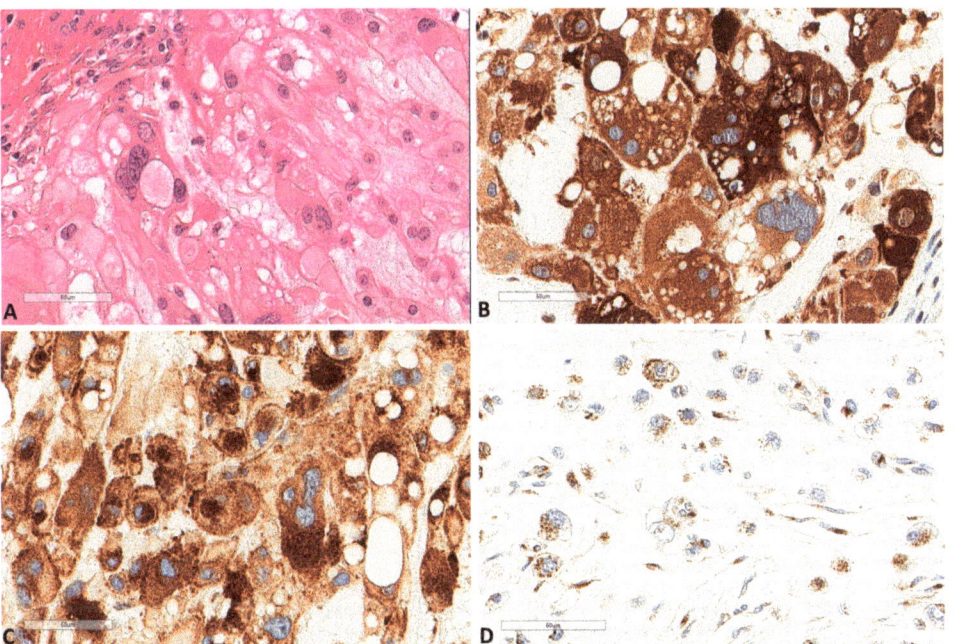

Figure 2. P62 and M6PR expression in chordomas. (**A**) The morphology of a chordoma tissue (×400). (**B**) P62 strong express Scheme 400. (**C**) Same focus for M6PR expression (×400). (**D**) Another chordoma with lower M6PR expression (×400).

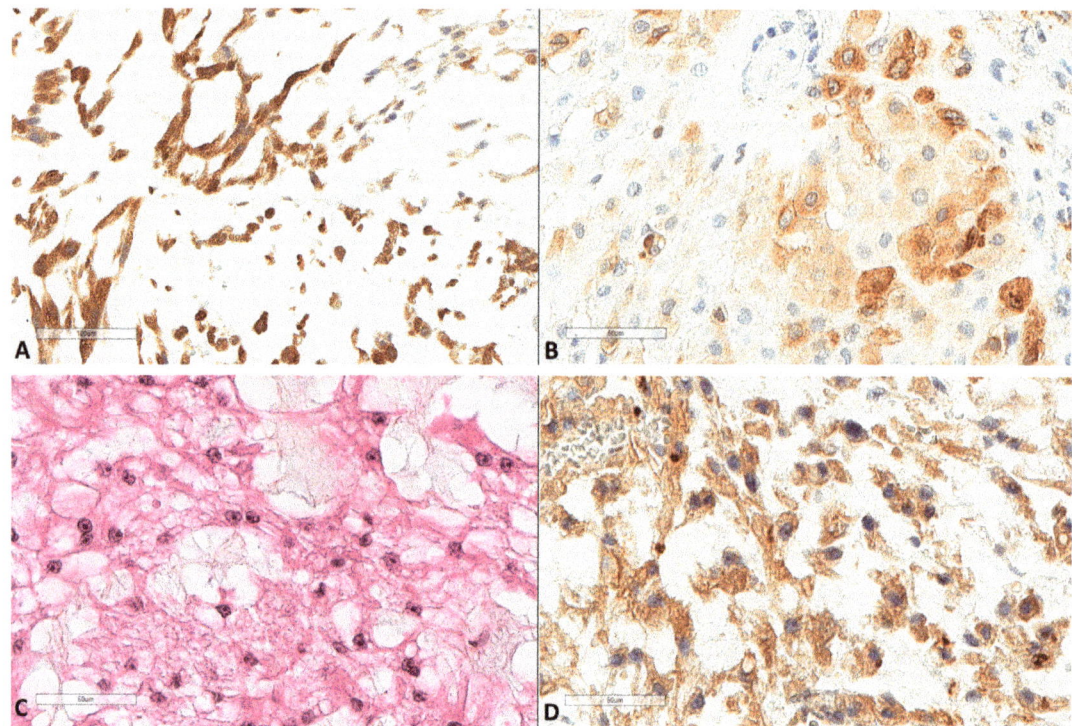

Figure 3. LC3B and ATG16L1 expression in chordomas. (**A**) LC3B strong expression of a chordoma (×200). (**B**) LC3B mild expression of another case (×400). (**C**) Another chordoma tissue (HES ×400). (**D**) ATG16L1 expression of the latter chordoma (×400).

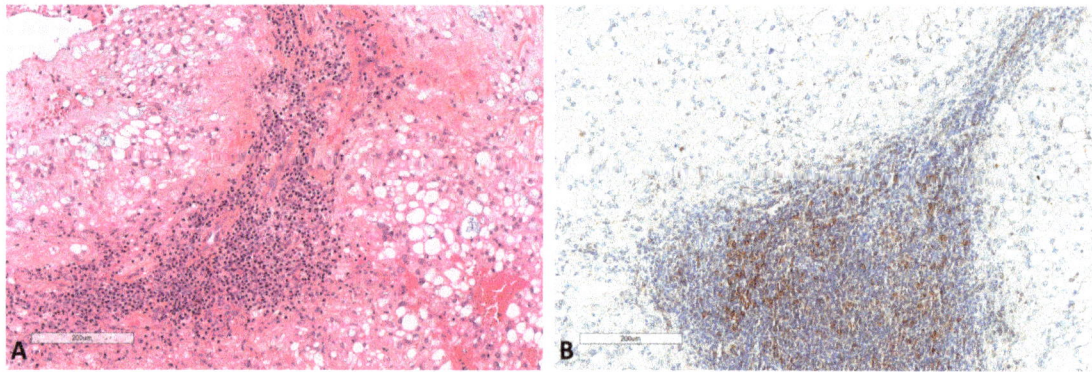

Figure 4. LC3B expression in immune cells of chordomas. (**A**) Immune cells in chordoma stromal tissue (HES ×100). (**B**) LC3B expression in immune cells at the same focus (×100).

We found that LC3B tumor cell expression (χ^2 test) was negatively associated with tumor size ($p = 0.03$, $\chi^2 = 4.5$), where tumor size was available for 29 tumors and the median tumor size (43 mm) was used as the cut-off value for the χ^2 test. Expression was marginally associated with localization, since it was less often found in sacral tumors ($p = 0.07$, $\chi^2 = 5.2$), but this probably reflected tumor size, because sacral tumors were larger than in other localizations ($p = 0.02$, $\chi^2 = 7$). None of the other parameters, such as age, sex, localization, or size were associated with the immunohistochemical factors studied.

Autophagic factors studied herein were compared (Figure 5 and Table 2) with our previous data regarding the immune micro-environment of chordomas (work under submission). The scheme of low/high expression, as mentioned above for each factor, was used for statistical analyses by χ^2 test. LC3B immune cell expression showed a marginal and negative association with CD20 B cells presence ($p = 0.07$, $\chi^2 = 3$). It showed a significant positive association with PD-L1+ immune cells ($p = 0.001$, $\chi^2 = 9.7$). It also showed a strong positive correlation with high vascular density as studied by CD34 ($p = 0.0004$, $\chi^2 = 12.4$). ATG16L1 expression was also positively associated with vascular density ($p = 0.01$, $\chi^2 = 6.4$), while no other association was found for this marker. The presence of CD163 positive macrophages was not associated with the present factors. The presence of high endothelial venules, assessed by the MECA-79 antibody, was not associated with any of the factors studied; however, it showed a trend ($p = 0.06$, $\chi^2 = 3.4$) for a negative association with p62 nuclear expression. A strong trend ($p = 0.05$, $\chi^2 = 3.7$) between p62 nuclear expression and the presence of lesser B cells was also noted.

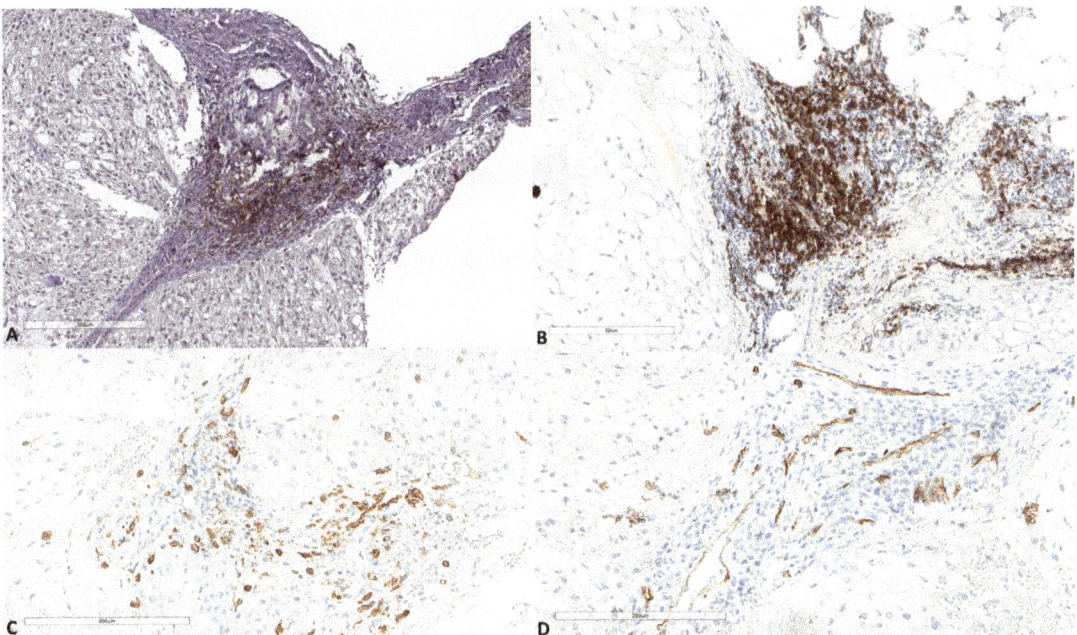

Figure 5. (**A**) PD-L1 expression in immune cells of chordomas (HES ×100, same focus as in Figure 4). (**B**) Another chordoma with high infiltration by B cells (×100, CD20+). (**C**) Infiltration by CD163+ macrophages (×200, same focus as in Figure 4). (**D**) Vascular channels as assessed by CD34 (×200, same focus as in Figure 4).

Table 2. Correlation between the immunohistochemical factors studied.

Variables	LC3B in Tumor Cells $n = 61$			LC3B in Immune Cells $n = 61$			ATG16L1 Expression $n = 55$			M6PR Expression $n = 61$				p62 Nuclear Expression $n = 61$		
	Low	High	p, χ^2	Low	High	p, χ^2	Low	High	p, χ^2	1	2	3	p, χ^2	No	Yes	p, χ^2
CD20 ($n = 60$)																
Low	35	18	0.7,	35	18	0.07,	34	14	0.9,	20	18	15	0.9,	41	12	0.05,
High	5	2	0.08	7	0	3	5	2	0.001	3	2	2	0.09	3	4	3.7
CD8 ($n = 61$)																
Low	25	11	0.7,	28	8	0.1,	26	7	0.1,	12	14	10	0.6,	29	7	0.1,
High	16	9	0.1	15	10	2.2	13	9	2.4	11	7	7	0.9	16	9	2
CD163 ($n = 61$)																
Low	23	12	0.7,	27	8	0.1,	25	7	0.1,	13	14	8	0.4,	25	10	0.6,
High	18	8	0.08	16	10	1.7	14	9	1.9	10	7	9	1.4	20	6	0.2
Vascular density ($n = 61$)																
Low	19	9	0.9,	26	2	**0.0004,**	22	3	**0.01,**	11	11	6	0.5,	22	6	0.4,
High	22	11	0.009	17	16	**12.4**	17	13	**6.4**	12	10	11	1.1	23	10	0.6
PD-L1+ immune cells ($n = 61$)																
No	32	12	0.1,	36	8	**0.001,**	30	9	0.1,	15	18	11	0.2,	33	11	0.7,
Yes	9	8	2.1	7	10	**9.7**	9	7	2.3	8	3	6	2.9	12	5	0.1
Tumor size ($n = 29$)																
<43 mm	7	7	**0.03,**	11	3	0.1,	7	6	0.6,	5	6	3	0.1,	11	3	0.7,
≥43 mm	13	2	**4.5**	9	6	1.7	8	5	0.1	9	2	4	3.2	11	4	0.1

Data presented in Table 2 were statistically calculated using the χ^2 test. Bold denotes statistical significance.

The immunohistochemical factors currently studied were not associated with each other (χ^2 test); however, a strong trend ($p = 0.05$, $\chi^2 = 5.7$) was found between M6PR and p62 nuclear expression: tumors with p62 nuclear expression showed milder M6PR expression.

Survival analysis showed no prognostic significance for the autophagic immunohistochemical factors studied.

Regarding notochords immunostaining (Figure 6), five notochords from fetal autopsies (ages of 14, 17, 23, 23 and 39 weeks of gestation) showed the same pattern in all cases: a very weak LC3B and M6PR expression, and no p62 expression.

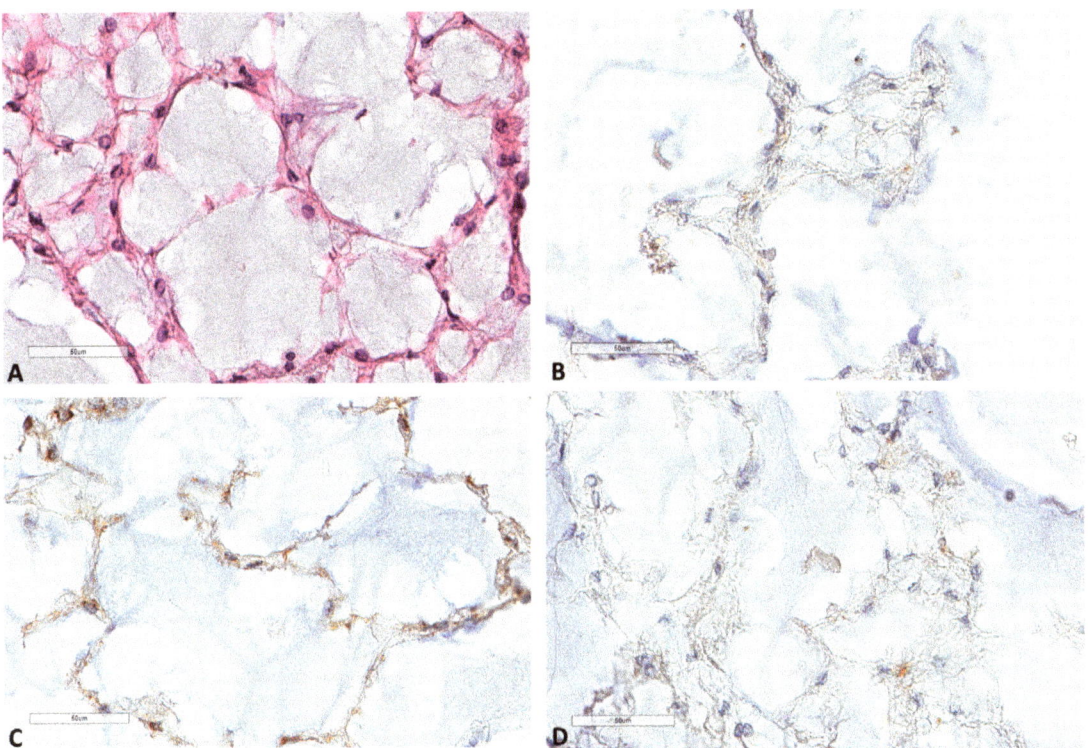

Figure 6. LC3B, M6PR and p62 expression in notochords. (**A**) Notochord morphology (39 weeks of gestation, HES ×400). (**B**) LC3B very mild expression at the same focus (×400). (**C**) M6PR mild expression at the same focus (×400). (**D**) p62 negative staining at the same focus (×400).

4. Discussion

This is the first study, to the best of our knowledge, examining the current immunohistochemical factors in chordoma tumor tissues. We found that all chordomas strongly and diffusely express p62, a receptor of autophagic cargos. This factor binds and transports the targets to the autophagosome by interacting with LC3, and then p62 itself is degraded during autophagolysosome cargo degradation; thus, reduced levels of p62 are typically used as a surrogate marker of an activated autophagy pathway [20]. Therefore, the constant and high expression of p62 in chordomas found herein probably reflect a blocked autophagic degradation. Simultaneously, we found that most tumors showed LC3B expression, which is used as a surrogate marker of autophagic vesicles. This combination of LC3B and p62 expression is suggested to represent activated but blocked, downstream autophagic machinery [15]. Similarly, the autophagy-related 16-like 1 (ATG16L1) protein was expressed in most tumors, further supporting the presence of autophagic factors in chordoma tissues. ATG16L1 is one of the critical initial steps of the autophagic activation, since it is the mediator that specifies the site of LC3 lipidation [21]. Additionally, it provides a link between autophagy and immune regulation, since it interacts with the cytokine receptor's intracellular domain [21]. Thus, our results are in favor of a probably activated but blocked autophagic mechanism in chordomas, resulting in accumulated autolysosomes in tumor cells cytoplasm. This could probably explain the chemoresistance of these cells. In line with this assumption, enhanced autophagy has been shown to protect osteosarcoma cells against chemotherapeutic stress [22,23]. Our results are also in line with previous studies in cell lines, where it was shown that lysosomal vacuoles in chordomas do not harbor acidic pH 7, and thus their function is impaired, which could explain the accumulation of p62. Furthermore, we show that staining of tumor tissues is different from staining seen in notochords, further supporting a dysregulated mechanism in the tumoral setting. The exact mechanism of activation of autophagy in chordomas is unknown, but a possible association with brachyury activation, which is the main pathogenetic molecular abnormality in chordomas, could be hypothesized since it induces autophagy in gliomas [8].

Mannose-6-phosphate receptor (M6PR), also called insulin-like growth factor-2 (IGF-2) receptor is a receptor that leads cell surface/cytoplasmic constituents to endosomal vesicles and to autophagosomes for degradation. The IGF-2R/M6PR, which is considered to act as a tumor growth suppressor, has two forms: a membrane-associated and a soluble one, both of which interact with several ligands, including IGF-2, TGFβ and lysosomal enzymes [24]. It was found in all chordomas, showing strong expression in almost one third of them. Another receptor of the same family, the IGF1R was also found to be expressed by most chordomas [25]. It has been shown that M6PR acts as a link between autophagy, chemotherapy and immunotherapy, since autophagy controls its traffic between the cytoplasm and the cell surface, where it augments T cell cytotoxic activity against tumor cells [26–28]. Furthermore, after chemotherapy, IGF2 confers resistance correlated with enhanced autophagy when expressed at elevated levels in osteosarcomas [23]. We did not find any association between M6PR and the immune microenvironment of chordomas, which could be explained by the cytoplasmic accumulation of this marker inside tumor cells. Interestingly, its expression was milder for tumors with p62 nuclear expression.

P62 harbors nuclear import/export signals, but the role of nuclear p62 is unknown [29]. Recent evidence suggests that p62 nuclear retention is favored by the inhibition of exportin 1, and that its nuclear retention enhances the expression of innate immune response related genes [29]. It has been also shown in virus-transformed cells that inhibition of autophagy leads to p62 nuclear accumulation, which in turn leads to reactive oxygen species (ROS)-induced DNA damage and proteasomal degradation of DNA repair proteins [30]. In previous immunohistochemical studies of p62 expression, nuclear expression has been also observed; in endometrial cancer, almost half of the cases showed nuclear expression, and with high cytoplasmic expression associated with absent p62 nuclear expression, denoted an adverse prognosis [16]. Similarly, lower p62 nuclear is associated with poorer survival in oral cancer patients [15]. In lung cancer, when both cytoplasmic and nuclear p62 expression were found, this signified adverse prognosis [20]. All these findings show that p62 nuclear expression is not a fortuitous event, rather, there is a pathophysiological importance for its nuclear accumulation that warrants further investigation. In the current study, its nuclear presence was marginally associated with lesser B cells and lesser high endothelial venules, suggesting a role in regulating this part of the immune microenvironment.

Another finding of our study is that some of the tumors harbored immune cells strongly expressing LC3B and that these cells were PD-L1+ immune cells. To the best of our knowledge, the role of autophagy inside the immune microenvironment of any tumor has not been yet elucidated. However, recent evidence suggests that autophagy is actively implicated in tumor infiltrating lymphocyte activity, and when T cells live inside tumors with elevated extracellular potassium, this reduces the uptake of local nutrients by these lymphocytes, leading to activation of their autophagy [14]. This autophagy activation in T cells, in turn, leads to less factors necessary for epigenetic remodeling, thus leading to a more stem cell-like and less differentiated/effector phenotype of these lymphocytes [14]. Moreover, LC3B+ autophagosomes released by tumor cells in the form of extracellular vesicles, correlate significantly with up-regulation of PD-L1 in matched monocytes from malignant effusions, also suggesting an immunosuppressive mechanism of autophagy in the tumor microenvironment [31]. Thus, our finding of LC3B expression in PD-L1+ immune cells in chordomas probably reflects starvation conditions and autophagic activation in these cellular subpopulations. It is worth noticing that autophagosomes and lysosomes have been found to contain major histocompatibility complex (MHC)-I molecules in pancreatic adenocarcinoma cells, preventing them from being expressed on the cell surface and thus from activating cytotoxic T cells [32,33]. Thus, our data add to the notion of autophagy being implicated in the immune tumor microenvironment and will prompt further investigation.

Our study has limitations associated with its retrospective nature. The main limitation is the investigation of these factors only by immunohistochemical means, where autophagy is a flow, and should also be studied functionally. However, our approach is warranted when a large tissue series of rare diseases, such as chordomas, are needed.

5. Conclusions

To conclude, we study for the first time, a large series of chordoma tissues for autophagic markers and compare them with their expression in notochords and with the tumor immune microenvironment. We show that autophagic factors, such as LC3B and ATG16L1, are often present in chordomas, associated with a strong and diffuse expression of p62, suggesting a blocked autophagic flow, in contrast to normal notochords. Furthermore, PD-L1+ immune cells also express LC3B, suggesting the need for further investigations between autophagy and the immune microenvironment.

Supplementary Materials: The following are available online at https://www.mdpi.com/article/10.3390/cancers13092169/s1.

Author Contributions: Conceptualization, G.K. and M.P.; Data curation, G.K., M.D., L.K.-D., F.V., E.J., T.J., C.B., J.M.P., J.M.D., D.M. and J.B.; Formal analysis, G.K., D.M., J.B. and M.P.; Funding acquisition, G.K.; Investigation, G.K., E.J., T.J., C.B., J.M.D., D.M., J.B. and M.P.; Methodology, G.K., J.M.D., D.M., J.B. and M.P.; Project administration, G.K. and M.P.; Resources, G.K., F.V., T.J., C.B. and M.P.; Software, G.K.; Supervision, G.K., F.V., E.J., T.J., J.M.D., D.M. and M.P.; Validation, J.M.D., D.M. and M.P.; Visualization, G.K.; Writing—original draft, G.K.; Writing—review & editing, M.D., F.V., E.J., T.J., C.B., J.M.P., J.M.D., D.M., J.B. and M.P. All authors have read and agreed to the published version of the manuscript.

Funding: Direction des Affaires Médicales et de la Recherche, CHU Saint-Etienne, France.

Institutional Review Board Statement: The local ethics committee approved the study (IRBN702020/CHUSTE); the acquisition of written informed consent was waived by the institutional review board given the retrospective nature of the study and the anonymization of all data. The study was performed according to the Declaration of Helsinki.

Informed Consent Statement: Patient consent was waived waived by the institutional review board given the retrospective nature of the study and the anonymization of all data.

Data Availability Statement: Data are available upon reasonable request.

Acknowledgments: The authors would like to thank Philippe Cosmo from the Tumorothèque/Centre de Ressources Biologiques de CHU Saint-Etienne (BRIF no. BB-0033-00041), as well as Isabelle Dumas and David Scaion for their excellent technical assistance.

Conflicts of Interest: The authors have no conflict of interest to declare.

References

1. Dridi, M.; Boutonnat, J.; Dumollard, J.M.; Peoc'H, M.; Karpathiou, G. The transcriptional factors CDX2 and FOXA1 in chordomas. *Pathol. Res. Pract.* **2020**, *216*, 153160. [CrossRef] [PubMed]
2. Karpathiou, G.; Dumollard, J.M.; Dridi, M.; Col, P.D.; Barral, F.-G.; Boutonnat, J.; Peoc'H, M. Chordomas: A review with emphasis on their pathophysiology, pathology, molecular biology, and genetics. *Pathol. Res. Pract.* **2020**, *216*, 153089. [CrossRef] [PubMed]
3. Karpathiou, G.; Sivridis, E.; Koukourakis, M.I.; Mikroulis, D.; Bouros, D.; Froudarakis, M.E.; Giatromanolaki, A. Light-Chain 3A Autophagic Activity and Prognostic Significance in Non-small Cell Lung Carcinomas. *Chest* **2011**, *140*, 127–134. [CrossRef] [PubMed]
4. Press Release. NobelPrize.Org. Nobel Media AB 2020. Available online: https://www.nobelprize.org/prizes/medicine/2016/press-release/ (accessed on 29 April 2021).
5. Levy, J.M.M.; Thorburn, A. Autophagy in cancer: Moving from understanding mechanism to improving therapy responses in patients. *Cell Death Differ.* **2020**, *27*, 843–857. [CrossRef]
6. Xu, J.; Patel, N.H.; Gewirtz, D.A. Triangular Relationship between p53, Autophagy, and Chemotherapy Resistance. *Int. J. Mol. Sci.* **2020**, *21*, 8991. [CrossRef] [PubMed]

7. Kolb-Lenz, D.; Fuchs, R.; Lohberger, B.; Heitzer, E.; Meditz, K.; Pernitsch, D.; Pritz, E.; Groselj-Strele, A.; Leithner, A.; Liegl-Atzwanger, B.; et al. Characterization of the endolysosomal system in human chordoma cell lines: Is there a role of lyso-somes in chemoresistance of this rare bone tumor? *Histochem. Cell Biol.* **2018**, *150*, 83–92. [CrossRef] [PubMed]
8. Pinto, F.; Ângela, M.C.; Santos, G.C.; Matsushita, M.M.; Costa, S.; Silva, V.A.O.; Miranda-Gonçalves, V.; Lopes, C.M.; Clara, C.A.; Becker, A.P.; et al. The T-box transcription factor brachyury behaves as a tumor suppressor in gliomas. *J. Pathol.* **2020**, *251*, 87–99. [CrossRef] [PubMed]
9. Petitprez, F.; De Reyniès, A.; Keung, E.Z.; Chen, T.W.-W.; Sun, C.-M.; Calderaro, J.; Jeng, Y.-M.; Hsiao, L.-P.; Lacroix, L.; Bougoüin, A.; et al. B cells are associated with survival and immunotherapy response in sarcoma. *Nature* **2020**, *577*, 556–560. [CrossRef]
10. Mathios, D.; Ruzevick, J.; Jackson, C.M.; Xu, H.; Shah, S.; Taube, J.M.; Burger, P.C.; McCarthy, E.F.; Quinones-Hinojosa, A.; Pardoll, D.M.; et al. PD-1, PD-L1, PD-L2 expression in the chordoma microenvironment. *J. Neurooncol.* **2015**, *121*, 251–259. [CrossRef]
11. Feng, Y.; Shen, J.; Gao, Y.; Liao, Y.; Côté, G.; Choy, E.; Chebib, I.; Mankin, H.; Hornicek, F.; Duan, Z. Expression of programmed cell death ligand 1 (PD-L1) and prevalence of tumor-infiltrating lymphocytes (TILs) in chordoma. *Oncotarget* **2015**, *6*, 11139–11149. [CrossRef]
12. Zou, M.; Pan, Y.; Huang, W.; Zhang, T.; Escobar, D.; Wang, X.; Jiang, Y.; She, X.; Lv, G.; Li, J. A four-factor immune risk score signature predicts the clinical outcome of patients with spinal chordoma. *Clin. Transl. Med.* **2020**, *10*, 224–237. [CrossRef]
13. Gill, C.M.; Fowkes, M.; Shrivastava, R.K. Emerging Therapeutic Targets in Chordomas: A Review of the Literature in the Ge-nomic Era. *Neurosurgery* **2020**, *86*, E118–E123. [CrossRef] [PubMed]
14. Vodnala, S.K.; Eil, R.; Kishton, R.J.; Sukumar, M.; Yamamoto, T.N.; Ha, N.-H.; Lee, P.-H.; Shin, M.; Patel, S.J.; Yu, Z.; et al. T cell stemness and dysfunction in tumors are triggered by a common mechanism. *Science* **2019**, *363*, eaau0135. [CrossRef] [PubMed]
15. Liu, J.-L.; Chen, F.-F.; Lung, J.; Lo, C.-H.; Lee, F.-H.; Lu, Y.-C.; Hung, C.-H. Prognostic significance of p62/SQSTM1 subcellular localization and LC3B in oral squamous cell carcinoma. *Br. J. Cancer* **2014**, *111*, 944–954. [CrossRef]
16. Iwadate, R.; Inoue, J.; Tsuda, H.; Takano, H.; Furuya, K.; Hirasawa, A.; Aoki, D.; Inazawa, J. High Expression of p62 Protein Is Associated with Poor Prognosis and Aggressive Phenotypes in Endome-trial Cancer. *Am. J. Pathol.* **2015**, *185*, 2523–2533. [CrossRef] [PubMed]
17. Camy, F.; Karpathiou, G.; Dumollard, G.M.; Magne, N.; Perrot, J.L.; Vassal, F.; Picot, T.; Mobarki, M.; Forest, F.; Casteillo, F.; et al. Brain metastasis PD-L1 and CD8 expression is dependent on primary tumor type and its PD-L1 and CD8 sta-tus. *J. Immunother.* **2020**, *8*, e000597.
18. Zou, M.-X.; Lv, G.-H.; Wang, X.-B.; Huang, W.; Li, J.; Jiang, Y.; She, X.-L. Clinical Impact of the Immune Microenvironment in Spinal Chordoma: Immunoscore as an Independent Favorable Prognostic Factor. *Neurosurgery* **2019**, *84*, E318–E333. [CrossRef] [PubMed]
19. Ruscetti, M.; Morris, J.P.; Mezzadra, R.; Russell, J.; Leibold, J.; Romesser, P.B.; Simon, J.; Kulick, A.; Ho, Y.-J.; Fennell, M.; et al. Senescence-Induced Vascular Remodeling Creates Therapeutic Vulnerabilities in Pancreas Cancer. *Cell* **2020**, *181*, 424–441.e21. [CrossRef] [PubMed]
20. Schläfli, A.M.; Adams, O.; Galván, J.A.; Gugger, M.; Savic, S.; Bubendorf, L.; Schmid, R.A.; Becker, K.-F.; Tschan, M.P.; Langer, R.; et al. Prognostic value of the autophagy markers LC3 and p62/SQSTM1 in early-stage non-small cell lung cancer. *Oncotarget* **2016**, *7*, 39544–39555. [CrossRef]
21. Serramito-Gómez, I.; Boada-Romero, E.; Villamuera, R.; Fernández-Cabrera, Á.; Cedillo, J.L.; Martín-Regalado, Á.; Carding, S.; Mayer, U.; Powell, P.P.; Wileman, T.; et al. Regulation of cytokine signaling through direct interaction between cytokine receptors and the ATG16L1 WD40 domain. *Nat. Commun.* **2020**, *11*, 5919. [CrossRef]
22. Chen, R.; Li, X.; He, B.; Hu, W. MicroRNA-410 regulates autophagy-related gene ATG16L1 expression and enhances chemosensi-tivity via autophagy inhibition in osteosarcoma. *Mol. Med. Rep.* **2017**, *15*, 1326–1334. [CrossRef]
23. Shimizu, T.; Sugihara, E.; Yamaguchi-Iwai, S.; Tamaki, S.; Koyama, Y.; Kamel, W.; Ueki, A.; Ishikawa, T.; Chiyoda, T.; Osuka, S.; et al. IGF2 Preserves Osteosarcoma Cell Survival by Creating an Autophagic State of Dormancy That Protects Cells against Chemotherapeutic Stress. *Cancer Res.* **2014**, *74*, 6531–6541. [CrossRef] [PubMed]
24. O'Gorman, D.B.; Weiss, J.; Hettiaratchi, A.; Firth, S.M.; Scott, C.D. Insulin-Like Growth Factor-II/Mannose 6-Phosphate Receptor Overexpression Reduces Growth of Choriocarcinoma Cells in Vitro and in Vivo. *Endocrinology* **2002**, *143*, 4287–4294. [CrossRef] [PubMed]
25. Scheipl, S.; Froehlich, E.V.; Leithner, A.; Beham, A.; Quehenberger, F.; Mokry, M.; Stammberger, H.; Varga, P.P.; Lazáry, A.; Windhager, R.; et al. Does insulin-like growth factor 1 receptor (IGF-1R) targeting provide new treatment options for chor-domas? A retrospective clinical and immunohistochemical study. *Histopathology* **2012**, *60*, 999–1003. [CrossRef]
26. Ramakrishnan, R.; Huang, C.; Cho, H.I.; Lloyd, K.; Johnson, J.; Ren, X.; Altiok, S.; Sullivan, D.; Weber, J.; Celis, E.; et al. Autophagy Induced by Conventional Chemotherapy Mediates Tumor Cell Sensitivity to Immuno-therapy. *Cancer Res.* **2012**, *72*, 5483–5493. [CrossRef]
27. Ramakrishnan, R.; Gabrilovich, D.I. The role of mannose-6-phosphate receptor and autophagy in influencing the outcome of combination therapy. *Autophagy* **2013**, *9*, 615–616. [CrossRef]
28. Wahba, J.; Natoli, M.; Whilding, L.M.; Parente-Pereira, A.C.; Jung, Y.; Zona, S.; Lam, E.W.-F.; Smith, J.R.; Maher, J.; Ghaem-Maghami, S. Chemotherapy-induced apoptosis, autophagy and cell cycle arrest are key drivers of synergy in chemo-immunotherapy of epithelial ovarian cancer. *Cancer Immunol. Immunother.* **2018**, *67*, 1753–1765. [CrossRef] [PubMed]

29. Meng, W.; Gao, S.-J. Targeting XPO1 enhances innate immune response and inhibits KSHV lytic replication during primary infection by nuclear stabilization of the p62 autophagy adaptor protein. *Cell Death Dis.* **2021**, *12*, 29. [CrossRef]
30. Wang, L.; Howell, M.E.A.; Sparks-Wallace, A.; Hawkins, C.; Nicksic, C.A.; Kohne, C.; Hall, K.H.; Moorman, J.P.; Yao, Z.Q.; Ning, S. p62-mediated Selective autophagy endows virus-transformed cells with insusceptibility to DNA damage under oxidative stress. *PLoS Pathog.* **2019**, *15*, e1007541. [CrossRef]
31. Wen, Z.-F.; Liu, H.; Gao, R.; Zhou, M.; Ma, J.; Zhang, Y.; Zhao, J.; Chen, Y.; Zhang, T.; Huang, F.; et al. Tumor cell-released autophagosomes (TRAPs) promote immunosuppression through induction of M2-like macrophages with increased expression of PD-L1. *J. Immunother. Cancer* **2018**, *6*, 151. [CrossRef]
32. Bozic, M.; Wilkinson, S. Selective Autophagy Conceals the Enemy: Why Cytotoxic T Cells Don't (MH)C Pancreatic Cancer. *Mol. Cell* **2020**, *79*, 6–8. [CrossRef] [PubMed]
33. Yamamoto, K.; Venida, A.; Yano, J.; Biancur, D.E.; Kakiuchi, M.; Gupta, S.; Sohn, A.S.W.; Mukhopadhyay, S.; Lin, E.Y.; Parker, S.J.; et al. Autophagy promotes immune evasion of pancreatic cancer by degrading MHC-I. *Nat. Cell Biol.* **2020**, *581*, 100–105. [CrossRef]

MDPI
St. Alban-Anlage 66
4052 Basel
Switzerland
Tel. +41 61 683 77 34
Fax +41 61 302 89 18
www.mdpi.com

Cancers Editorial Office
E-mail: cancers@mdpi.com
www.mdpi.com/journal/cancers

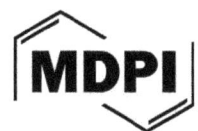

www.ingramcontent.com/pod-product-compliance
Lightning Source LLC
LaVergne TN
LVHW070632100526
838202LV00012B/787